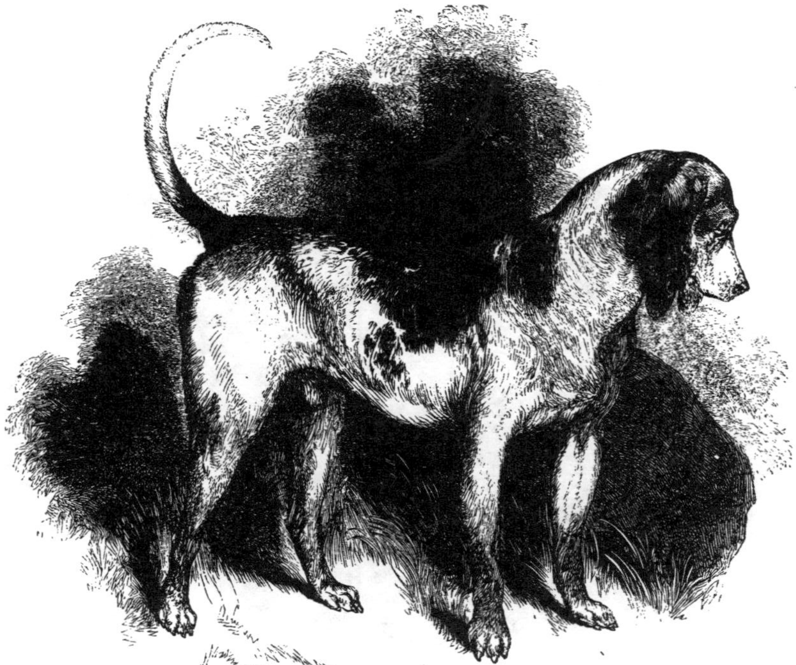

THE SOUTHERN HOUND.

THE DOG,

BY WILLIAM YOUATT.

WITH ILLUSTRATIONS

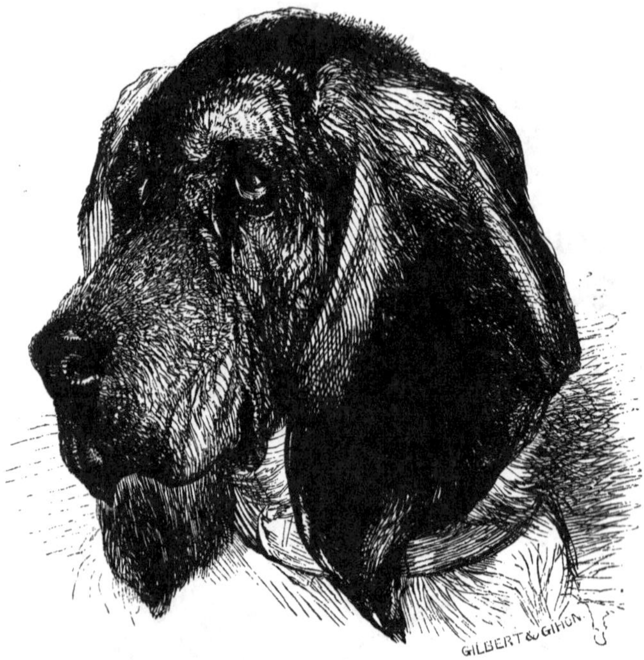

HEAD OF BLOODHOUND

EDITED, WITH ADDITIONS,

BY E. J. LEWIS, M.D.

Member of the Academy of Natural Sciences of Philadelphia; of the Philadelphia Medical Society:
of the Parisian Medical Society, &c. &c.

PHILADELPHIA:
LEA AND BLANCHARD.
1852.

THE DOG,

BY WILLIAM YOUATT.

EDITED, WITH ADDITIONS,

BY E. J. LEWIS, M.D.

MEMBER OF THE ACADEMY OF NATURAL SCIENCES OF PHILADELPHIA;
OF THE PHILADELPHIA MEDICAL SOCIETY; OF THE
PARISIAN MEDICAL SOCIETY, ETC.

PHILADELPHIA:
BLANCHARD AND LEA.
1852.

STEREOTYPED BY J. FAGAN.
PRINTED BY C. SHERMAN.

LIST OF ILLUSTRATIONS.

PREFACE OF THE EDITOR.

The Editor, having been called upon by the American publishers of the present volume to see it through the press, and add such matter as he deemed likely to increase its value to the sportsman and the lover of dogs in this country, the more readily consented to undertake the task, as he had previously, during the intervals of leisure left by professional avocations, paid much attention to the diseases, breeding, rearing, and peculiarities of the canine race, with a view to the preparation of a volume on the subject.

His design, however, being in a great measure superseded by the enlarged and valuable treatise of Mr. Youatt, whose name is a full guarantee as to the value of whatever he may give to the world, he found that not much remained to be added. Such points, however, as he thought might be improved, and such matter as appeared necessary to adapt the volume more especially to the wants of this country, he has introduced in the course of its pages. These additions, amounting to about sixty pages, will be found between brackets, with the initial of the Editor appended. He trusts they will not detract from the interest of the volume, while he hopes that its usefulness may be thereby somewhat increased.

With this explanation of his connexion with the work, he leaves it in the hope that it may prove of value to the sportsman from its immediate relation to his stirring pursuits; to the general reader, from the large amount of curious information collected in its pages, which is almost inaccessible in any other form; and to the medical student, from the light it sheds on the pathology and diseases of the dog, by which he will be surprised to learn how many ills that animal shares in common with the human race.

The editor will be satisfied with his agency in the publication of this volume, if it should be productive of a more extended love for this brave, devoted, and sagacious animal, and be the means of improving his lot of faithful servitude. It is with these views that the editor has occasionally turned from more immediate engagements to investigate his character, and seek the means of ameliorating his condition.

PHILADELPHIA, *October*, 1846.

TABLE OF CONTENTS.

THE DOG.

CHAPTER I.

THE EARLY HISTORY AND ZOOLOGICAL CLASSIFICATION OF THE DOG.

THE Dog, next to the human being, ranks highest in the scale of intelligence, and was evidently designed to be the companion and the friend of man. We exact the services of other animals, and, the task being performed, we dismiss them to their accustomed food and rest; but several of the varieties of the dog follow us to our home; they are connected with many of our pleasures and wants, and guard our sleeping hours.

The first animal of the domestication of which we have any account, was the sheep. "Abel was a keeper of sheep."[a] It is difficult to believe that any long time would pass before the dog—who now, in every country of the world, is the companion of the shepherd, and the director or guardian of the sheep—would be enlisted in the service of man.

From the earliest known history he was the protector of the habitation of the human being. At the feet of the *lares*, those household deities who were supposed to protect the abodes of men, the figure of a barking dog was often placed. In every age, and almost in every part of the globe, he has played a principal part in the labours, the dangers, and the pleasures of the chase.

In process of time, man began to surround himself with many servants from among the lower animals, but among them all he had only one friend—the dog; one animal only whose service was voluntary, and who was susceptible of disinterested affection and gratitude. In every country, and in every time, there has existed between man and the dog a connection different from that which is observed between him and any other animal. The ox and the sheep submit to our control, but their affections are principally, if not solely, confined to themselves. They submit to us, but they can rarely be said to love, or even to recognise us, except as connected with the supply of their wants.

The horse will share some of our pleasures. He enjoys the

[a] Gen. iv. 2.

chase as much as does his rider; and, when contending for vic tory on the course, he feels the full influence of emulation. Remembering the pleasure he has experienced with his master, or the daily supply of food from the hand of the groom, he often exhibits evident tokens of recognition; but that is founded on a selfish principle—he neighs that he may be fed, and his affections are easily transferred.

The dog is the only animal that is capable of disinterested affection. He is the only one that regards the human being as his companion, and follows him as his friend; the only one that seems to possess a natural desire to be useful to him, or from a spontaneous impulse attaches himself to man. We take the bridle from the mouth of the horse, and turn him free into the pasture, and he testifies his joy in his partially recovered liberty. We exact from the dog the service that is required of him, and he still follows us. He solicits to be continued as our companion and our friend. Many an expressive action tells us how much he is pleased and thankful. He shares in our abundance, and he is content with the scantiest and most humble fare. He loves us while living, and has been known to pine away on the grave of his master.

[It is stated that the favourite lap-dog of Mary, Queen of Scots, that accompanied her to the scaffold, continued to caress the body after the head was cut off, and refused to relinquish his post till forcibly withdrawn, and afterwards died with grief in the course of a day or two.

The following account is also an authentic instance of the inconsolable grief displayed by a small cur-dog at the death of his master:—A poor tailor in the parish of St. Olave, having died, was attended to the grave by his dog, who had expressed every token of sorrow from the instant of his master's death, and seemed unwilling to quit the corpse even for a moment. After the funeral had dispersed, the faithful animal took his station upon the grave, and was with great difficulty driven by the sexton from the church ground; on the following day he was again observed lying on the grave of his master, and was a second time expelled from the premises. Notwithstanding the harsh treatment received on several succeeding days by the hands of the sexton, this little creature would persist in occupying this position, and overcame every difficulty to gain access to the spot where all he held most dear was deposited. The minister of the parish, learning the circumstances of the case, ordered the dog to be carried to his house, where he was confined and fed for several days, in hopes of weaning him by kind treatment to forget his sorrow occasioned by the loss of his master. But all his benevolent efforts were of no utility, as the dog availed himself of the first opportunity to escape, and immediately repaired to his chosen spot over the grave.

This worthy clergyman now allowed him to follow the bent of his own inclinations; and, as a recompense for true friendship and unfeigned sorrow, had a house built for him over this hallowed spot, and daily supplied him with food and water for the space of two years, during which time he never wandered from his post, but, as a faithful guardian, kept his lonely watch day and night, till death at last put an end to his sufferings, and laid him by the side of his long-expected master.—L.]

As an animal of draught the dog is highly useful in some countries. What would become of the inhabitants of the northern regions, if the dog were not harnessed to the sledge, and the Laplander, and the Greenlander, and the Kamtschatkan drawn, and not unfrequently at the rate of nearly a hundred miles a day, over the snowy wastes? In Newfoundland, the timber, one of the most important articles of commerce, is drawn to the water-side by the docile but ill-used dog; and we need only to cross the British Channel in order to see how useful, and, generally speaking, how happy a beast of draught the dog can be.

[Large mongrel dogs are very extensively used on the Continent in pulling small vehicles adapted to various purposes. In fact, most of the carts and wagons that enter Paris, or are employed in the city, have one of these animals attached to them by a short strap hanging from the axle-tree. This arrangement answers the double purpose of keeping off all intruders in the temporary absence of the master, and, by pushing himself forward in his collar, materially assists the horse in propelling a heavy load up-hill, or of carrying one speedily over a plain surface. It is quite astonishing to see how well broken to this work these dogs are, and at the same time to witness with what vigour and perseverance they labour in pushing before them, in this way, enormous weights.—L.]

Though, in our country, and to its great disgrace, this employment of the dog has been accompanied by such wanton and shameful cruelty, that the Legislature—somewhat hastily confounding the abuse of a thing with its legitimate purpose—forbade the appearance of the dog-cart in the metropolitan districts, and were inclined to extend this prohibition through the whole kingdom, it is much to be desired that a kindlier and better feeling may gradually prevail, and that this animal, humanely treated, may return to the discharge of the services of which nature has rendered him capable, and which prove the greatest source of happiness to him while discharging them to the best of his power.

In another and very important particular,—as the preserver of human life,—the history of the dog will be most interesting. The writer of this work has seen a Newfoundland dog who, on five distinct occasions, preserved the life of a human being; and it is said of the noble quadruped whose remains constitute one of the most interesting specimens in the museum of Berne, that forty persons were rescued by him from impending destruction.

When this friend and servant of man dies, he does not or may not cease to be useful; for in many countries, and to a far greater extent than is generally imagined, his skin is useful for gloves, or leggings, or mats, or hammercloths; and, while even the Romans occasionally fattened him for the table, and esteemed his flesh a dainty, many thousands of people in Asia, Africa, and America, now breed him expressly for food.

If the publication of the present work should throw some additional light on the good qualities of this noble animal; if it should enable us to derive more advantage from the services that he can render—to train him more expeditiously and fully for the discharge of those services—to protect him from the abuses to which he is exposed, and to mitigate or remove some of the diseases which his connection with man has entailed upon him; if any of these purposes be accomplished, we shall derive considerable "useful knowledge" as well as pleasure from the perusal of the present volume.

Some controversy has arisen with regard to the origin of the dog. Professor Thomas Bell, to whom we are indebted for a truly valuable history of the British quadrupeds, traces him to the wolf. He says, and it is perfectly true, that the osteology of the wolf does not differ materially from that of the dog more than that of the different kinds of dogs differs; that the cranium is similar, and they agree in nearly all the other essential points; that the dog and wolf will readily breed with each other, and that their progeny, thus obtained, will again mingle with the dog. [The relative length of the intestines is a strong distinctive mark both as to the habits and species of animals; those of a purely carnivorous nature are much shorter than others who resort entirely to an herbaceous diet, or combine the two modes of sustenance according to circumstances. The dog and wolf have the intestines of the same length. (See Sir Everard Home on Comparative Anatomy.)—L.] There is one circumstance, however, which seems to mark a decided difference between the two animals; the eye of the dog of every country and species has a circular pupil, but the position or form of the pupil is oblique in the wolf. Professor Bell gives an ingenious but not admissible reason for this. He attributes the forward direction of the eyes in the dog to the constant habit, "for many successive generations, of looking towards their master, and obeying his voice:" but no habit of this kind could by possibility produce any such effect. It should also be remembered that, in every part of the globe in which the wolf is found, this form of the pupil, and a peculiar setting on of the curve of the tail, and a singularity in the voice, cannot fail of being observed; to which may be added, that the dog exists in every latitude and in every climate, while the habitation of the wolf is confined to certain parts of the globe.

There is also a marked difference in the temper and habits of the two. The dog is, generally speaking, easily manageable, but nothing will, in the majority of cases, render the wolf moderately tractable. There are, however, exceptions to this. The author remembers a bitch wolf at the Zoological Gardens that would always come to the front bars of her den to be caressed as soon as any one that she knew approached. She had puppies while there, and she brought her little ones in her mouth to be noticed by the spectators; so eager, indeed, was she that they should share with her in the notice of her friends, that she killed them all in succession against the bars of her den as she brought them forcibly forward to be fondled.

M. F. Cuvier gives an account of a young wolf who followed his master everywhere, and showed a degree of affection and submission scarcely inferior to the domesticated dog. His master being unavoidably absent, he was sent to the menagerie, where he pined for his loss, and would scarcely take any food for a considerable time. At length, however, he attached himself to his keepers, and appeared to have forgotten his former associate. At the expiration of eighteen months his master returned, and, the moment his voice was heard, the wolf recognised him, and lavished on his old friend the most affectionate caresses. A second separation followed, which lasted three years, and again the long-remembered voice was recognised, and replied to with impatient cries; after which, rushing on his master, he licked his face with every mark of joy, menacing his keepers, towards whom he had just before been exhibiting fondness. A third separation occurred, and he became gloomy and melancholy. He suffered the caresses of none but his keepers, and towards them he often manifested the original ferocity of his species.

These stories, however, go only a little way to prove that the dog and the wolf have one common origin. [There are some naturalists that even go so far as to state that the different varieties of dogs are sprung from, or compounded of, various animals, as the hyæna, jackal, wolf, and fox. The philosophic John Hunter commenced a series of experiments upon this interesting subject, and was forced to acknowledge that "the dog may be the wolf tamed, and the jackal may probably be the dog returned to his wild state."

The ancient Cynegetical writers were not only acquainted with the cross between the wolf and dog, but also boasted the possession of breeds of animals, supposed to have been derived from a connection with the lion and tiger. The Hyrcanian dog, although naturally a savage and powerful beast, was rendered much more formidable in battle, or in conflict with other animals, by his fabled cross with the tiger. In corroboration of this singular, but not less fabulous belief, Pliny states that the inhabitants of India take pleasure in having their dog bitches lined by the wild tigers, and to facilitate this union, they are in the habit of tieing them when in heat out in the woods, so that the male tigers may visit them. (See L. 8, c. xl.)

There is, however, but little doubt that the wolf and dog are varieties of the same family, as they can be bred together, and their offspring continuing the cross thus formed, will produce a race quite distinct from the original. French writers do not hesitate at all upon this point, but even assert that it is very difficult to take a she-wolf with male dogs during the period of oestrum, parceque la veulent saillir et covrir comme une chienne.

Baudrillart, in the "dictionaire des chasses," further remarks that the mongrels produced by this connection are very viciously disposed and inclined to bite.

The period of utero-gestation, and the peculiar mode of copulation in the wolf, is the same as that of the canine family, which two circumstances are certainly very strong presumptive evidences of the similarity of the species. The dogs used by our northern Indians resemble very much, in their general appearance, the wolves of that region, and do not seem very far removed from that race of animals, notwithstanding they have been in a state of captivity, or domestication, beyond the traditionary chronicles of this rude people.

Another strong circumstance in favour of the common origin of these two quadrupeds, is the existence in our own country of the Canis Latrans, or prairie wolf, who whines and barks in a manner so similar to the smaller varieties of dogs, that it is almost impossible to distinguish his notes from those of the terrier.

Major Long remarks, that "this animal, which does not seem to be known to naturalists, unless it should prove to be the Mexicanus, is most probably the original of the domestic dog, so common in the villages of the Indians of this region, some of the varieties of which still retain much of the habit and manners of this species." (Vol. i, page 174.)

If further proof be necessary to establish the identity of the dog and wolf, the circumstances related by Captain Parry in his first voyage of discovery, ought to be sufficient to convince every mind that the wolf, even in its wild state, will seek to form an alliance or connection with one of our domestic dogs. "About this time it had been remarked that a white setter dog, belonging to Mr. Beverly, had left the Griper for several nights past at the same time, and had regularly returned after some hours absence. As the daylight increased we had frequent opportunities of seeing him in company with a she-wolf, with whom he kept up an almost daily intercourse for several weeks, till at length he returned no more to the ships; having either lost his way by rambling to too great a distance, or what is more likely, perhaps, been destroyed by the male wolves. Some time after a large dog of mine, which was also getting into the habit of occasionally remaining absent for some time, returned on board a good deal lacerated and covered with blood, having, no doubt, maintained a severe encounter with a male wolf, whom we traced to a considerable distance by the tracks on the snow. An old dog, of the Newfoundland breed, that we had on board the Hecla, was also in the habit of remaining out with the wolves for a day or two together, and we frequently watched them keeping company on the most friendly terms." (Page 136, 1st voyage.)

In volume 1st, page 111, of the Menageries, it is stated that Mr. Wombwell exhibited in October, 1828, two animals from a cross between the wolf and the domestic dog, which had been bred in that country. They were confined in the same den with a female setter, and were likely again to multiply the species. Mr. Daniel remarks that Mr. Brook, famous for his menagerie, turned a wolf to a Pomeranian bitch at heat; the congress was immediate, and, as usual between the dog and bitch, ten puppies were the produce. These animals strongly resembled their sire both in appearance and disposition, and one of them being let loose at a deer, instantly caught at the animal's throat and killed it. (See Daniel's Rural Sports, vol. i, page 14.—L.]

It may appear singular that in both the Old Testament and the New the dog was spoken of almost with abhorrence. He ranked among the unclean beasts. The traffic in him and the price of him were considered as an abomination, and were forbidden to be offered in the sanctuary in the discharge of any vow.[a]

One grand object in the institution of the Jewish ritual was to preserve the Israelites from the idolatry which at that time prevailed among every other people. Dogs were held in considerable veneration by the Egyptians, from whose tyranny the Israelites had just escaped. Figures of them appeared on the friezes of most of the temples,[b] and they were regarded as emblems of the Divine Being. Herodotus, speaking of the sanctity in which some animals were held by the Egyptians, says that the people of every family in which a dog died, shaved themselves—their expression of mourning—and he adds, that "this was a custom existing in his own time."[c]

---

[a] Deut. xxiii. 18.

[b] In some of Belzoni's beautiful sketches of the frieze-work of the old Egyptian temples, the dog appears, with his long ears and broad muzzle, not unlike the old Talbot hound.

[c] Herodotus, lib. ii. c. 66.

The cause of this attachment to and veneration for the dog is, however, explained in a far more probable and pleasing way than many of the fables of ancient mythology. The prosperity of Lower Egypt, and almost the very subsistence of its inhabitants, depended on the annual overflowing of the Nile; and they looked for it with the utmost anxiety. Its approach was announced by the appearance of a certain star—SIRIUS. As soon as that star was seen above the horizon, they hastened to remove their flocks to the higher ground, and abandoned the lower pastures to the fertilizing influence of the stream. They hailed it as their guard and protector; and, associating with its apparent watchfulness the well-known fidelity of the dog, they called it the "dog-star," and they worshipped it. It was in far later periods and in other countries that the appearance of the dog-star was regarded as the signal of insufferable heat or prevalent disease.

One of the Egyptian deities—Anubis—is described as having the form and body of a man, but with a dog's head. These were types of sagacity and fidelity.

["Who knows not that infatuate Egypt finds
Gods to adore in brutes of basest kinds?
This at the crocodile's resentment quakes,
While that adores the ibis, gorged with snakes!
And where the radiant beam of morning rings
On shattered Memnon's still harmonious strings;
And Thebes to ruin all her gates resigns,
Of huge baboon the golden image shines!
To *mongrel curs* infatuate cities bow,
And cats and fishes share the frequent vow!"
Juvenal, Sat. xv.—Badham's Trans.—L.]

In Ethiopia, not only was great veneration paid to the dog, but the inhabitants used to elect a dog as their king. He was kept in great state, and surrounded by a numerous train of officers and guards. When he fawned upon them, he was supposed to be pleased with their proceedings: when he growled, he disapproved of the manner in which their government was conducted. These indications of his will were implicitly obeyed, or rather, perhaps, were translated by his worshippers as their own caprice or interest dictated.

[Among the many strange and wonderful things mentioned by Pliny as being discovered in Africa, is a people called Ptœmbati or Ptremphanæ, whose principal city is Aruspi, where they elect a dog for their king and obey him most religiously, being governed entirely by the different motions of his body, which they interpret according to certain signs. (See Pliny, lib. vi, c. xxx.)—L.]

Even a thousand years after this period the dog was highly esteemed in Egypt for its sagacity and other excellent qualities; for, when Pythagoras, after his return from Egypt, founded a new sect in Greece, and at Croton, in southern Italy, he taught, with the Egyptian philosophers, that, at the death of the body, the soul entered into that of different animals. He used, after the decease of any of his favourite disciples, to cause a dog to be held to the mouth of the dying man, in order to receive his departing spirit; saying, that there was no animal that could perpetuate his virtues better than that quadruped.

It was in order to preserve the Israelites from errors and follies like these, and to prevent the possibility of this species of idolatry being established, that the dog was afterward regarded with utter abhorrence among the Jews.[a] This feeling prevailed during the continuance of the Israelites in Palestine. Even in the New Testament the Apostle warns those to whom he wrote to "beware of dogs and evil-workers;"[b] and it is said in The Revelations that "without are dogs and sorcerers," &c.[c] Dogs were, however, employed even by the Jews. Job says, "Now they that are younger than I have me in derision, whose fathers I would have disdained to have set with the dogs of my flock."[d] Dogs were employed either to guide the sheep or to protect them from wild beasts; and some prowled about the streets at night, contending with each other for the offal that was thrown away.

To a certain degree this dislike of the dog continues to the present day; for, with few exceptions, the dog is seldom the chosen companion of the Jew, or even the inmate of his house. Nor was it originally confined to Palestine. Wherever a knowledge of the Jewish religion spread, or any of its traditions were believed, there arose an abhorrence of the dog. The Mohammedans have always regarded him as an unclean animal, that should never be cherished in any human habitation—belonging to no particular owner, but protecting the street[e] and the district rather than the house of a master.

The Hindoos regard him likewise as unclean, and submit to various purifications if they accidentally come in contact with him, believing that every dog was animated by a wicked and malignant spirit, condemned to do penance in that form for crimes committed in a previous state of existence. If by chance a dog passed between a teacher and his pupil during the period of instruction, it was supposed that the best lesson would be completely poisoned, and it was deemed prudent to suspend the tuition for at least a day and a night. Even in Egypt, dogs are now as much avoided as they were venerated. In every Mohammedan and Hindoo

[a] No dog was suffered to come within the precints of the Temple at Jerusalem. Εξω κυνες was a prevalent expression among the Jews. Bryant's Mythology, vol. ii. p. 42.

[b] Phil. iii. 2.

[c] Rev. xxii. 15.

[d] Job xxx. 1. See also Isaiah lvi 10, 11.

[e] Psalm lix. 6.

country, the most scurrilous epithet bestowed on a European or a Christian is—"a dog!"[a]

This accounts for the singular fact that in the whole of the Jewish history there is not a single allusion to hunting with dogs. Mention is made of nets and snares, but the dog seems to have been never used in the pursuit of game.

In the early periods of the history of other countries this seems to have been the case even where the dog was esteemed and valued, and had become the companion, the friend, and the defender of man and his home. So late as the second century of the Christian era, the fair hunting of the present day needed the eloquent defence of Arrian, who says that "there is as much difference between a fair trial of speed in a good run, and ensnaring a poor animal without an effort, as between the secret piratical assaults of robbers at sea, and the victorious naval engagements of the Athenians at Artemisium and at Salamis."[b] The first hint of the employment of the dog in the pursuit of other animals is given by Oppian in his Cynegeticus, who attributes it to Pollux, about 200 years after the promulgation of the Levitical law.

Of the precise species of dog that prevailed or was cultivated in Greece at this early period, little can with certainty be affirmed. One beautiful piece of sculpture has been preserved, and is now in the possession of Lord Feversham at Duncombe Hall. It is said to represent the favourite dog of Alcibiades, and to have been the production of Myson, one of the most skilful artists of ancient times. It differs but little from the Newfoundland dog of the present day. He is represented as sitting on his haunches, and earnestly looking at his master. Any one would vouch for the sagacity and fidelity of that animal.

The British Museum contains a group of greyhound puppies of more recent date, from the ruins of the villa of Antoninus, near Rome. One is fondling the other; and the attitude of both, and the characteristic puppy-clumsiness of their limbs, which indicate, nevertheless, the beautiful proportions that will soon be developed, are an admirable specimen of ancient art. (See cut on page 23.)

The Greeks, in the earlier periods of their history, depended too much on their nets; and it was not until later times that they pursued their prey with dogs, and then not with dogs that ran by

---

[a] Carpenter's Scripture Natural History, p. 109. It is a remarkable fact that from this faithful animal, the companion of man, and the guardian of his person and property, should originate so many terms of reproach as "dog," "cur," "hound," "puppy," "dog-cheap," "a dog's trick," "dog sick," "dog-weary," "to lead the life of a dog," "to use like a dog." All this probably originated in the East, where the dog was held in abhorrence as the common scavenger of the streets.

[b] Arrian's Cynegeticus, cap. 26.

[c] New Sporting Magazine, vol. xiv. p. 97.

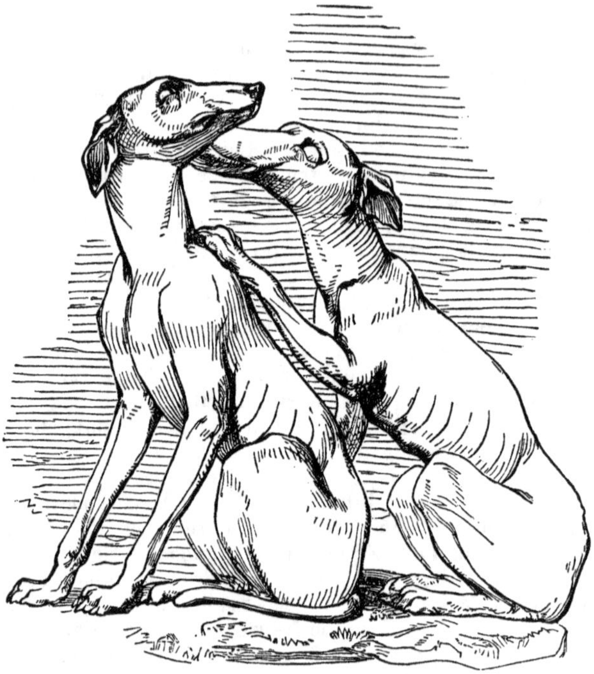

sight, or succeeded by their swiftness of foot, but by beagles very little superior to those of modern days.[a] Of the stronger and more ferocious dogs there is, however, occasional mention. The bull-dog of modern date does not excel the one (possibly of nearly the same race) that was presented to Alexander the Great, and that boldly seized a ferocious lion, or another that would not quit his hold, although one leg and then another was cut off.

It would be difficult and foreign to the object of this work fully to trace the early history of the dog. Both in Greece and in Rome he was highly estimated. Alexander built a city in honour of a dog; and the Emperor Hadrian decreed the most solemn rites of sepulture to another on account of his sagacity and fidelity.

The translator of Arrian imagines that the use of the *pugnaces* (fighting) and the *sagaces* (intelligent)—the more ferocious dogs, and those who artfully circumvented and caught their prey—was known in the earlier periods of Greek and Roman history, but that the *celeres*, the dogs of speed, the greyhounds of every kind,

[a] New Sporting Magazine, vol. xiv. p. 97.

were peculiar to the British islands, or to the western and northern continents of Europe, the interior and the produce of which were in those days unknown to the Greeks and Romans. By most authors who have inquired into the origin of these varieties of the dog, the *sagaces* have been generally assigned to Greece—the *pugnaces* to Asia—and the *celeres* to the Celtic nations.

[The vertragi, *canes celeres*, or dogs that hunted by sight alone, were not known to the ancients previous to the time of the younger Zenophon, who then describes them as novelties just introduced into Greece:—

"But the swift-footed Celtic hounds are called in the Celtic tongue οὐέρτραγοι; not deriving their name from any particular nation, like the Cretan, Carian, or Spartan dogs, but, as some of the Cretans are named διαπονοι from working hard, ἰταμαὶ from their keenness, and mongrels from their being compounded of both, so these Celts are named from their swiftness. In figure, the most high-bred are a prodigy of beauty; their eyes, their hair, their colour, and bodily shape throughout. Such brilliancy of gloss is there about the spottiness of the parti-coloured, and in those of uniform colour, such glistening over the sameness of tint, as to afford a most delightful spectacle to an amateur of coursing."

It is probable these dogs were carried, about this time, into the southern parts of Europe by the various tribes of Celts who overran the continent, and also occupied Ireland, Britain, and the other western islands, and ultimately took possession of Gaul.—L.]

Of the aboriginal country of the latter there can be little doubt; but the accounts that are given of the English mastiff at the invasion of Britain by the Romans, and the early history of the English hound, which was once peculiar to this country, and at the present day degenerates in every other, would go far to prove that these breeds also are indigenous to our island.

Oppian thus describes the hunting dog as he finds him in Britain:—"There is, besides, an excellent kind of scenting dogs, though small, yet worthy of estimation. They are fed by the fierce nation of painted Britons, who call them *agasæi*. In size they resemble worthless greedy house-dogs that gape under tables. They are crooked, lean, coarse-haired, and heavy-eyed, but armed with powerful claws and deadly teeth. The *agasæus* is of good nose and most excellent in following scent.[a]"

Among the savage dogs of ancient times were the Hyrcanian, said, on account of their extreme ferocity, to have been crossed with the tiger[b],—the Locrian, chiefly employed in hunting the

[a] Oppian's Cynegeticus, lib. i. v. 468—480.

[b] ["At contrà facilēs, magnique Lycaones armis.
Sed non Hyrcanæ satis est vehementia genti

boar,—the Pannonian, used in war as well as in the chase, and by whom the first charge on the enemy was always made,—and the Molossian, of Epirus, likewise trained to war as well as to the honours of the amphitheatre and the dangers of the chase. This last breed had one redeeming quality—an inviolable attachment to their owners. This attachment was reciprocal; for it is said that the Molossi used to weep over their faithful quadruped companions slain in war.

[Of all the dogs of the ancients, those bred on the continent of Epirus were the most esteemed, and more particularly those from a southern district called Molossia, from which they received their name.

These animals are described as being of enormous size, great courage and powerful make, and were considered worthy not only to encounter the wolf, bear, and boar, but often overcame the panther, tiger, and lion, both in the chase and amphitheatre. They also, being trained to war, proved themselves most useful auxiliaries to this martial people.

The learned translator of Arrian states that "the fabled origin of this breed is consistent with its high repute; for, on the authority of Nicander, we are told by Julius Pollux, that the Epirote was descended from the brazen dog which Vulcan wrought for Jupiter, and animated with all the functions of canine life." These were not the only dogs fashioned by the skilful hands of the Olympic artist, as we find Alcinous, king of the Phæacians, possessing golden dogs also wrought at the celestial forge.

Pliny states that a dog of enormous magnitude was sent as a present by the king of Albania to Alexander the Great when on his march to India; and "that this monarch being delighted at the sight of so huge and fair a dog, let loose unto him first bears, then wild boars, and lastly fallow deer, all of which animals he took no notice of, but remained perfectly unconcerned. This great warrior being a man of high spirit and wonderful courage, was greatly displeased at the apparent cowardice and want of energy in so powerful an animal, and ordered him to be slain. This news was speedily carried to the king of Albania, who thereupon sent unto him a second dog, stating that he should not make trial of his courage with such insignificant animals, but rather with a lion or elephant, and if he destroyed this one also, he need not expect to obtain any other of this breed, as these two were all he possessed.

Tanta: suis petiere ultro fera semina sylvis,
Dat Venus accessus, et blando fœdere jungit.
Tunc et mansuetis tuto ferus erat adulter
In stabulis, ultroque gravis succedere tigrim
Ausa canis, majore tulit de sanguine foetum.
Gratii Falisci Cyneget., liv. 1. v. 160.—L.]

Alexander being much surprised, made immediate preparations for a trial, and soon saw the lion prostrate, with his back broken, and his body torn in pieces by the noble dog. Then he ordered an elephant to be produced; and in no fight did he take more pleasure than in this. For the dog, with his long, rough, shaggy hair, that covered his whole body, rushed with open mouth, barking terribly, and thundering, as it were, upon the elephant. Soon after he leaps and flies upon him, advancing and retreating, now on one side, now on the other, maintaining an ingenious combat; at one time assailing him with all vigour, at another shunning him. So actively did he continue this artificial warfare, causing the huge beast to turn around so frequently on every side to avoid his attacks, that he ultimately came down with a crash that made the earth tremble with his fall." Book viii. chap. 40.

The Molossian dogs were at a later period much esteemed by the Romans as watch dogs, not only of their dwellings, but also to guard their flocks against the incursions of wild animals. Horace, in the following lines, passes a just tribute to the worth of this animal, when referring to his watchfulness, and the ardour with which he pursues those wild animals, even '*per altas nives,*' that threaten the flocks entrusted to his care.

> "Quid immerentes, hospites vexas canis,
> Ignarus adversum lupos?
> Quin huc inanes, si potes, vertis minas,
> Et me remorsurum petis?
> Nam, qualis aut Molossus, aut fulvus Lacon,
> Amica vis pastoribus,
> Agam per altas aure sublatâ nives,
> Quæcunpue præcedet fera." *Epode* vi.—L.]

Ælian relates that one of them, and his owner, so much distinguished themselves at the battle of Marathon, that the effigy of the dog was placed on the same tablet with that of his master.

Soon after Britain was discovered, the *pugnaces* of Epirus were pitted against those of our island, and, according to the testimony of Gratius, completely beaten. A variety of this class, but as large and as ferocious, was employed to guard the sheep and cattle, or to watch at the door of the house, or to follow the owner on any excursion of business or of pleasure. Gratius says of these dogs, that they have no pretensions to the deceitful commendation of form; but, at the time of need, when courage is required of them, most excellent mastiffs are not to be preferred to them.

The account of the British *pugnaces* of former times, and also of the *sagaces* and *celeres*, will be best given when treating of their present state and comparative value. In describing the different breeds of dogs, some anecdotes will be related of their sagacity and fidelity; a few previous remarks, however, may be admissible.

A young man lost his life by falling from one of the precipices of the Helvellyn mountains. Three months afterwards his remains were discovered at the bottom of a ravine, and his faithful dog, almost a skeleton, still guarding them. Sir Walter Scott beautifully describes the scene:

Dark-green was the spot, 'mid the brown mountain heather,
Where the pilgrim of nature lay stretched in decay;
Like the corpse of an outcast, abandoned to weather,
Till the mountain winds wasted the tenantless clay;
Nor yet quite deserted, though lonely extended,
For, faithful in death, his mute favourite attended,
The much-loved remains of her master defended,
And chased the hill-fox and the raven away.
How long didst thou think that his silence was slumber?
When the wind waved his garments, how oft didst thou start?
How many long days and long weeks didst thou number
Ere he faded before thee, the friend of thy heart?

Burchell, in his Travels in Africa, places the connexion between man and the dog, and the good qualities of this animal, in an interesting point of view. A pack of dogs of various descriptions formed a necessary part of his caravan, occasionally to provide him with food, but oftener to defend him from wild beasts or robbers. "While almost every other quadruped fears man as his most formidable enemy," says this interesting traveller, "there is one who regards him as his companion, and follows him as his friend We must not mistake the nature of the case. It is not because we train him to our use, and have made choice of him in preference to other animals, but because this particular species of animal feels a natural desire to be useful to man, and, from spontaneous impulse, attaches himself to him. Were it not so, we should see in various countries an equal familiarity with other quadrupeds, according to their habits, and the taste or caprices of different nations; but, everywhere, it is the dog only that takes delight in associating with us, and in sharing our abode. It is he who knows us personally, watches over us, and warns us of danger. It is impossible for the naturalist not to feel a conviction that this friendship between creatures so different from each other must be the result of the laws of nature; nor can the humane and feeling mind avoid the belief that kindness to those animals, from which he derives continued and essential assistance, is part of the moral duty of man.

"Often in the silence of the night, when all my people have been fast asleep around the fire, have I stood to contemplate these faithful animals watching by their side, and have learned to esteem them for their social inclination towards mankind. When, wandering over pathless deserts, oppressed with vexation and distress at the conduct of my own men, I have turned to these as my only friends, and felt how much inferior to them was man when actuated only by selfish views."

Of the stanchness and incorruptible fidelity of the dog, and his disregard of personal inconvenience and want, when employed in our service, it is impossible to entertain a doubt. We have sometimes thought that the attachment of the dog to its master was increased, or, at least, the exhibition of it, by the penury of the owner. At all events one fact is plain enough, that, while poverty drives away from us many a companion of our happier hours, it was never known to diminish the love of our quadruped friend.

The early history of the dog has been described, and the abomination in which he was held by the Israelites. At no great distance of time, however, we find him, almost in the neighbourhood of Palestine, in one of the islands of the Ionian Sea, the companion and the friend of princes, and deserving their regard. The reader will forgive a somewhat abbreviated account of the last meeting of Ulysses and his dog.

Twenty years had passed since Argus, the favourite dog of Ulysses, had been parted from his master. The monarch at length wended his way homewards, and, disguised as a beggar, for his life would have been sacrificed had he been known, stood at the entrance of his palace-door. There he met with an old dependant, who had formerly served him with fidelity and who was yet faithful to his memory; but age and hardship and care, and the disguise which he now wore, had so altered the wanderer that the good Eumæus had not the most distant suspicion with whom he was conversing; but—

Near to the gates, conferring as they drew,
Argus the dog his ancient master knew,
And, not unconscious of the voice and tread
Lifts to the sound his ears, and rears his head.
He knew his lord, he knew, and strove to meet;
In vain he strove to crawl and kiss his feet:
Yet, all he could, his tail, his ears, his eyes
Salute his master, and confess his joys.[a]

[Lord Byron, who had much experience and acquaintance with the canine family, was rather sceptical as regards the memory of this animal, having been, on one occasion, entirely forgotten by a favourite dog from whom he was separated some considerable time, and in fact was most savagely assailed by him, when on his return he attempted to caress him as he was wont to do in former times.

This unkind reception at Newstead Abbey, on the part of his pampered pet, may have given rise to the poet's feelings as embodied in the following misanthropic lines:—

[a] Pope's Odyssey, xvii.

"And now I'm in the world alone,
Upon the wide, wide sea:
But why should I for others groan,
When none will sigh for me?
Perchance my dog will whine in vain,
Till fed by stranger hands;
But long ere I come back again,
He'd tear me where he stands."—L.]

In Daniel's Rural Sports, the account of a nobleman and his dog is given. The nobleman had been absent two years on foreign service. On his return this faithful creature was the first to recognise him, as he came through the court-yard, and he flew to welcome his old master and friend. He sprung upon him; his agitation and his joy knew not any bounds; and at length, in the fulness of his transport, he fell at his master's feet and expired.

[An interesting circumstance, strongly exhibiting canine fidelity and attachment in a large mastiff, came under the Editor's own eye during his childhood, and which, from its striking character, deserves to be recorded on the page of history as another testimony to the high moral worth of these useful animals.

A gentleman of Baltimore, with his family, lived during a portion of the year a short distance in the country, and was in the habit of returning to the city late in the fall to pass the winter. On his estate there was a fine young mastiff, who though extremely cross to strangers, exhibited at all times a great degree of tenderness and affection for the younger branches of the family;—more particularly for the younger son, his most constant companion, and who would often steal secretly away to share his daily meal with this affectionate participator in his childish sports: or, when fatigued with romping together, would retire to the well-kept kennel, and recruit his limbs in a refreshing sleep, while reclining upon the body of the faithful dog. If the little truant should now be missed by those having him in charge, the most natural question to ask was, "Where is Rolla?" knowing full well that wherever this honest brute was, there might his young master be found also. On such occasions, however, this trusty guardian would refuse all solicitations to abandon his post, and express great dissatisfaction at any attempt to arouse or carry off his young charge, whom he continued to watch over till he awoke, refreshed from his slumber and eager again to resume their frolics.

The period of returning to the city at last arrived, and the dog exhibited marked signs of uneasiness, while the bustling preparations for this end were going on, as if conscious of the separation that was about to take place between his young master and himself, as also the other children, who had been his constant companions for so many joyful months.

Everything being completed, the childish group bid an affectionate adieu to the downcast Rolla, whom they left standing on the hill-top, watching the carriage as it disappeared in the wood. A few days after their departure, and when this poor animal was forgotten in the new scenes around them, a communication was received from the overseer of the farm, in which he stated that the favourite dog appeared much grieved since the family had left for the city, and was fearful that he might die if he continued in the same condition. Little attention, however, was given to these remarks, all imagining that the dog's melancholy was only the result of temporary distress, owing to his secluded life, so different from that which he had led when surrounded by the various members of a large family. Little did any one suppose that this poor neglected brute was suffering the acutest pangs of mental distress, even sufficient to produce death.

Two weeks had now elapsed since the separation from Rolla, when another message came from the overseer, stating that the dog would surely die with grief, if not removed to the city, as he had refused all sustenance for several days, and did nothing but wander about from place to place, formerly frequented by the children, howling and moaning in the most piteous manner.

Orders were now given, much to the children's delight, for the conveyance of the favourite to the city; but, alas! this arrangement came too late, as the poor creature sank from exhaustion, while in the wagon on his way to join those beloved companions whose short absence had broken his heart and grieved him even unto death.—L.]

We will not further pursue this part of our subject at present. We shall have other opportunities of speaking of the disinterested and devoted affection which this noble animal is capable of displaying when he occupies his proper situation, and discharges those offices for which nature designed him. It may, however, be added that this power of tracing back the dog to the very earliest periods of history, and the fact that he then seemed to be as sagacious, as faithful, and as valuable as at the present day, strongly favour the opinion that he descended from no inferior and comparatively worthless animal,—that he was not the progeny of the wolf, the jackal, or the fox, but he was originally created, somewhat as we now find him, the associate and the friend of man.

If, within the first thousand years after the Deluge, we observe that divine honours were paid to him, we can scarcely be brought to believe his wolfish genealogy. The most savage animals are capable of affection for those to whom they have been accustomed, and by whom they have been well treated, and therefore we give full credit to several accounts of this sort related of the wolf, the lion, and even the cat and the reptile: but in no other animal—in no other, even in the genus *Canis*—do we find the qualities of the domestic dog, or the slightest approach to them. "To his master he flies with alacrity," says the eloquent Buffon, "and submissively lays at his feet all his courage, strength, and talent. A glance of the eye is sufficient; for he understands the smallest indications of his will. He has all the ardour of friendship, and fidelity and constancy in his affections, which man can have. Neither interest nor desire of revenge can corrupt him, and he has no fear but that of displeasing. He is all zeal and obedience. He speedily forgets ill-usage, or only recollects it to make returning attachment the stronger. He licks the hand which causes him pain, and subdues his anger by submission. The training of the dog seems to have been the first art invented by man, and the fruit of that art was the conquest and peaceable possession of the earth." "Man," says Burns, "is the God of the dog; he knows no other; and see how he worships him. With what reverence he crouches at his feet—with what reverence he looks up to him—with what delight he fawns upon him, and with what cheerful alacrity he obeys him!"

If any of the lower animals bear about them the impress of the Divine hand, it is found in the dog: many others are plainly and decidedly more or less connected with the welfare of the human being; but this connexion and its effects are limited to a few points, or often to one alone. The dog, different, yet the same, in every region, seems to be formed expressly to administer to our comforts and to our pleasure. He displays a versatility, and yet a perfect unity of power and character, which mark him as our destined servant, and, still more, as our companion and friend. Other animals may be brought to a certain degree of familiarity, and may display much affection and gratitude. There was scarcely an animal in the menagerie of the Zoological Society that did not acknowledge the superintendent as his friend; but it was only a casual intercourse, and might be dissolved by a word or look. At the hour of feeding, the brute principle reigned supreme, and the companion of other hours would be sacrificed if he dared to interfere; but the connexion between man and the dog, no lapse of time, no change of circumstances, no infliction of evil can dissolve. We must, therefore, look far beyond the wolf for the prototype of the dog.

Cuvier eloquently states that the dog exhibits the most complete and the most useful conquest that man has made. Each individual is entirely devoted to his master, adopts his manners, distinguishes and defends his property, and remains attached to him even unto death; and all this springing not from mere necessity, or from constraint, but simply from gratitude and true friendship. The swiftness, the strength, and the highly developed power of smelling of the dog, have made him a powerful ally of man against the other animals; and, perhaps, these qualities in the dog were necessary to the establishment of society. It is the only animal that has followed the human being all over the earth.

There is occasionally a friendship existing between dogs resembling that which is found in the human being. The author pledges himself as to the accuracy of the following little anecdote. Two dogs, the property of a gentleman at Shrewsbury, had been companions for many years, until one of them died of old age. The survivor immediately began to manifest an extraordinary degree of restless anxiety, searching for his old associate in all his former haunts, and refusing every kind of food. He gradually wasted away, and, at the expiration of the tenth day, he died, the victim of an attachment that would have done honour to man.

The Dog belongs to the division of animals termed VERTEBRATED, (see 'The Horse, 2d edition, page 106), because it has a cranium or skull, and a spine or range of VERTEBRÆ proceeding from it. It ranks under the *class* MAMMALIA, because it has teats, by which the female suckles her young; the *tribe* UNGUICULATA, because its extremities are armed with nails; the *order* DIGITIGRADES, because it walks principally on its toes. The *genus* CANIS has two tubercular teeth behind the large carnivorous tooth in the upper jaw; and the *sub-genus familiaris*, the DOG, has the pupils of the eye circular, while those of the wolf are oblique, and those of the fox upright and long.

There has been some dispute whether the various species of dogs are of different origin, or sprung from one common source. When we consider the change that climate and breeding effect in the same species of dog, and contrast the rough Irish or Highland greyhound with the smoother one of the southern parts of Britain, or the more delicate one of Greece, or the diminutive but beautifully formed one of Italy, or the hairless one of Africa or Brazil—or the small Blenheim spaniel with the magnificent Newfoundland; if also we observe many of them varied by accident, and that accidental variety diligently cultivated into a new species, altogether different in form or use, we shall find no difficulty in believing that they might be derived from one common origin.

One of the most striking proofs of the influence of climate on the form and character of this animal, occurs in the bull-dog. When transported to India he becomes, in a few years, greatly altered in form, loses all his former courage and ferocity, and becomes a perfect coward.

It is probable that all dogs sprang from one common source, but climate, food, and cross-breeding caused variations of form, which suggested particular uses; and these being either designedly or accidentally perpetuated, the various breeds of dogs thus arose, and they have become numerous in proportion to the progress of civilization. Among the ruder, or savage tribes, they possess but one form; but the ingenuity of man has devised many inventions to increase his comforts: he has varied and multiplied the characters and kinds of domestic animals for the same purpose, and hence the various breeds of horses, and cattle, and dogs.

The parent stock it is now impossible to trace; but the wild dog, wherever found on the continent of Asia, or Northern Europe, has nearly the same character, and bears no inconsiderable resemblance to the British fox-dog, while many of those from the Southern Ocean can scarcely be distinguished from the English lurcher. There is, however, no more difficulty in this respect with regard to the dog, than any other of our domesticated animals. Climate, or chance, produced a change in certain individuals, and the sagacity of man, or, perhaps, mere chance, founded on these accidental varieties numerous breeds possessed of certain distinct characteristic properties. The degeneracy of the dog, also, in different countries, cannot for a moment be disputed.

The most natural arrangement of all the varieties of the dog is according to the development of the frontal sinus and the cerebral cavity, or, in other words, the power of scent, and the degree of intelligence. This classification originated with M. F. Cuvier, and has been adopted by most naturalists. He reckoned three divisions of the dog:—

I. Those having the head more or less elongated, and the parietal bones of the skull widest at the base, and gradually approaching towards each other as they ascend, the condyls of the lower jaw being on the same line with the upper molar teeth. The *Greyhound* and all its varieties belong to this class.

II. The head moderately elongated, and the parietals diverging from each other for a certain space as they rise upon the side of the head, enlarging the cerebral cavity and the frontal sinus. To this class belong our most valuable dogs,—the *Spaniel*, *Setter*, *Pointer*, *Hound*, and the *Sheep-dog*.

III. The muzzle more or less shortened, the frontal sinus enlarged, and the cranium elevated, and diminished in capacity. To this class belong some of the *Terriers*, and a great many dogs that might very well be spared.

This division of the different species of the dog is adopted here as being the most simple, intelligible, and satisfactory.

CHAPTER II.

THE VARIETIES OF THE DOG.

FIRST DIVISION.

The head more or less elongated, the parietal bones widest at the base and gradually approaching to each other as they ascend, and the condyls of the lower jaw being on the same line with the upper molar teeth.

To this division belong the greater number of the

WILD DOGS.

The wild dog, as existing in considerable numbers or communities, seems to be nearly extirpated in the southern parts of Europe; but there are several cases on record, of dogs having assumed the character of the wild race from which they had descended, abandoning their state of domestication, and reasserting their native independence. A black greyhound bitch, belonging to a gentleman in Scarisbrick, in Lancashire, though she had apparently been well broken in, and always well used, ran away from the habitation of her master, and betook herself to the woods. She killed a great number of hares and made free with the sheep, and became an intolerable nuisance to the neighbourhood. She was occasionally seen, and the depredations that were committed were brought home to her. Many were the attempts made to entrap or destroy her, but in vain: for more than six months she eluded the vigilance of her pursuers. At length she was observed to creep into a hole in an old barn. She was caught as she came out, and the barn being searched three whelps were found, which, very foolishly, were destroyed.

The bitch evinced the utmost ferocity, and, although well secured, attempted to seize every one who approached her. She was, however, dragged home and treated with kindness. By degrees her ferocity abated. In the course of two months, she became perfectly reconciled to her original abode, and, a twelvemonth afterwards (1822), she ran successfully several courses. There was still a degree of wildness in her appearance; but, although at perfect liberty, she seemed to be altogether reconciled to a domestic life.

In 1784 a dog was left by a smuggling vessel on the coast of Northumberland. He soon began to worry the sheep for his subsistence, and did so much mischief that he caused very considerable alarm. He was frequently pursued by hounds and greyhounds;

but when the dogs came up he lay upon his back as if supplicating for mercy, and in that position they would never hurt him. He therefore lay quietly until the hunters approached, when he made off without being followed by the hounds until they were again excited to the pursuit. He one day led them 30 miles in this way. It was more than three months before he was caught, and was then shot.[a]

A dog with every character of the wild one has occasionally been seen in some of the forests of Germany, and among the Pyrenean mountains; but he has rarely been found gregarious there. In the country on the eastern side of the Gulf of Venice wild dogs are more frequent. They increase in the Austrian and Turkish dominions, and are found on almost every part of the coast of the Black Sea, but even there they rarely gather in flocks: they do not howl in concert, as the wolf; nor are they the precursors of other and larger beasts, like the jackal. Most of these dogs have the muzzle and head elongated, the ears erect, triangular, and small, the body and neck large and muscular, and the tail short, but with a brush of crisped hair. In many parts of Arabia the wild dog—or *dakhun*—is occasionally found. In Persia, they are most decidedly congregated together, and still more so in almost every part of India.[b]

Mr. Hodgson has favoured the Zoological Society with an account of

THE WILD DOG OF NEPAL,

the *búánsú*, and, finding it more or less prevailing through the whole of Northern India, and even southward of the coast of Coromandel, he thought that he had discovered the primitive race of the dog. This is a point that can never be decided. "These dogs hunt their prey by night, as well as by day, in packs of from

[a] Annals of Sporting, vol. vi. p. 99.

[b] The superstition of the Arabians and Turks with regard to dogs is somewhat singular: neither have they much affection for these animals, or suffer them to be in or near the camp, except to guard it in the night. They have, however, some charity for the females that have whelps. As for other dogs, they feed them well, and give them good words, but never touch them nor go near them, because dogs are regarded as unclean animals. They particularly drive them away in wet weather; for, if one drop of water from a dog should fall on their raiment, their devotion would be interrupted and useless. They who are fond of hunting make their religion subservient to their pleasure, and say that greyhounds and setters are excepted from the general rule, because when not running these dogs are tied up where nothing unclean can reach them, and they are never suffered to eat any thing unclean. Their opinion is the same with regard to small dogs, which are kept with great care, and no one willingly injures a dog, or, if he should injure purposely, or destroy one of them, the law would punish him. Chevalier Darvieux's Travels in Arabia Deserta, 1718, p. 155.

six to ten individuals, maintaining the chase more by the scent than by the eye, and generally succeeding by dint of strength and perseverance. While hunting, they bark like the hound, yet the bark is peculiar, and equally unlike that of the cultivated breeds of dogs, and the cries of the jackal and the fox." Bishop Heber gives the following account of them. "They are larger and stronger than a fox, which in the circumstances of form and fur they much resemble. They hunt, however, in packs, give tongue like dogs, and possess an exquisite scent. They make of course tremendous havoc among the game in these hills; but that mischief they are said amply to repay by destroying wild beasts, and even tigers."[a]

Wild dogs are susceptible of certain social combinations. In Egypt, Constantinople, and throughout the whole of the East, there are in every village troops of wandering dogs who belong to no particular person. Each troop has its own quarter of the place; and if any wander into a quarter which does not belong to him, its inhabitants unite together and chase him out. At the Cape of Good Hope there are many dogs half-starved. On going from home the natives induce two or more of these animals to accompany them, warn them of the approach of any ferocious animal, and if any of the jackals approach the walls during the night, they utter the most piercing cries, and at this signal every dog sallies out, and, uniting together, put the jackals to speedy flight.[b]

The wild Nepâl dogs caught when at an adult age make no approach towards domestication; but a young one, which Mr. Hodgson obtained when it was not more than a month old, became sensible to caresses, and manifested as much intelligence as any sporting dog of the same age.[c]

Captain T. Williamson gives an interesting account of the ferocious character of some of these wild dogs. "They have considerable resemblance to the jackal in form. They are remarkably savage, and frequently will approach none but their *doonahs* or keepers, not allowing their own masters to come near them. Some of them are very fleet; but they are not to be depended upon in coursing; for they are apt suddenly to give up the chase when it is a severe one, and, indeed, they will too often prefer a sheep or a goat to a hare. In hog-hunting they are more valuable. It seems to suit their temper, and they appear to enjoy the snapping and the snarling, incident to that species of sports."

He says that many persons affect to treat the idea of degenera tion in quadrupeds with ridicule; but all who have been any considerable time resident in India must be satisfied that dogs of Eu

---

[a] Heber's Narrative, p. 500.

[b] Histoire du Chien, par Elzear Blaze, p. 54.

[c] Proceedings of the Zoological Society, Part I. 833.

ropean breed become, after every successive generation, more and more similar to the pariah, or indigenous dog of that country. The hounds are the most rapid in their decline, and, except in the form of their ears, they are very much like many of the village curs. Greyhounds and pointers also rapidly decline, although with occasional exceptions. Spaniels and terriers deteriorate less, and spaniels of eight or nine generations, and without a cross from Europe, are not only as good as, but far more beautiful than, their ancestors. The climate is too severe for mastiffs, and they do not possess sufficient stamina; but, crossed by the East Indian greyhound, they are invaluable in hunting the hog.[a]

Colonel Sykes, at one of the meetings of the Zoological Society, produced a specimen of

THE WILD DOG OF DAKHUN

or Deccan, a part of India far to the south of Nepâl, and gave the following description of this supposed primitive dog:—"Its head is compressed and elongated, but its muzzle not very sharp. The eyes are oblique, the pupils round, and the *irides* light-brown. The expression of the countenance is that of a coarse ill-natured Persian greyhound, without any resemblance to the jackal, the fox, or the wolf. The ears are long, erect, and somewhat rounded at the top. The limbs remarkably large and strong in relation to the bulk of the animal. The size is intermediate between the wolf and the jackal. The neck long, the body elongated, and the entire dog of a red-brown colour. None of the domesticated dogs of Dakhun are common in Europe, but those of Dakhun and Nepâl are very similar in all their characters. There is also a dog in Dakhun with hair so short as to make him appear naked. It is called the *polugar* dog.

THE WILD DOG OF THE MAHRATTAS

possesses a similar conformation; and the fact is, that the East Indian wild dog is essentially the same in every part of that immense extent of country. There is no more reason, however, for concluding that it was the primitive dog, than for conferring on the Indian cattle the same honour among the ruminants. The truth of the matter is that we have no guide what was the original breed in any country. The lapse of 4000 years would effect strange alterations in the breeds. The common name of this dog, in the track lying between South Bahar and the Mahratta frontier towards Maghore, is

DHOLE,

the *Chryseus Scylex* of Hamilton Smith.

[a] Williamson's Oriental Field Sports.

Captain Williamson, in his Oriental Field Sports, gives the following account of the Dholes:—

"They are to be found chiefly, or only, in the country from Midnapore to Chamu, and even there are not often to be met with. They are of the size of a small greyhound. Their countenance is enlivened by unusually brilliant eyes. Their body, which is slender and deep-chested, is thinly covered by a coat of hair of a reddish-brown or bay colour. The tail is dark towards its extremity. The limbs are light, compact, and strong, and equally calculated for speed and power. They resemble many of the common pariah dogs in form, but the singularity of their colour and marks at once demonstrates an evident distinction.

"These dogs are said to be perfectly harmless if unmolested. They do not willingly approach persons; but, if they chance to meet any in their course, they do not show any particular anxiety to escape. They view the human race rather as objects of curiosity, than either of apprehension or enmity. The natives who reside near the Ranochitty and Katcunsandy passes, in which vicinity the *dholes* may frequently be seen, describe them as confining their attacks entirely to wild animals, and assert that they will not prey on sheep, goats, &c.; but others, in the country extending southward from Jelinah and Mechungunge, maintain that cattle are frequently lost by their depredations. I am inclined to believe that the *dhole* is not particularly ceremonious, but will, when opportunity offers, and a meal is wanting, obtain it at the expense of the neighbouring village.

"The peasants likewise state that the *dhole* is eager in proportion to the size and powers of the animal he hunts, preferring the elk to every other kind of deer, and particularly seeking the royal tiger. It is probable that the *dhole* is the principal check on the multiplication of the tiger; and, although incapable individually, or perhaps in small numbers, to effect the destruction of so large and ferocious an animal, may, from their custom of hunting in packs, easily overcome any smaller beast found in the wilds of India.

"They run mute, except that they sometimes utter a whimpering kind of note, similar to that sometimes expressed by dogs when approaching their prey. This may be expressive of their own gratification, or anxiety, or may serve as a guide to other *dholes* to join in the chase. The speed of the *dhole* is so strongly marked in his form as to render it probable no animal in the catalogue of game could escape him for any distance. Many of the *dholes* are destroyed in these contests; for the tiger, the elk, and the boar, and even many of the smaller classes of game are capable of making a most obstinate defence. Hence the breed of the *dholes* is much circumscribed."

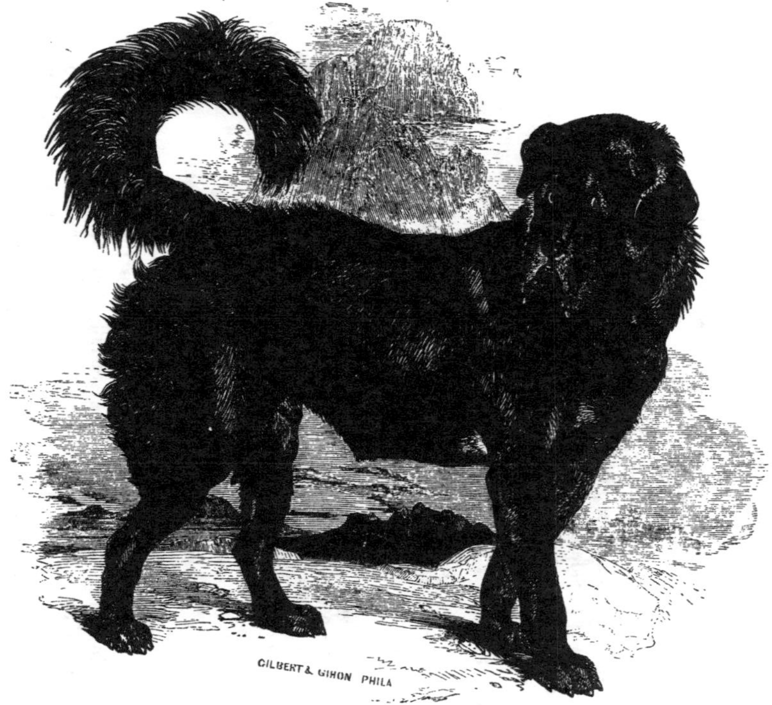

THE THIBET DOG.

THE THIBET DOG.

Mr. Bennett, in his scientific and amusing description of the Zoological Gardens, gave the best account we have of this noble dog, and our portrait is a most faithful likeness of him. He is bred in the table-land of the Himalaya mountains bordering on Thibet. The Bhoteas, by whom many of them are carefully reared, come down to the low countries at certain seasons of the year to sell their borax and musk. The women remain at home, and they and the flocks are most sedulously guarded by these dogs. They are the defenders of almost every considerable mansion in Thibet. In an account of an embassy to the court of the Teshoo Llama in Thibet, the author says, that he had to pass by a row of wooden cages containing a number of large dogs, fierce, strong, and noisy. They were natives of Thibet, and, whether savage by nature or soured by confinement, they were so impetuously furious that it was unsafe even to approach their dens. Every writer who describes these dogs, speaks of their noble size, and their ferocity, and antipathy to strangers.

It is said, however, that the Thibet dog rapidly degenerates when removed from its native country, and certainly the specimens which have reached the Zoological Gardens exhibited nothing of ferocity. The one that was in that menagerie had a noble and commanding appearance; but he never attempted to do any injury.

The colour of the Thibet dog is of a deep black, slightly clouded on the sides, his feet alone and a spot over each eye being of a full tawny or bright brown hue. He has the broad short truncated muzzle of the mastiff, and the lips are still more deeply pendulous. There is also a singular general looseness of the skin on every part of him.

THE PARIAH.

There are several varieties of this dog. There is a wild breed very numerous in the jungles and in some of the lower ranges of the Himalaya mountains. They usually hunt in packs, and it is not often that their prey escapes them. They generally are very thin, and of a reddish-brown colour, with sharp-pointed ears, deep chest, and tucked-up flanks. Many persons hunt with these dogs singly, and they are very useful. They bring the hog to bay, or indicate the course that he has taken, or distract his attention when the sportsman is at hand.

There is also in every inhabited part of the country the poor desolate pariah,—unowned by any one,—daring to enter into no house, but wandering about, and picking up a living in any way that he can. He is, however, of a superior race to the wild dog, and belongs to the second class of the dog, although mentioned here in order that we may altogether quit the dog of India. They are neglected by the Hindoos; but the Mohammedans of India, and other strangers, consider it an act of charity to throw out occasionally a morsel of food to them. They are most of them mongrels; but the benevolent Bishop Heber does them no more than justice when he says that he "was forcibly struck at finding the same dog-like and amiable qualities in these neglected animals as in their more fortunate brethren in Europe."

Colonel Sykes says of these outcasts that among the pariahs is frequently found the turnspit-dog. There is also a small petted variety of the pariah, usually of a white colour, and with long silky hair. This animal is taught to carry flambeaux and lanterns.

According to Captain Williamson, in some of the ditches of the Carnatic forts, alligators are purposely kept, and all the pariah dogs found in the forts are thrown into the ditches as provision for these monsters. Some persons who have kept tigers in cages have adopted the same means of supply for their royal captives, putting the poor pariah through an aperture made for the purpose in the cage; and they justify themselves by asserting that they thus get rid of a troublesome breed of curs, most of which are unappropriated, and which being numerous are very troublesome to passengers, often wantonly biting them, and raising a yelling noise at night, that sets all attempts to rest at defiance.

It did not always happen that the tiger killed the pariah put into his cage. "I knew an instance," says Captain Williamson, "of one that was destined for the tiger's daily meal, standing on the defensive in a manner that completely astonished both the tiger and the spectator. He crept into a corner, and whenever the tiger approached seized him by the lip or the neck, making him roar most piteously. The tiger, however, impelled by hunger,—for all supply of food was purposely withheld,—would renew the attack. The result was ever the same. At length the tiger began to treat the dog with more deference, and not only allowed him to partake of the mess of rice and milk furnished daily for his subsistence, but even refrained from any attempt to disturb him. The two animals at length became reconciled to each other, and a strong attachment was formed between them. The dog was then allowed ingress and egress through the aperture; and, considering the cage as his own, he left it and returned to it just as he thought proper. When the tiger died he moaned the loss of his companion for a considerable period."

A wild variety exists in Sumatra. It is described by Cuvier as "possessing the countenance of a fox, the eyes oblique, the ears rounded and hairy, the muzzle of a foxy-brown colour, the tail bushy and pendulous, very lively, running with the head lifted high, and the ears straight." This animal can scarcely be rendered tractable, and even when he is apparently tamed can rarely be depended upon.

As we proceed through the Indian Archipelago, towards Australasia, we skirt the coast of Java. Every Javanese of rank has large packs of dogs with which he hunts the muntjak, the deer of that country. The dogs are led in strings by the attendants until they scent the prey: they are then unloosed, while the sportsmen follow, but not at the speed which would distinguish the British sportsman. The animal is generally found at bay. The male muntjak usually exhibits considerable courage, and probably several of the dogs have been wounded by his tusks. As soon as they come up every gun is discharged, and the animal almost immediately drops. At other times the mounted sportsmen attack them with a spear or sword. Generally, the muntjak does not go off like the stag in any direct track, but takes a circular course, and soon returns to the spot whence it was started. It perhaps makes several of these circles, and at length entangles itself in a thicket, where it is secured.

These dogs are the indigenous breed of the island, the body lank, the ears erect, ferocious in their disposition, and with very little attachment to their masters. Such is the account given of them by Dr. Horsfield.

THE DINGO, AUSTRALASIAN, OR NEW HOLLAND DOG.

The newly discovered southern continent was, and some of it still continues to be, overrun by the native wild dogs. Dampier describes them, at the close of the last century, as "beasts like the hungry wolves, lean like so many skeletons, and being nothing but skin and bone." It was not until the publication of Governor Phillip's voyage to Botany Bay, that any accurate description or figure of this dog could be obtained. He approaches in appearance to the largest kind of shepherd's dog. The head is elongated, the forehead flat, and the ears short and erect, or with a slight direction forwards. The body is thickly covered with hair of two kinds—the one woolly and gray, the other silky and of a deep yellow or fawn colour. The limbs are muscular, and, were it not for the suspicious yet ferocious glare of the eye, he might pass for a handsome dog. The Australasian dog, according to M. Desmarest, resembles in form and in the proportion of his limbs the common shepherd's dog. He is very active and courageous, covered in some parts with thick hair woolly and gray, in other parts becoming of a yellowish-red colour, and under the belly having a whitish hue. When he is running, the head is lifted more than usual in dogs, and the tail is carried horizontally. He seldom barks Mr. Bennett observes that "dogs in a state of nature never bark. They simply whine, howl, or growl. The explosive noise of the bark is only found among those that are domesticated." Sonini speaks of the shepherds' dogs in the wilds of Egypt as not having this faculty; and Columbus found the dogs which he had previously carried to America, almost to have lost their propensity to bark.

He does, however, occasionally bark, and has the same kind of snarling voice which the larger dogs generally have. The Australasian dogs that have been brought to Europe have usually been of a savage and untractable disposition.

There are several of the Australasian dogs in the gardens of the Zoological Society of London. One of them has been an inmate of that establishment nine years, others more than five years; but not an individual has acquired the bark of the other dogs by which they are surrounded. When a stranger makes his appearance, or when the hour of feeding arrives, the howl of the Australasian is the first sound that is heard, and it is louder than all the rest.

If some of them have thrown off a portion of their native ferocity, others retain it undiminished. A bitch and two of her whelps, nearly half grown—a male and female—had inhabited the same cage from the time that the young ones were born. Some cause of quarrel occurred on a certain night, and the two bitches fell upon the dog and perfectly destroyed him. There was not a limb left whole. A stronger instance of the innate ferocity of this breed could scarcely be given. Even in their native country all attempts perfectly to domesticate them have failed; for they never lose an opportunity to devour the poultry or attack the sheep. Every domesticated dog coming within their reach was immediately destroyed. One that was brought to England broke his chain—scoured the surrounding country—and, before dawn, had destroyed several sheep; and another attacked, and would have destroyed, an ass, if he had not been prevented.

Mr. Oxley, Surveyor-General of New South Wales, however, gives an interesting account of the mutual attachment between two of the native and wild New Holland dingos. "About a week ago we killed a native dog, and threw his body on a small bush. On returning past the same spot to-day, we found the body removed three or four yards from the bush, and the female in a dying state lying close beside it: she had apparently been there from the day the dog was killed. Being now so weakened and emaciated as to be unable to move on our approach, it was deemed a mercy to despatch her."

When Van Diemen Land began to be colonized by Europeans, the losses sustained by the settlers by the ravages of the wild dogs were almost incredible. The districts infested by these animals

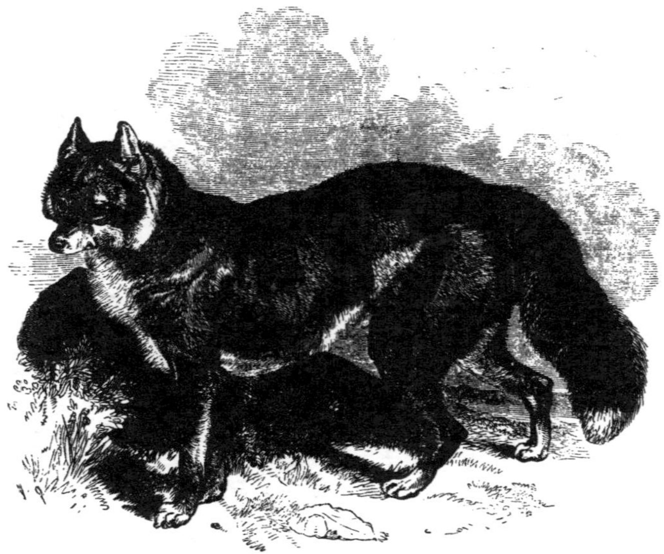

THE DINGO, OR NEW HOLLAND DOG.

were principally those appropriated to sheep, and there was scarcely a flock that did not suffer. It was in vain to double the number of shepherds, to watch by night and by day, or to have fires at every quarter of the fold; for these animals would accomplish their object by stratagem or by force. One colony lost no fewer than 1200 sheep and lambs in three months; another colony lost 700.

The ravagers were either the native wild dogs of the island, or those that had escaped from their owners. They seemed to have apportioned the country into different districts, each troop having its allotted range. At length the evil became so great that a general meeting of the colonists was convened. The concluding sentences of the speech of Lieutenant Hill forcibly express the extent of the evil. "The country is free from bush-rangers: we are no longer surrounded and threatened by the natives. We have only one enemy left in the field; but that enemy strikes at the very root of our welfare, and through him the stream of our prosperity is tainted at its very source." The colonists were then few, but they cordially united in the endeavour to extirpate this formidable enemy; and, although the wild dog is still found in the interior of the island, he is comparatively seldom seen, and his ravages have nearly ceased.

THE CANIS AUSTRALIS—KARÁRAHÉ, NEW ZEALAND DOG.

A tradition exists in New Zealand of this dog having been given to the natives two or three centuries ago by a number of divinities who made their descent on these shores, probably Juan Fernandez and his companions. The sagacious animal has, however, dwindled down to the lowest rank of his family, but ill usage has not altogether destroyed his worth. In New Zealand he is the safeguard of every village. Should the slightest alarm exist, he is the first to ascertain the cause of it, and many families have saved themselves by flight, or have taken arms in self-defence against the incursions of predatory bands. The New Zealanders are therefore kind in their treatment of the dog, except that they occasionally destroy him for his hide.

The name formerly given to the New Zealand dog was *pero*, which in some measure substantiates the supposition of Juan Fernandez having visited the country—*perro*, in the Spanish language, being the name of a dog.

We will now turn to the northern parts of America. The races of wild dogs are there considerably limited, both in number and the districts which they occupy.

In the elevated sandy country north of the source of the Missouri, inhabited by the "Stone" and the "Black Foot" Indians, is a doubtful species of dogs—wolves they used to be called—who hunt in large packs and are exceedingly swift; whose bark is similar to that of the domestic dog, but who burrow in the ground, and eagerly run to their holes, when the gun of the hunter is heard. [Our author evidently, in the above remarks, confounds the Louisiana marmot, Arctomys Ludovicianus or Prairie dog, with the Canis Latrans of Say, as he certainly would not make us believe that such harmless animals as the marmot should associate themselves in packs to hunt the deer or other quadrupeds; neither would he tell us that so different an animal as the Canis Latrans could burrow in the ground and retreat to their holes when surprised by the hunter. The Louisiana Marmot, improperly called Prairie dog, is about sixteen inches long, and lives in extended villages or excavations surmounted by mounds. These communities often comprise several thousand inhabitants, whose sole food consists in the scanty herbage surrounding the settlement, as they seldom extend their excursions beyond a half-mile from their burrows for fear of the wolves, and many other enemies

The Canis Latrans, on the other hand, is quite a large and savage animal, and frequently unites in bands to run down deer or buffalo calves, but as for living under ground in burrows, it is quite out of reason to suppose such a thing possible with this quadruped, who secretes himself in the depths of the forest, and appears on the open plain only when in pursuit of game.—L.] The habit of selecting large, open, sandy plains, and burrowing there, extends to the greater part of the American wild dogs.

[We have been credibly informed by several gentlemen, familiar with the country of Mexico, that there is a diminutive species of dog running wild, and burrowing in the ground as rabbits, in the neighbourhood of Santa Fe and Chihuahua. A gentleman who has seen these animals, states that there is no doubt as to their identity, having met with them in a state of domestication, when they exhibited all the actions and manners of a French lap dog, such as come from Cuba or other West India Islands.

They are of every variety of hue, and resort to their burrows whenever disturbed in their natural haunts. What they subsist on it is difficult to say, as they are too harmless and insignificant to attack any other animal beyond a mouse or a snail. They are represented as being very difficult to tame, but when domesticated show no disposition to return to their former mode of life. The lady of the Mexican Minister, when in this city, had one of these dogs as a boudoir pet; it was lively and barked quite fiercely. We have not been able to ascertain whether they bark in their natural state. The breed of dog cultivated in China for food alone, are fed entirely upon rice meal and other farinaceous articles, having no relish whatever for flesh or other strong aliment.—L.]

In some parts of North America whole troops of horses are guarded and kept together by dogs. If any of the troop attempt to steal away, the dog will immediately fly after the horse, head him, and bring him back to his companions.

[To show the necessity of having dogs for this purpose, as well as to guard the flocks of sheep, we need only mention that it is no uncommon thing for a Mexican to own several thousand horses, besides an immense number of cattle.

Mr. Kendall, in his Santa Fé expedition, states that the proprietress of one hacienda, a widow, and comparatively poor when the wonderful wealth of her ancestors is considered, now owns fifty thousand horses and mules, beside herds of cattle and sheep, and that the pasture ground extended for fifty miles on either side of the road.

One of the former owners of this immense estate, a short time previous to the revolution, sent as a present to a Spanish colonel, just arrived with his regiment of dragoons, a thousand white horses, nearly all of the same age, and every one raised on this prolific hacienda.—L.]

The wild dogs abound in many parts of South America. In some of the forests on the banks of the Oronoko they multiply to an annoying degree. The Cayotte of Mexico, described by some as a wolf, and bearing no slight resemblance to that animal, belongs to the South American wild dogs, as do also the Aguara dogs of every kind. These wanderers of the woods are, however, diminished in numbers in every part of that continent, and are replaced by other kinds, many of which have been imported from Europe and domesticated.

[There is no country in the world more cursed with worthless curs than that of Mexico and the other southern republics; the cities and villages actually swarm with these animals, and produce no little vexation to travellers, who speak of their eternal yelping and barking in the most indignant terms.

Mr. Kendall, on entering San Antonio, says, "From every house some half dozen Mexican curs would jump forth and greet us with a chorus of yelps and barks, and before we had fairly entered the town the canine hue and cry was general. Those who have for the first time entered a Mexican town or city must have been struck with the unusual number of dogs, and annoyed by their incessant barking; but the stranger soon learns that they spend all their courage in barks—they seldom bite."—L.]

Many of the Indian tribes have succeeded in reclaiming the dog of the woods, and have made him a useful although not a perfectly attached servant.

The dogs of the Falkland Islands, and the Indian North American dogs generally, are brown or gray-coloured varieties of the wild dog; but they are nearly exterminated.

The history of the

WILD DOG OF AFRICA

will occupy little space. It has already been stated that in Egypt and in Nubia we have the first records of the dog. Many superstitious notions were connected with him, and divine honours were paid to him. Those times are passed away, and he is regarded with aversion by the Moslem of the present day. He is an outcast. He obtains a scanty living by the offal which he gathers in the towns, or he is become a perfect wild dog, and scours the country for his prey. His modern name is the *deab.* He is of considerable size, with a round muzzle, large head, small erect ears, and long and hairy tail, spotted with black, white, and yellow, and having a fierce wolfish aspect. These dogs are not, however, numerous; but the mischief which they do is often great, whether in pairs they burrow in the earth, or associate with others and hunt in troops.[a]

In Nubia is a smaller dog of the same kind, which never burrows. It lives on small animals and birds, and rarely enters any of the towns. A similar dog, according to Colonel Hamilton Smith, inhabits the neighbourhood of the Cape, and particularly the Karroo or Wilderness. It is smaller than either of the others, and lives among bushes or under prominent rocks. Others, although not identified with the jackal, yet associating with him, inhabit the Uplands of Gambia and Senegal.

On the Gold Coast, the dog is used and prized as an article of food. He is fattened and driven to market as the European drives his sheep and hogs. The dog is even more valued than the sheep for human subsistence, and is deemed the greatest luxury that can be placed even on the royal table.

In Loango, or Lower Guinea, is a town from which the African wild dogs derive their name — the *dingo.* They hunt in large packs. They fearlessly attack even the elephant, and generally

[a] Poiret, in his Travels in Barbary, asserts that "the dog loses in the East a great part of those good qualities that make him the friend of man. He is no longer a faithful domesticated animal, faithfully attached to his master, and ever ready to defend him even at the expense of his own life. He is cruel and blood-thirsty, his look is savage, and his appearance revolting; carrion, filth, anything is good enough for him if he can but appease his hunger. They seldom bite one another, but they unite against a stranger who approaches the Arab tents, and would tear him to pieces if he did not seek his safety in flight."—Vol. i. p. 353.

Denon, when in the city of Alexandria, in Egypt, says, "I have no longer recognised the dog, that friend of man, the attached and faithful companion — the lively and honest courtier. He is here a gloomy egotist, and cut off from all human intercourse without being the less a slave. He does not know him whose house he protects, and devours his corpse without repugnance." — Travels in Lower Egypt, p. 32.

destroy him. In the neighbourhood of the Cape, the country is nearly cleared of wild beasts; but in Cape Town there are a great number of lean and miserable dogs, who howl about the streets at night, quitting their dens and lurking-places, in quest of offal. No great while ago, the wolves and hyænas used to descend and dispute the spoil with the dogs, while the town resounded with their hideous howlings all the night long.

This will be a proper place to refer to the numerous accounts that are given both in ancient and modern times of the immolation of dogs, and of their being used for food. They were sacrificed at certain periods by the Greeks and Romans to almost all their deities, and particularly to Mars, Pluto, and Pan, to Minerva, Proserpine, and Lucina, and also to the moon, because the dog by his barking disturbed all charms and spells, and frightened away all spectres and apparitions. The Greeks immolated many dogs in honour of Hecate, because by their baying the phantoms of the lower world were disturbed. A great number of dogs were also destroyed in Samothrace in honour of the same goddess Dogs were periodically sacrificed in February, and also in April and in May; also to the goddess Rubigo, who presided over the corn, and the Bona Dea, whose mysterious rites were performed on Mount Aventine. The dog Cerberus was supposed to be watching at the feet of Pluto, and a dog and a youth were periodically sacrificed to that deity. The night when the Capitol had nearly been destroyed was annually celebrated by the cruel scourging of a dog in the principal public places, even to the death of the animal.

[As on a certain occasion, the dogs who had the Capitol in custody, did not bark and give warning when the Gauls attempted to scale the walls, there is a custom annually observed at Rome, to transfix certain dogs to forkes, and thus crucified, hang them on an elder tree as examples of justice. (Book 29, chap. IV. Pliny.)—L.]

Many of the Greek and Roman epicures were strangely fond of the flesh of the dog, and those who ought to have known much better encouraged the use of this food. Galen speaks of it in the strongest terms of praise. Hippocrates says that the meat of old dogs is of a warm and dry quality, giving strength to the eater. Ananias, the poet, speaks of dog's flesh served up with that of the hare and fox. Virgil recommends that the fatted dog should be served up with whey or butter; and Dioscorides, the physician, says that they should be fed on the whey that remains after the making of cheese.

[Independent of the many useful and interesting qualities that necessarily endeared this animal to the ancients, he had yet stronger claims upon them, in the prophylactic properties of dif ferent portions of his body. Pliny, Hippocrates, Aristotle and others, speak of various preparations made of his flesh, for the cure of many distempers. The first-mentioned writer observes, that the ashes of burnt dogs, made into a liniment, with oil, will make an excellent application to the eye-brows, to turn them black. We doubt not that an analogous compound, if proved to be really efficacious, might be introduced to the notice of the belles of our own time, or meet with extensive sale for dyeing the pagoties and mustachios of the modern dandy. This quaint philosopher also recommends the same substance as a healing salve, for malignant wounds, and the internal use of the same article as a preventive or cure of hydrophobia and other distempers. (Book 28, chap. XI. and X.)—L.]

Before Christianity was established among the Danes, on every ninth year at the winter solstice, a monstrous sacrifice of 99 dogs was effected. In Sweden the sacrifice was still worse. On each of 9 successive days, 99 dogs were destroyed. This sacrifice of the dog, however, gave way to one as numerous and as horrible. On every 9th year, 99 human victims were immolated, and the sons of the reigning tyrant among the rest, in order that the life of the monarch might be prolonged.[a]

On the other hand, the dog was frequently the executioner; and, from an early period, whether in the course of war or the mock administration of justice, thousands of poor wretches were torn to pieces by animals trained to that horrible purpose.

Many of the Indians of North America, and almost of the present day, are fond of the flesh of the dog.

Captain Carver, in his Travels in North America in 1766, 1767, and 1768, describes the admission of an Indian into one of the horrible societies of that country. "The dishes being brought near to me," says he, "I perceived that they consisted of dog's flesh, and I was informed that at all their grand feasts they never made use of any other food. The new candidate provides fat dogs for the festival, if they can be procured at any price. They ate the flesh; but the head and the tongue were left sticking on a pole with the front towards the east. When any noxious disease appeared among them, a dog was killed, the intestines were wound between two poles, and every man was compelled to pass between them."

The Nandowepia Indians also eat dog's flesh as an article of luxury, and not from any want or scarcity of other animal food; for they have the bear, buffalo, elk, deer, beaver, and racoon.

Professor Keating, in his interesting work on the expedition to Peter's River, states that he and a party of American officers

---

Histoire du Chien, p. 200. The Voyage of Dumont d'Urville, vol. ii. p. 474.

were regaled in a large pavilion on buffalo meat, and *tepsia*, a vegetable boiled in buffalo grease, and the flesh of three dogs kept for the occasion, and without any salt. They partook of the flesh of the dogs with a mixture of curiosity and reluctance, and found it to be remarkably fat, sweet, and palatable, divested of any strong taste, and resembling the finest Welsh mutton, but of a darker colour. So strongly rooted, however, are the prejudices of education, that few of them could be induced to eat much of it.

The feast being over, great care was taken to replace the bones in their proper places in the dish, after which they were carefully washed and buried, as a token of respect to the animals generally, and because there was the belief among them that at some future time they would return again to life. Well-fattened puppies are frequently sold; and an invitation to a feast of dog's meat is the greatest distinction that can be offered to a stranger by any of the Indian nations east of the Rocky Mountains.

[Notwithstanding the Indians occasionally eat their dogs either through necessity or when they wish to pay a marked tribute of respect to their gods, or prepare a feast of friendship with strangers, they value them very highly, and do not by any means consider their flesh superior to that of the buffaloes or other animals of the chase. Mr. Catlin remarks, that "the dog, amongst all Indian tribes, is more esteemed and more valued than amongst any part of the civilized world: the Indian, who has more time to devote to his company, and whose untutored mind more nearly assimilates to that of his faithful domestic, keeps him closer company and draws him nearer his heart: they hunt together, and are equal sharers in the chase—their bed is one; and on the rocks and on their coats of arms they carve his image as the symbol of fidelity." (Vol. I., p. 230.)

On visiting the Sioux, they prepared for this gentleman as a token of regard a dog feast, previous to partaking of which they addressed him in a manner that plainly exhibits the veneration in which they held these faithful animals, at the same time forcibly demonstrating the peculiar circumstances under which they alone are willing to destroy them:

"My father, I hope you will have pity upon us; we are very poor. We offer you to-day not the best we have got; for we have a plenty of good buffalo hump and marrow; but we give you our hearts in this feast, we have killed our faithful dogs to feed you, and the Great Spirit will seal our friendship. I have no more to say." (Vol. I., p. 229.)—L.]

As a counterpart to much of this, the ancient Hyrcanians may be mentioned, who lived near the Caspian Sea, and who deemed it one of the strongest expressions of respect to leave the corpse of their deceased friends to be torn and devoured by dogs. Every

5

man was provided with a certain number of these animals, as a living tomb for himself at some future period, and these dogs were remarkable for their fierceness.

[Not only the Hyrcanians but most of the people dwelling on or near the Caspian sea, preserved this race or a similarly formidable one, more particularly to devour their dead; it being considered more propitiatory to the Gods, and more flattering to the spirits of the deceased, to make this disposition of the corpse, than consigning it to the gloomy grave or funeral pile.

This custom is noticed by Theodoret as being pursued by the inhabitants of those parts, and was not abolished till after their adherence to Christianity.—L.]

DOMESTICATED DOGS OF THE FIRST DIVISION.

Some of the readers of this work may possibly recollect three beautiful dogs of this species in the gardens of the Zoological Society of London, which afforded a perfect illustration of the elongated head of the dogs belonging to Cuvier's first section. Mr. Bennett, the Secretary of the Society, gave an interesting account of them in 1835, derived from the observation of Sir John Franklin and Dr. Richardson.

The elongation and sharpness of the muzzle, and the small capacity of the skull, first attract attention. The dog was doubtless fitted for its situation, where its duty is to hunt by sight after the moose or rein-deer, but would have been comparatively worthless if he was to be guided by the scent. Its erect ears, widened at the base and pointed at the top, gave it an appearance of vivacity and spirit. Its depth of chest, and tucked-up flank, and muscular quarters, marked it as a dog of speed, while its light frame, and the length of the toes, and wideness of web between them, seem to depict the kind of surface over which it was to bound. It is not designed to seize and to hold any animal of considerable bulk; it bounds over the snow without sinking, if the slightest crust is formed upon it, and eagerly overtakes and keeps at bay the moose or the rein-deer until the hunters arrive. This animal furnishes a beautiful illustration of adaptation for a particular purpose.

The hair of these dogs is white, with patches of grayish-black and brown. They are known only in the neighbourhood of the Mackenzie River and of the Great Bear Lake in North America They appear to be good-tempered and easily manageable, and soon become familiar even with strangers. They are most valuable to the Indians, who live almost entirely on the produce of the chase. In their native country they never bark, but utter a whine and howl resembling that of the Esquimaux dog; yet one of the three, who was born a few days after its parents arrived at the gardens,

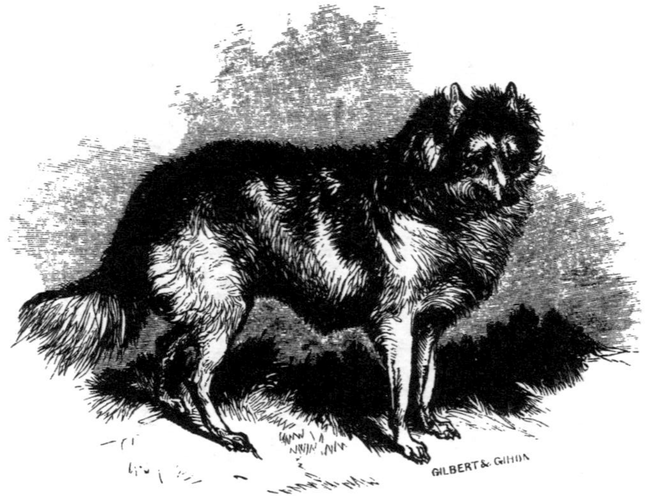

THE HARE INDIAN DOG.

while it whined and howled occasionally with its parents, at other times uttered the perfect bark of its companions of various breeds around it.

[It is the general belief among the Indians and others who are familiar with this dog, that his origin is connected, in some way, with the Arctic Fox, Canis Lagopus, as he so much resembles this animal in his general appearance and habits.

This fox when taken is easily tamed, a few days of captivity being often sufficient to render him quite docile, and ample opportunities have thus been afforded for studying his peculiarities.

Although the cross between the wolf and dog may be considered established beyond controversy, the testimony is not so very conclusive as regards the fox. The most authentic instances on record are perhaps those mentioned by Mr. Daniel, who states that Mr. Tattersall had a terrier bitch, who bred by a fox, and the produce again had whelps by dogs, also that the woodman of Mongewell manor had a bitch, the offspring of a tame dog-fox, by a shepherd's cur, and she again had puppies by a dog; he does not state, however, that he knew these facts personally; but concludes from these two instances, that the fox species may be fairly added to the other supposed original stocks of dogs. (Daniel's Rural Sports, vol. 1. p. 15.)

Mr. Collinson also states, that it is certain that the Siberian dog not only copulates with the wolf, but with the fox also. Notwithstanding this assertion, he is not able to cite a single instance, but on the other hand is forced to acknowledge, that he never met with any person who had seen the coupling of these two animals. The peasants of that country have a small dog, which, from their foxy appearance, they term fox-dogs. Our Indian dogs, also, resemble somewhat the wolves and foxes, the original inhabitants of this continent, while the canine family throughout the east is strongly marked with the jackal, the wild aboriginees of that portion of the world.

These dogs, when fighting, do not shake their antagonists, like the perfectly domesticated dog; their teeth are extremely sharp, and when snarling, the skin is drawn from the mouth; their bite is more severe, and they show but little disposition to attack the wolves, although quite eager in the pursuit of all other game. The Indians had no dogs previous to the coming of the whites, but depended in a great measure, when hunting, upon the presence of the wolves, who, by their howlings, indicated the position of the herds of buffalo or deer, knowing full well that after the general carnage, they would come in for a full share of the garbage of these animals.

Harlan, in his Fauna Americana, says, "we have very little doubt that the various species of domestic dogs are mere varieties of prolific hybrids, produced by the union of the wolf with the fox or jackal. A prolific hybrid of this kind once produced, the progeny would more readily unite with the congeners of either parent, and with each other, and in this manner give rise to the innumerable varieties which at the present day are found scattered over the face of the earth." (Page 77.)

It is somewhat strange, that no naturalist has, as yet, succeeded in causing a union between the fox and dog, if the thing be possible. We ourselves are cognizant of an instance, where every effort was made to produce an offspring from such a connexion, but to no purpose, although the terrier bitch was thrice in heat while confined with the fox, and lived on the most amicable terms with him. We agree with Doct. Godman, that if a litter has ever been generated by these two animals, they were hybrids, as nothing to the contrary of an authentic character has been brought forward, whereas it is well known that the fox always exhibits a great antipathy and instinctive repugnance to such an union. It is also reasonable to suppose that if prolific hybrids had at any time been produced, the breed, from its singular character, would have been propagated by the fortunate possessor, either from curiosity or utility. The intestines of the fox are shorter than those of the dog or wolf.—L.]

THE ALBANIAN DOG

can be traced to a very remote period of history. Some of the old authors speak of it as the dog which in the times of ancient mythology Diana presented to Procris. Pliny describes in enthusiastic terms the combat of one of them with a lion, and afterwards with an elephant. A dog very much resembling the ancient stories is yet found in Albania, and most of the districts of Greece. He is almost as large as a mastiff, with long and silky hair, the legs being shorter and stronger than those of the greyhound. He is gentle and tractable with those whom he knows, and when there is no point of duty at stake; but no bribe can seduce him from his post when any trust is committed to him.

[This dog, it is very probable, was highly impregnated with molossian blood, and like that animal, was trained both for war and the chase. It is rather doubtful, whether the dogs presented to Alexander the Great by the king of Albania, were those of his own country or some that he had obtained from other parts. We are inclined to believe that they were imported dogs, for Pliny distinctly states, that these two were all that the generous monarch possessed, and if destroyed could not be replaced. From this circumstance it is natural to suppose, that, if these dogs had been native Albanians, the king would have been able to supply any reasonable quantity of them, and, therefore, not necessitated to

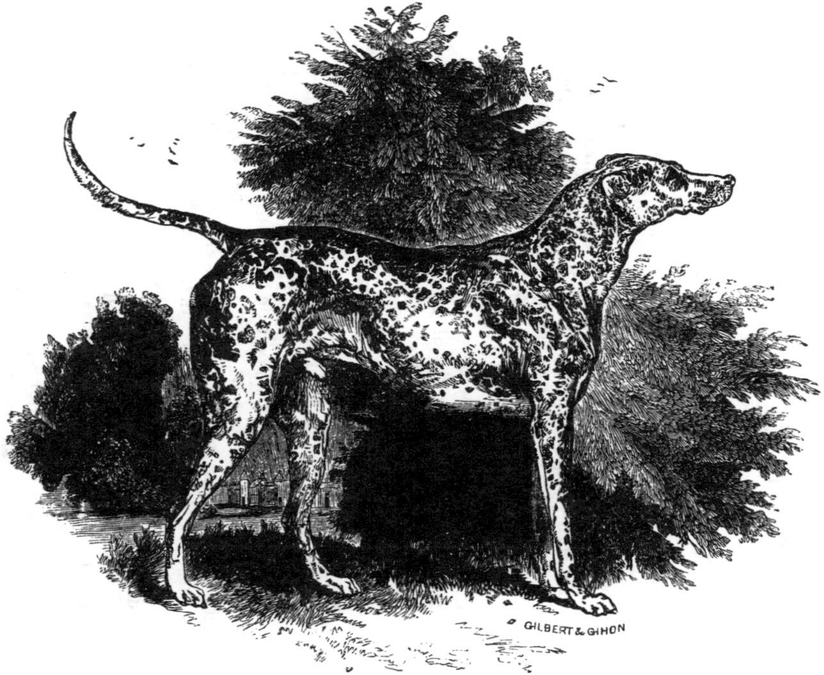

THE DANISH, OR DALMATIAN DOG.

send this message to Alexander. On the other hand, if these dogs had been of the pure molossian type, such as were raised in Epirus, it is probable that their huge dimensions would not have surprised this monarch so much, as it is reasonable to believe that Alexander would certainly have seen, if not heard, of dogs so remarkable, belonging to a kingdom in immediate contiguity with his own. We are, therefore, forced to look to some other source, from whence came these proud dogs, who alone deigned to contend with the lion and elephant, and must yield to Strabo, who states that these animals were of the Indian breed.—L. 15.]

THE GREAT DANISH DOG, CALLED ALSO THE DALMATIAN OR SPOTTED DOG.

The difference between these two breeds consists principally in the size, the Dalmatian being much smaller than the Danish. The body is generally white, marked with numerous small round black or reddish-brown spots. The Dalmatian is said to be used in his native country for the chase, to be easily broken, and stanch to his work. He has never been thus employed in England, but is chiefly distinguished by his fondness for horses, and as being the frequent attendant on the carriages of the wealthy. To that its office seems to be confined; for it rarely develops sufficient sense or sagacity to be useful in any of the ordinary offices of the dog.

[This dog is, perhaps, the tallest of the canine species in existence; the smaller Dane, or "le braque de Bengal," of the French writers, is perhaps a cross of this animal with the pointer or hound, or the original dog degenerated by removal from his native soil. Although these dogs generally display little or no intelligence, and are, in fact, denounced by many writers as being incapable of acquiring sufficient knowledge to make them in any way serviceable for hunting, still we are led to believe that these latent qualities might be developed in this breed as well as any other of his particular physical construction.

We had a little Dane in our possession, whom we instructed, with little trouble, in a variety of tricks; although at first surly and stupid, he soon exhibited great aptness and pleasure in repeating the various lessons which we taught him. If he had been younger we might have given him an opportunity of displaying himself in the field, as we are confident, from his tractable disposition, that he might have been tutored, with perseverance, even sufficiently well to stand upon game. The dogs of Epirus were supposed to have been spotted like the Dalmatian, if not of the same breed. These dogs may also be the "spotted hounds" given by Pan to Diana.

Let the little Dane's intellectual abilities be what they may, long habit and association have so intimately connected him with the stable and its occupants that he seems no longer fit for any other purpose than that of following in the wake of the carriages of the wealthy. This he does with peculiar fondness and singular ingenuity; for, although constantly by the side or at the heels of the horses, or under the tongue of the vehicle, his sure retreat when attacked by other dogs, who seem to have an antipathy for these pampered and fancy attendants on the affluent, he seldom or never is trod upon, or otherwise injured.

The little Dane is often a good ratter; and a gentleman of this city informs me that his dogs not only exhibit an attachment to horses in general, but that one of them has a particular partiality for an old carriage-horse, with whom he has been intimately associated for many years, and always greets his return to the stable with every demonstration of delight, by jumping up and kissing him, &c.—L.]

THE FRENCH MATIN.

(*Canis laniarius*). There is considerable difficulty in describing this variety. The French consider it as the progenitor of all the breeds of dogs that resemble and yet cannot be perfectly classed with the greyhound. It should rather be considered as a species in which are included a variety of dogs,—the Albanian, the Danish, the Irish greyhound, and almost the pure British greyhound. The head is elongated and the forehead flat, the ears pendulous towards the tips, and the colour of a yellowish fawn. This is the usual sheep-dog in France, in which country he is also employed as a house-dog. He discharges his duty most faithfully; and, notwithstanding his flat forehead, shows himself to possess a very high degree of intelligence.

[The French matin we have seen of every variety of colour, being mostly patched with brown, yellow, grey, black, or white. He is employed both in France and Germany in hunting the boar and wolf; which savage animals he fearlessly attacks with courage equal to any dog they possess.—L.]

THE GREYHOUND.

We find no mention of this dog in the early Grecian records. The *pugnaces* and the *sagaces* are mentioned; but the *celeres*—the swift-footed—are not spoken of as a peculiar breed. The Celtic nations, the inhabitants of the northern continent of Europe and the Western Islands, were then scarcely known, and the swift-footed dogs were peculiar to those tribes. They were not, however, introduced into the more southern parts of Europe until after the dissolution of the Roman commonwealth.

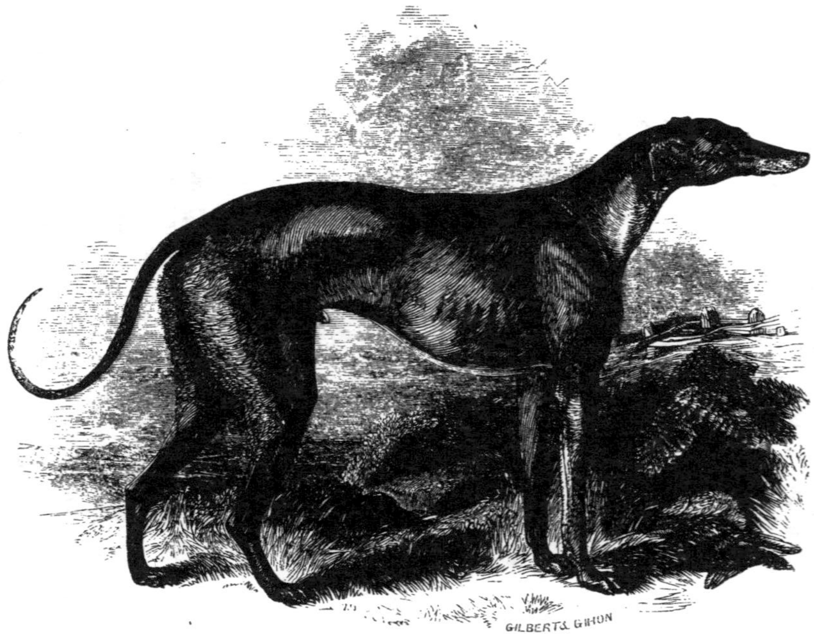

THE GREYHOUND.

The dog is, however, mentioned by Ovid; and his description of coursing the hare is so accurate that we cannot refrain from inserting it. We select a translation of it from Golding.

> "I gat me to the knap
> Of this same hill, and there behelde of this strange course the hap,
> In which the beaste seemes one while caught, and ere a man would thinke
> Doth quickly give the grewnd[a] the slip, and from his biting shrinke;
> And, like a wilie fox, he runs not forth directly out,
> Nor makes a winlas over all the champion fields about,
> But, doubling and indenting, still avoydes his enemie's lips,
> An turning short, as swift about as spinning-wheele he wips,
> To disappoint the snatch. The grewnd, pursuing at an inch,
> Doth cote[b] him, never loosing. Continually he snatches
> In vaine, but nothing in his mouth, save only hair, he catches."

There is another sketch by the same poet:

> "As when th' impatient greyhound, slipped from far,
> Bounds o'er the glade to course the fearful hare,
> She in her speed does all her safety lay,
> And he with double speed pursues the prey;
> O'erruns her at the sitting turn, but licks
> His chaps in vain, yet blows upon the flix;
> She seeks the shelter, which the neighbouring covert gives,
> And, gaining it, she doubts if yet she lives."[c]

The English, Scotch, and Irish greyhounds were all of Celtic derivation, and their cultivation and character correspond with the civilization of the different Celtic tribes. The dogs that were exported from Britain to Rome were probably of this kind. Mr. Blaine gives an account of the progress of these dogs, which seems to be evidently founded on truth. "Scotland, a northern locality, has long been celebrated for its greyhounds, which are known to be large and wiry-coated. They are probably types of the early Celtic greyhounds, which, yielding to the influences of a colder climate than that they came from, became coated with a thick and wiry hair. In Ireland, as being milder in its climate, the frame expanded in bulk, and the coat, although not altogether, was yet less crisped and wiry. In both localities, there being at that time boars, wolves, and even bears, powerful dogs were required. In England these wild beasts were more early exterminated, and consequently the same kind of dog was not retained, but, on the contrary, was by culture made finer in coat, and of greater beauty in form."

[The canis leporarius, or greyhound of the present day, is quite an inferior animal in point of size, when compared with his forefathers, who alone were occupied in the chase of the boar, wolf, bear, deer, and other animals both powerful and savage.

As these wild animals gradually disappeared under the hand of

---

[a] Greyhound. [b] Overcast, or overrun. [c] Ovid, Metamorph., lib. i. v. 353.

civilization, these hardy dogs were less wanted; and thus, by slow degrees, have degenerated into the less powerful, but more beautiful and symmetrical proportions that we now see. This change, however, has better adapted him for speed, and the coursing of such quadrupeds as depend upon nimbleness and activity of motion, to secure their escape.

Owing, in some measure, to the climate, but more particularly to the inactive life that they lead in this country, so much at variance with that of England, we can lay claim to but few dogs that would be considered above mediocrity among British sportsmen. We have seen several of these dogs which, living in a state of idle luxury, have degenerated considerably even in the third generation; and we cannot now recall but one dog, in the possession of a young lady in Philadelphia, that would at all come up to the English standard of perfection; and this one is a descendant from a fine imported stock in the second generation. The ancient Greeks were much devoted to coursing, but previous to the time of Arrian, their hounds were not a sufficient match, in point of speed, for the hare, and it was seldom that their sports were attended with success in the actual capture of this fleet animal by the dogs alone. If taken at all, it was generally by running them down in a long chase, or driving them into nets, toils, and other similar contrivances, as forcibly described in the following lines of the ancient poet, when extolling the pleasures of a country life.

"Aut trudit acres hinc et hinc multâ cane
Apros in obstante plagas,
Aut amite levi rara tendit retia,
Turdis edacibus dólos;
Pavidumve leporem, et advenam laqueo gruem,
Jucunda captat prœmia."—*Horace, Epode* ii., v. 31.

Even after the introduction of the Celtic hound, who, as before stated, was far inferior as regards speed to the present race, it was no easy matter to take the hare, it being necessary to carry several couples of dogs into the field, and let them slip at certain intervals in the chase, so that the fresh dogs might, in this way, overtake the little animal, already frightened and fatigued by previous exertion.

In reference to this mode of coursing, the younger Xenophon particularly enjoins that to prevent confusion in the field, naturally arising from the hunters letting their dogs loose at improper intervals, from eagerness to see them run, "that a steward should be appointed over the sport, should match the dogs, and give orders to the field:—if the hare start on this side, you and you are to slip, and nobody else; but if on that side, you and you: and let strict attention be paid to the orders given." Arrian, chap. xx.

Alciphron, in his familiar epistles descriptive of the domestic manners of the Greeks, gives a lively description of a course not very different from those of the present day, as will be seen in the following extract:—

"In trying whether the young dogs were fit for the chase, I started a hare from a little bush; my sons loosed the dogs from the slips. They frightened her confoundedly, and were very near taking the game. The hare, in her flight, climbed a steep place, and found a retreat in some burrow. One of the more spirited of the dogs, pressing close upon her, gasping, and expecting to take her in his gripe, went down with her into the hole. In endeavouring to pull out the hare, he broke one of his fore-legs. I lifted up my good dog, with his lame leg, and found the hare half devoured: thus, when I hoped to get something, I encountered a serious loss." Letter ix.

We will close our remarks upon this subject by introducing a few descriptive lines, selected from one of the very rare English authors who have attempted a versification of this exciting sport.

> "Yet if for silvan sport thy bosom glow,
> Let thy fleet greyhound urge his flying foe.
> With what delight the rapid course I view!
> How does my eye the circling race pursue!
> He snaps deceitful air with empty jaws;
> The suttle hare darts swift beneath his paws;
> She flys, he stretches, now with nimble bound
> Eager he presses on, but overshoots his ground:
> She turns, he winds, and soon regains the way,
> Then tears with goary mouth the screaming prey."
>
> *Gay's Poems*, vol i.—*Rural Sports*, v. 290.—L.]

Mr. Richardson, in his History of the Greyhound, gives a different derivation of the name of this dog. He says that the greyhound was of Grecian origin—*canis Græcus*,—that *Græcus* was not unfrequently written *Græius*, and thence was derived the term *greyhound*. This derivation, however, is somewhat too far-fetched.

Mention occurs of the greyhound in a very early period of the British history. He was an inmate of the Anglo-Saxon kennels in the time of Elfric, king of Mercia. There are paintings of him that can be satisfactorily traced to the ninth century. In the time of Canute he was reckoned first in degree of rank among the canine species, and no one under the degree of a gentleman, *liberalis*, or more properly, perhaps, a *freeholder*, was allowed by the forest laws to keep them. Even he could not keep them within two miles of a royal forest, unless two of the toes were cut off, and for every mile that an uncut dog was found within this distance a fine of a shilling was levied on the owner. The nobleman was rarely seen abroad without his hawk upon his fist, and his greyhound at his side.

Henry II. was passionately fond of them. John spared no expense to procure good horses and swift hounds, and appears frequently to have received greyhounds in lieu of money on the issue or removal of grants. For the renewal of a grant in the year 1203 he received five hundred marks, ten horses, and ten leashes of greyhounds, and for another, in 1210, one swift running horse and six greyhounds.

The Isle of Dogs, now devoted to purposes of commerce, derived its name from its having been, at this period, the receptacle of the greyhounds and spaniels of this monarch. It was selected on account of its contiguity to Waltham and the other royal forests where coursing was a frequent amusement. For the same purpose he often took up his abode at Greenwich.[a]

Blount's Ancient Tenures abound with instances of the high repute in which this dog has ever been held in Great Britain. The holders of land in the manor of Setene in Kent were compelled, as the condition of their tenure to Edward I. and II., to lend their greyhounds, when this king went into Gascony, "so long as a pair of shoes of 4*d* price would last." Edward III. was partial to greyhounds; for when he was engaged in war with France he took with him sixty couples of them, besides other large hunting dogs.

Charles I. was as fond of the greyhound as his son Charles II. was of the spaniel. Sir Philip Warwick thus writes of that unfortunate monarch: "Methinks, because it shows his dislike of a common court vice, it is not unworthy the relating of him, that one evening, his dog scratching at his door, he commanded me to let in Gipsy; whereupon I took the boldness to say, Sir, I per-

---

[a] A singular story is told of Richard II., and one of these dogs. It is given in the language of Froissart. "A grayhounde called Mithe, who always wayted upon the kynge, and woulde knowe no man els. For when so ever the kynge did ryde, he that kept the grayhounde dyd lette him lose, and he wolde streyght runne to the kynge and faune uppon hym, and leape with his fore fete uppon the kynge's shoulders. And, as the kynge and the Erle of Derby talked togyder in the courte, the grayhounde, who was wonte to leape uppon the kynge, left the kynge and came to the Erle of Derby, Duke of Lancastre; and made to him the same friendly continuance and chere as he was wonte to do to the kynge. The duke, who knewe not the grayhounde, demanded of the kynge what the grayhounde wolde do? 'Cousin,' quod the kynge, 'it is a greate goode token to you, and an evyl signe to me.' 'How knowe you that?' quod the duke. 'I knowe it well,' quod the kynge. 'The grayhounde acknowledgeth you here this daye as Kynge of England, as ye shall be, and I shal be deposed; the grayhounde hath this knowledge naturally: therefore take hym to you, he wyll followe you and forsake me.' The duke understood well those words, and cheryshed the grayhounde, who wolde never after followe kynge Richarde, but followed the duke of Lancastre."

ceive you love a greyhound better than you do a spaniel. Yes, says he, for they equally love their masters, and yet do not flatter them so much."

On most of the old tombs in the sculpture of which the dog is introduced, the greyhound is represented lying at the feet of his master; and an old Welsh proverb says that a gentleman may be known by his hawk, his horse, and his greyhound.

The following poetical record of the fidelity, prowess, and ill-fate of Gêlert, the favourite greyhound of Llewellyn Prince of Wales, and son-in-law to King John, will be read with interest:—

The spearman heard the bugle sound
  And cheerly smiled the morn,
And many a brach and many a hound
  Obeyed Llewellyn's horn.

And still he blew a louder blast,
  And gave a louder cheer,
"Come, Gêlert! why art thou the last
  Llewellyn's horn to hear?"

"Oh, where does faithful Gêlert roam?
  The flower of all his race!
So true, so brave; a lamb at home,
  A lion in the chase?"

'Twas only at Llewellyn's board
  The faithful Gêlert fed,
He watched, he served, he cheered his lord,
  And sentinel'd his bed.

In sooth he was a peerless hound,
  The gift of royal John;
But now no Gêlert could be found,
  And all the chase rode on.

And now as over rocks and dells
  The gallant chidings rise,
All Snowdon's craggy chaos yells
  With many mingled cries.

That day Llewellyn little loved
  The chase of hart or hare;
And scant and small the booty proved,
  For Gêlert was not there.

Unpleased Llewellyn homeward hied.
  When near the portal seat
His truant Gêlert he espied,
  Bounding his lord to greet.

But when he gained the castle-door,
  Aghast the chieftain stood;
The hound was smeared with gouts of gore—
  His lips and fangs ran blood.

Llewellyn gazed with wild surprise:
  Unused such looks to meet,
His favourite check'd his joyful guise
  And crouched and licked his feet.

Onward in haste Llewellyn pass'd,
  And on went Gêlert too;
And still where'er his eyes he cast,
  Fresh blood-gouts shocked his view.

O'erturned his infant's bed he found,
  The blood-stained covert rent;
And all around the walls and ground,
  With recent blood besprent.

He called his child—no voice replied—
  He searched with terror wild:
Blood! blood! he found on every side,
  But nowhere found the child.

'Hellhound! by thee my child's devoured!'
  The frantic father cried;
And to the hilt his vengeful sword
  He plunged in Gélert's side.

His suppliant, as to earth he fell,
  No pity could impart;
But still his Gêlert's dying yell
  Passed heavy o'er his heart.

Aroused by Gêlert's dying yell,
  Some slumberer wakened nigh:
What words the parent's joy can tell
  To hear his infant cry!

Concealed beneath a mangled heap
  His hurried search had missed,
All glowing from his rosy sleep,
  His cherub boy he kissed.

Nor scratch had he, nor harm, nor dread,
  But the same couch beneath,
Lay a great wolf, all torn and dead,
  Tremendous still in death.

Ah, what was then Llewellyn's pain!
  For now the truth was clear:
The gallant hound the wolf had slain,
  To save Llewellyn's heir.

Vain, vain was all Llewellyn's wo:
  "Best of thy kind, adieu!
The frantic deed which laid thee low,
  This heart shall ever rue."

And now a gallant tomb they raise,
  With costly sculpture decked;
And marbles, storied with his praise,
  Poor Gêlert's bones protect.

Here never could the spearman pass,
  Or forester, unmoved;
Here oft the tear-besprinkled grass
  Llewellyn's sorrow proved.

And here he hung his horn and spear;
  And oft, as evening fell,
In fancy's piercing sounds would hear
  Poor Gêlert's dying yell!

It will be evident, however, from the story of the noble hound whose history is just related, that the greyhounds of the time were very different from those which are used at the present day. There are no Gêlerts now to combat successfully with the wolf, if these ferocious animals were yet to be met with in our forests. The greyhound of this early period must have resembled the Irish wolf-dog of the present day, a larger, stronger, fiercer dog than we are accustomed to see.

The owner of Gêlert lived in the time of John, in the early part of the thirteenth century; but, at the latter part of the fifteenth century, the following singular description is given of the greyhound of that period. It is extracted from a very curious work entitled "The Treatise perteynynge to Hawkynge, Huntynge, &c., emprynted at Westmestre, by Wynkyn de Werde, 1496."

A greyhounde should be headed lyke a snake,
And neckyd lyke a drake,
Fotyd lyke a cat,
Tayled lyke a ratte,
Syded like a teme
And chyned like a bream.
The fyrste yere he must lerne to fede,
The seconde yere to feld him lede.
The thyrde yere he is felow lyke.
The fourth yere there is none syke.
The fifth yere he is good ynough.
The syxth yere he shall hold the plough,
The seventh yere he will avaylle
Grete bytches for assayle.
But when he is come to the ninth yere
Have him then to the tannere;
For the best hounde that ever bytch had
At the ninth yere is full bad.

As to the destiny of the poor animal in his ninth year, we differ from the author; but it cannot be denied that few dogs retain their speed beyond the eighth or ninth year.

There can scarcely be a better description of the greyhound of the present day; but it would not do for the antagonist of the wolf. The breed had probably begun to degenerate, and that process would seem to have slowly progressed. Towards the close of the last century, Lord Orford, a nobleman enthusiastically devoted to coursing, imagined, and rightly, that the greyhound of his day was deficient in courage and perseverance. He bethought himself how this could best be rectified, and he adopted a plan which brought upon him much ridicule at the time, but ultimately redounded to his credit. He selected a bull-dog, one of the smooth rat-tailed species, and he crossed one of his greyhound bitches with him. He kept the female whelps and crossed them with some of his fleetest dogs, and the consequence was, that, after the sixth or seventh generation, there was not a vestige left of the form of the bulldog; but his courage and his indomitable perseverance remained, and, having once started after his game, he did not relinquish chase until he fell exhausted or perhaps died. This cross is now almost universally adopted. It is one of the secrets in the breeding of the greyhound.

Of the stanchness of the well-bred greyhound, the following is a satisfactory example. A hare was started before a brace of greyhounds, and ran by them for several miles. When they were found, both the dogs and the hare lay dead within a few yards of each other. A labouring man had seen them turn her several times; but it did not appear that either of them had caught her, for there was no wound upon her.

A favourite bitch of this breed was Czarina, bred by Lord Or ford, and purchased at his decease by Colonel Thornton: she won every match for which she started, and they were no fewer than forty-seven. Lord Orford had matched her for a stake of considerable magnitude; but, before the appointed day arrived, he became seriously ill and was confined to his chamber. On the morning of the course he eluded the watchfulness of his attendant, saddled his favourite piebald pony, and, at the moment of starting, appeared on the course. No one had power to restrain him, and all entreaties were in vain. He peremptorily insisted on the dogs being started, and he would ride after them. His favourite bitch displayed her superiority at every stroke; she won the stakes: but at the moment of highest exultation he fell from his pony, and, pitching on his head, almost immediately expired. With all his eccentricities, he was a kind, benevolent, and honourable man.

In the thirteenth year of her age, and in defiance of the strange verses just now quoted, Czarina began to breed, and two of her progeny, Claret and young Czarina, challenged the whole kingdom and won their matches. Major, and Snowball, without a white spot about him, inherited all the excellence of their dam. The former was rather the fleeter of the two, but the stanchness of Snowball nothing could exceed. A Scotch greyhound, who had beaten every opponent in his own country, was at this time brought to England, and challenged every dog in the kingdom. The challenge was accepted by Snowball, who beat him in a two-mile course. Snowball won the Malton cup on four successive years, was never beaten, and some of his blood is now to be traced in almost every good dog in every part of the kingdom, at least in all those that are accustomed to hunt in an open country. The last match run by Snowball was against Mr. Plumber's celebrated greyhound Speed; and, so severely contested was it, that Speed died soon afterwards. A son of the old dog, called Young Snowball, who almost equalled his father, was sold for one hundred guineas.

The speed of the greyhound has been said to be equal to that of the fleetest horse. A singular circumstance, which occurred at Doncaster, proved that it was not much inferior. A mare cantering over the Doncaster course, her competitor having been withdrawn, was joined by a greyhound bitch when she had proceeded about a mile. She seemed determined to race with the mare, which the jockey humoured, and gradually increased his pace, until at the distance they put themselves at their full speed. The mare beat her antagonist only by a head. The race-horse is, perhaps, generally superior to the greyhound on level ground, but the greyhound would have the advantage in a hilly country.

Lord Rivers succeeded to Major Topham and Colonel Thornton, the owners of Major and Snowball, as the leading man on the course. His kennels at Strathfieldsaye were the pride of the neighbouring country. At first he bore away almost every prize, but breeding too much in and in, and for speed more than for stoutness, the reputation of his kennel considerably declined before his death.

In 1797 a brace of greyhounds coursed a hare over the edge of a chalk-pit at Offham, in Sussex. The hare and both the dogs were found dead at the bottom of the pit.

On another occasion a hare was chased by a brace of greyhounds: she was killed at the distance of seven miles from the place at which they started. Both of the dogs were so exhausted, that every possible assistance being given, they were with difficulty recovered.

The English greyhound hunts by sight alone; not because he is altogether devoid of scent, but because he has been taught to depend upon his speed, and that degree of speed which is utterly incompatible with the searching out of the scent. It is like a pack of hounds, running breast high, with the game in view. They are then running by sight, and not by scent, almost doubling their usual pace, and sometimes, from an unexpected turning of the fox or hare, thrown out for a little while. The hound soon recovers the track by his exquisite sense of smell. The English greyhound is never taught to scent his game, but, on the contrary, is called off the moment he has lost sight of the hare, the re-starting of which is left to the spaniel.

The English greyhound is distinguished by its peculiarly long and attenuated head and face, terminating in a singular sharpness of the nose, and length of the muzzle or mouth. There are two results from this: the length of the mouth gives a longer grasp and secures the prey, but, as the nasal cavities and the cavity of the skull are proportionately diminished, there is not so much room for the expansion of the membrane of the nose, there is less power of scent, and less space for the development of the brain.

There is little want of extraordinary acute hearing, and the ears of the greyhound are small compared with his bulk. Markham recommends the ears to be close, sharp, and drooping, neither protruding by their bulk, nor tiring by their weight.

The power of the eye is but of little consequence, for the game is rarely distant from the dog, and, therefore, easily seen.

The neck is an important portion of the frame. It should be long, in order to correspond with the length of the legs, and thus enable the dog to seize and lift the game, as he rapidly pursues his course, without throwing any undue or dangerous weight on the fore extremities. In the act of seizing the hare the short-necked dog may lose the centre of gravity and fall.

The chest is a very important part of the greyhound, as well as of every other animal of speed. It must be capacious: this capacity must be obtained by depth rather than by width, in order that the shoulders may not be thrown so far apart as to impede progression.

The form and situation of the shoulders are of material consequence; for on them depends the extent of the action which the animal is capable of exerting. The shoulders should be broad and deep, and obliquely placed. They are so in the horse, and the action of the dog depends entirely on this conformation.

The fore legs should be set on square at the shoulder: bulging out at the elbow not only gives a clumsy appearance, but makes the dog slow. The legs should have plenty of bone, and be straight, and well set on the feet, and the toes neither turned out nor in. The fore arm, or that portion of the leg which is between the elbow and the knee, should be long, straight, and muscular. These are circumstances that cannot be dispensed with. The length of the fore arm, and the low placing of the pastern, are of essential importance.

With regard to the form of the back and sides of the greyhound, Mr. Thacker says, with much truth, that "It is the strength of the back which is brought into requisition, in particular, in running over hilly ground. Here may be said to rest the distinction between long and short backs, supposing both to be good and strong. The more lengthy the back, and proportionately strong, the more the greyhound is calculated to beat the shorter-backed dog on the flat; but on hilly ground one with a shorter back will have the advantage."[a]

The ribs should also be well arched. We would perhaps avoid him with sides too decidedly outswelling, but still more would we avoid the direct flat-sided dog.

Without really good haunches and muscular thighs, it has been well remarked that the odds are against any dog, be his other points whatever they may. It is by the propulsatory efforts of the muscles of the loins and thighs that the race is won. The thighs should be large, and muscularly indented; the hocks broad, and, like the knee, low placed. These are very important points; for, as Mr. Blaine has properly remarked, "on the extent of the angles formed between these several portions of the hinder limbs, depends the extent of the space passed over at each bound."

The colour of the greyhound varies exceedingly. Some are perfectly black and glossy. In strength and endurance, the brindled dog, or the brown or fawn-coloured one, is the best. The white greyhound, although a beautiful animal and swift, is not, perhaps, quite so much to be depended on.

The greyhound is said to be deficient in attachment to his master and in general intelligence. There is some truth in the imputation; but, in fact, the greyhound has, far less than even the hound, the opportunity of forming individual attachments, and no other exercise of the mind is required of him than to follow the game which starts up before him, and to catch it if he can. If, however, he is closely watched he will be found to have all the intellect that his situation requires.[b]

As to the individual attachment which the greyhound may form,

---

[a] Thacker on Sporting.

[b] The writer of this work had a brace of greyhounds as arrant thieves as ever lived. They would now and then steal into the cooking-room belonging to the kennel, lift the lid from the boiler, and, if any portion of the joint or piece of meat projected above the water, suddenly seize it, and before there was time for them to feel much of its heat, contrive to whirl it on the floor, and eat it at their leisure as it got cold. In order to prevent this, the top of the boiler was secured by an iron rod passing under its handle, and tied to the handle of the boiler on each side; but not many days passed ere they discovered that they could gnaw the cords asunder, and displace the rod, and fish out the meat as before. Small chains were then substituted for the cords, and the meat was cooked in safety for nearly a week, when they found that, by rearing themselves on their hind legs, and applying their united strength towards the top of the boiler, they could lift it out of its bed and roll it along the floor, and so get at the broth, although the meat was out of their reach. The man who looked after them expressed himself heartily glad when they were gone; for, he said, he was often afraid to go into the kennel, and was sure they were devils, and not dogs.

he has not always or often the opportunity to acquire or to exhibit it. The keeper exercises over him a tyrannical power, and the owner seldom notices him in the manner which excites affection, or scarcely recognition; but, as a plea for the seeming want of fondness, which, compared with other breeds, he exhibits, it will be sufficient to quote the testimony of the younger Xenophon, who had made the greyhound his companion and his friend.

"I have myself bred up," says he, "a swift, hard-working, courageous, sound-footed dog. He is most gentle and kindly affectioned, and never before had I any such a dog for myself, or my friend, or my fellow-sportsman. When he is not actually engaged in coursing, he is never away from me. On his return he runs before me, often looking back to see whether I had turned out of the road, and as soon as he again catches sight of me, showing symptoms of joy, and once more trotting away before me. If a short time only has passed since he has seen me or my friend, he jumps up repeatedly by way of salutation, and barks with joy as a greeting to us. He has also many different tones of speech, and such as I never heard from any other dog. Now really I do not think that I ought to be ashamed to chronicle the name of this dog, or to let posterity know that Xenophon the Athenian had a greyhound, called Hormé, possessed of the greatest speed, and intelligence, and fidelity, and excellent in every point."

[The Greek sportsmen held their dogs in peculiar estimation; they were not only their attendants in the field, but their constant companions in their houses, were fed from their tables, and even shared their beds. It is with some degree of pleasure that the patrons of this noble animal will witness, in the following remarks, the tender solicitude with which this people watched over their dogs.

"There is nothing like a soft and warm bed for greyhounds, but it is best for them to sleep with men, as they become thereby affectionately attached, pleased with the contact of the human body, and as fond of their bed-fellow as of their feeder. If any ailing affect the dog the man will perceive it, and will relieve him in the night, when thirsty, or urged by any call of nature. He will also know how the dog has rested. For if he has passed a sleepless night, or groaned frequently in his sleep, or thrown up any of his food, it will not be safe to take him out coursing. All these things the dog's bed-fellow will be acquainted with." (Arrian, chap. ix. Trans.)

It was also not an unusual circumstance for the most polished Greeks, when sending notes of invitation to their friends, requesting their presence in celebration of some festive occasion, to extend the same civilities to their favourite dogs, by desiring them to be brought along, as will be seen by the following paragraph selected from a letter of this kind addressed by one friend to another.

"I am about to celebrate the birth-day of my son, and I invite you, my Pithacion, to the feast. But come not alone; bring with you your wife, children, and your brother. If you will bring also your bitch, who is a good guard, and by the loudness of her voice drives away the enemies of your flocks, she will not, I warrant, disdain to be partaker of our feast, &c." (Letter xviii., Alciphron's Epistles.)—L.]

The greyhound has within the last fifty years assumed a somewhat different character from that which he once possessed. He is distinguished by a beautiful symmetry of form, of which he once could not boast, and he has even superior speed to that which he formerly exhibited. He is no longer used to struggle with the deer, but he contends with his fellow over a shorter and speedier course.

The rules for breeding and breaking-in of greyhounds are very simple. The utmost attention should be paid to the qualities of the parents; for it is as certain in these dogs as in the horse that all depends upon the breeding. The bitch should be healthy and of good size; the dog muscular, stanch, and speedy, and somewhat larger than the bitch. Both should have arrived at their full vigour, and with none of their powers beginning to fail. Those as much as possible should be selected whose peculiar appearance bids fair to increase the good qualities and diminish the bad ones on either side. The best blood and the best form should be diligently sought. Breeding from young dogs on either side should, generally speaking, be avoided. With regard to older dogs, whether male or female, there may be less care. Many greyhounds, both male and female, eight, nine, and ten years of age, have been the progenitors of dogs possessing every stanch and good quality.

On no consideration, however, should the bitch be put to the dog before she is two years old. Little can be done to regulate the period of œstrum; but the most valuable breed will be almost invariably that which is produced during the spring, because at that time there will often be opportunity for that systematic exercise on which the growth and powers of the dog so materially depend. A litter of puppies in the beginning or even the middle of winter will often be scarcely worth the trouble or expense of rearing.

The age of the greyhound is now taken from the first day in the year; but the conditions of entry are fixed at different periods. It seems, however, to be agreed that no dog or bitch can qualify for a puppy cup after two years of age.

One principle to be ever kept in mind is a warm and comfortable situation, and a plentiful supply of nourishment for the mother and for the puppies from the moment of their birth. The dog that is stinted in his early growth will never do its owner credit. The bitch should be abundantly supplied with milk, and the young ones with milk and bread, and oatmeal, and small portions of flesh as soon as they are disposed to eat it; great care, however, being taken that they are not over-gorged. Regular and proper feeding, with occasional exercise, will constitute the best preparation for the actual training. If a foster-mother be required for the puppies, it should, if possible, be a greyhound; for it is not at all impossible that the bad qualities of the nurse may to a greater or less degree be communicated to the whelps. Bringing up by hand is far preferable to the introduction of any foster-mother. A glass or Indian-rubber bottle may be used for a little while, if not until the weaning. Milk at first, and afterwards milk and sop alternately, may be used.

There is a difference of opinion whether the whelp should be kept in the kennel and subjected to its regular discipline, or placed at walk in some farm-house. In consequence of the liberty he will enjoy at the latter, his growth will probably be more rapid; but, running with the farmers' dogs, and probably coursing many hares, he will acquire, to a certain degree, a habit of wildness. It is useless to deny this; but, on the other hand, nothing will contribute so much to the development of every power as a state of almost unlimited freedom when the dogs are young. The wildness that will be exhibited can soon be afterwards restrained so far as is necessary, and the dog who has been permitted to exert his powers when young will manifest his superiority in more advanced age, and in nothing more than his dexterity at the turn.

When the training actually commences, it should be preceded by a couple of doses of physic, with an interval of five or six days, and, probably, a moderate bleeding between them; for, if the dog begins to work overloaded with flesh and fat, he will suffer so severely from it that possibly he will never afterwards prove a game dog. In the course of his training he should be allowed every advantage and experience every encouragement. His courses should be twice or thrice a-week, according to their severity, and as often as it can be effected he should be rewarded with some mark of kindness.

In the 'Sportsman' for April, 1840, is an interesting account of the chase of the hare. It is said that, in general, a good greyhound will reach a hare if she runs straight. He pursues her eagerly, and the moment he is about to strike at her she turns short, and the dog, unable to stop himself, is thrown from ten to twenty yards from her. These jerking turns soon begin to tell upon a dog, and an old well-practised hare will seldom fail to make her escape. When, however, pursued by a couple of dogs, the hare has a more difficult game to play, as it frequently happens that when she is turned by the leading dog she has great difficulty in avoiding the stroke of the second.

It is highly interesting to witness the game of an old hare. She has generally some brake or thicket in view, under the cover of which she means to escape from her pursuers. On moving from her seat she makes directly for the hiding-place, but, unable to reach it, has recourse to turning, and, *wrenched* by one or the other of her pursuers, she seems every moment almost in the jaws of one of them, and yet in a most dexterous manner she accomplishes her object. A greyhound, when he perceives a hare about to enter a thicket, is sure to strike at her if within any reasonable distance. The hare shortens her stride as she approaches the thicket, and at the critical moment she makes so sudden, dexterous, and effectual a spring, that the dogs are flung to a considerable distance, and she has reached the cover and escaped.

The isle of Cyprus has for many years been celebrated for its breed of the greyhound. On grand days, or when the governor is present, the sport is conducted in a curious manner. When the hare is ready to become the prey of its enemies, the governor rushes forwards, and, throwing before the greyhounds a stick which he carries, they all instantaneously stop. The hare now runs a little distance; but one of the swiftest greyhounds is then let loose. He pursues the hare, and, having come up with it, carries it back, and, springing on the neck of the governor's horse, places it before him. The governor delivers it to one of his officers, who sends it to the park, where he maintains many prisoners of the same kind; for he will not destroy the animal that has contributed to his amusement.[a]

The following, according to Mr. Blaine, an ardent courser in his youth, is the best mode of feeding greyhounds at regular work: —"The dogs had a full flesh meal every afternoon or evening, as more nutriment is derived from night-feeding than by day, and when sleeping than when waking. In the morning they were let out, and either followed the keeper about the paddock, or the groom in his horse exercise, and then had a trifling meal of mixed food, as a quieting portion, until the evening full meal. Such was our practice on the days when no coursing was contemplated, and, with the exception of lowering the quantity and quality of the evening meal, the same plan was pursued throughout the year. On the day previous to coursing, if we intended anything like an exhibition of our dogs before company engaged to meet us on the marshes, we gave a plentiful meal early the previous day, some

[a] Scott's Sportsman's Repository, p. 97.

exercise also in the afternoon, and a light supper at night, of meal with either broth or milk, with a man on horseback going a gentle trot of six or seven miles an hour."[a]

Mr. Thacker orders the greyhounds out on the fore part of every day; but, instead of being loose and at liberty, they would be much better two and two; then, when he meets with a proper field to loose them in, to give them a good gallop. This will be a greater novelty than if they had been loose on the road, and they will gallop with more eagerness. Four days in a week will be enough for this exercise. On one day there should be a gallop of one or two miles, or even a course for each brace of dogs.

The young dog has usually an older and more experienced one to start with him. That which is of most importance is, that his leader should be a thoroughly stout and high-mettled dog. If he shrinks or shies at any impediment, however formidable, the young one will be sure to imitate him, and to become an uncertain dog, if not a rank coward. Early in November is the time when these initiatory trials are to be made. It is of consequence that the young one should witness a death as soon as possible. Some imagine that two old dogs should accompany the young one at its first commencement. After the death of the leveret, the young dog must be coaxed and fondled, but never suffered to taste the blood.

In kennels in which the training is regularly conducted, the dog should be brushed all over twice every day. Few things contribute so much to health as general cleanliness, and friction applied to the skin. Warmth is as necessary for greyhounds as for horses, and should not be forgotten in cold weather. Body-clothing is a custom of considerable antiquity, and should not be abandoned. The breeder of greyhounds for the purpose of coursing must reckon upon incurring considerable expense; but, if he loves the sport, he will be amply remunerated by the speed and stoutness of his dogs.

A question has arisen whether, on the morning of the coursing, any stimulant should be given to the dog. The author of this work would unhesitatingly approve of this practice. He has had abundant experience of the good effect of it; but the stimulus must be that which, while it produces the desired effect, leaves no exhaustion behind.[b]

THE SCOTCH GREYHOUND

has the same sharpness of muzzle, length of head, lightness of ear, and depth of chest, as the English dog; but the general frame is stronger and more muscular, the hind quarters more prominent,

[a] Blaine's Encyclopedia of Sporting.

[b] For a set of laws for Coursing Matches, see Appendix.

there is evident increase of size and roughness of coat, and there is also some diminution of speed. If it were not for these points, these dogs might occasionally be taken for each other. In coursing the hare, no north-country dog will stand against the lighter southern, although the southern would be unequal to the labour often required from the Highlander.

The Scotch greyhound is said—perhaps wrongly—to be oftenest used by those who look more to the quantity of game than to the fairness and openness of the sport, and in some parts of the country this dog is not permitted to be entered for a sweepstakes, because, instead of depending on his speed alone, as does the English greyhound, he has recourse to occasional artifices in order to intercept the hare. In sporting language he runs sly, and, therefore, is sometimes excluded.

THE HIGHLAND GREYHOUND, OR DEER-HOUND,

is a larger, stronger, and fiercer dog, and may be readily distinguished from the Lowland Scotch greyhound by its pendulous, and, generally, darker ears, and by the length of hair which almost covers his face. Many accounts have been given of the perfection of its scent, and it is said to have followed a wounded deer during two successive days. He is usually two inches taller than the Scotch greyhound. The head is carried particularly high, and gives to the animal a noble appearance. His limbs are exceedingly muscular, his back beautifully arched. The tail is long and curved, but assumes the form of an almost straight line when he is much excited. The only fault which these dogs have is their occasional ill-temper, or even ferocity; but this does not extend to the owner and his family.

It appears singular that the English greyhound exhibits so little power of scent; but this is simply because he has never been taught to use it, or has been cruelly corrected when he has attempted to exercise it.

Holinshed relates the mischief that followed the stealing of one of these dogs: — "Divers of the young Pictesh nobilitye repaired unto Craithlint, King of the Scots, for to hunt and make merie with him; but, when they should depart homewards, perceiving that the Scotish dogs did far excel theirs, both in fairnesse, swiftnesse, and hardinesse, and also in long standing up and holding out, they got diverse both dogs and bitches of the best kind for breed, to be given them by the Scotish Lords; and yet not so contented, they stole one belonging to the King from his keeper, being more esteemed of him than all the others which he had about him. The maister of the leash, being informed hereot pursued after them that had stolen the dog, thinking, indeed, to have taken him from them; but they not being to part with him fell at altercation, and at the end chanced to strike the maister of the leash through with their horse spears, so that he did die presently. Whereupon noise and crie being raised in the country by his servantes, divers of the Scots, as they were going home from hunting, returned, and falling upon the Picts to revenge the death of their fellow, there ensued a shrewed bickering betwixt them; so that of the Scots there died three score gentlemen, besides a great number of the commons, not one of them understanding what the matter meant. Of the Picts there were about 100 slaine."

Mr. H. D. Richardson describes a cross between the greyhound and British bloodhound:—"It is a tall muscular raw-boned dog, the ears far larger, and more pendulous, than those of the greyhound or deer-hound. The colour is generally black, or black and tan; his muzzle and the tips of the ears usually dark. He is exceedingly swift and fierce; can pull down a stag single-handed; runs chiefly by sight, but will also occasionally take up the scent. In point of scent, however, he is inferior to the true deer-hound. This dog cannot take a turn readily, but often fails at the double."[a]

THE IRISH GREYHOUND.

This dog differs from the Scotch, in having shorter and finer hair, of a pale fawn colour, and pendent ears. It is, compared with the Scotch dog, gentle and harmless, perhaps indolent, until roused. It is a larger dog than the Scottish dog, some of them being full four feet in length, and proportionately muscular. On this account, and also on account of their determined spirit when roused, they were carefully preserved by some Irish gentlemen. They were formerly used in hunting the wolf when that animal infested the forests of Ireland. Mr. Bell says that the last person who kept the pure breed was Lord Altamont, who in 1780 had eight of them.[b]

THE GASEHOUND,

the *agasæus* of former times, was probably allied to, or connected with, the Irish greyhound. It hunted entirely by sight, and, if its prey was lost for a time, it could recover it by a singular distinguishing faculty. Should the deer rejoin the herd, the dog would unerringly select him again from all his companions:

> "Seest thou the gasehound how with glance severe
> From the close herd he marks the destined deer?"[c]

There is no dog possessed of this quality at present known in Europe; but the translator of Arrian thinks that it might be produced between the Irish greyhound and the bloodhound.

---

[a] Sportsman, vol. xi. p. 314. [b] Bell's British Quadrupeds, p. 241.
[c] Tickell's Miscellanies.

THE IRISH WOLF-DOG.

This animal is nearly extinct, or only to be met with at the mansions of one or two persons by whom he is kept more for show than use, the wild animals which he seemed powerful enough to conquer having long disappeared from the kingdom. The beauty of his appearance and the antiquity of his race are his only claims, as he disdains the chase of stag, fox, or hare, although he is ever ready to protect the person and the property of his master. His size is various, some having attained the height of four feet, and Dr. Goldsmith states that he saw one as large as a yearling calf. He is shaped like a greyhound, but stouter; and the only dog which the writer from whom this account is taken ever saw approaching to his graceful figure, combining beauty with strength, is the large Spanish wolf-dog: concerning which he adds, that, showing one of these Spanish dogs to some friends, he leaped through a window into a cow-house, where a valuable calf was lying, and seizing the terrified animal, killed it in an instant; some sheep having in the same way disappeared, he was given away. The same writer says that his grandfather had an Irish wolf-dog which saved his mother's life from a wolf as she was paying a visit attended by this faithful follower. He rushed on his foe just when he was about to make his spring, and after a fierce struggle laid him dead at his mistress's feet. His name was Bran.[a]

THE RUSSIAN GREYHOUND

is principally distinguished by its dark-brown or iron-grey colour —its short semi-erect ears—its thin lanky body—long but muscular legs—soft thick hair, and the hair of its tail forming a spiral twist, or fan, (thence called the fan-tailed dog,) and as he runs having a very pleasing appearance. He hunts by scent as well as by sight, and, therefore, small packs of this kind are sometimes kept, against which the wolf, or even the bear, would stand little chance. He is principally used for the chase of the deer or the wolf, but occasionally follows the hare. The deer is the principal object of pursuit, and for this he is far better adapted than to contend with the ferocious wolf. His principal faults are want of activity and dexterity. He is met with in most parts of Russia, where his breed is carefully preserved by the nobility, with whom coursing is a favourite diversion.

Some dogs of this breed were not long ago introduced into Ireland.

---

[a] Sporting Mag. 1837, p. 156.

THE GRECIAN GREYHOUND.

The author is glad that he is enabled to present his readers with the portrait of one now in the menagerie of the Zoological Society of London. It is the dog whose image is occasionally sculptured on the friezes of some of the ancient Grecian temples, and was doubtless a faithful portrait of one of the dogs which Xenophon the Athenian valued, and was the companion of the heroes of Greece in her ancient glory.

The principal difference between the Grecian and the English greyhound is, that the former is not so large, the muzzle is not so pointed, and the limbs are not so finely framed.

THE TURKISH GREYHOUND

is a small-sized hairless dog, or with only a few hairs on his tail. He is never used in the field, and bred only as a spoiled pet, yet not always spoiled, for anecdotes are related of his inviolable attachment to his owner. One of them belonged to a Turkish Pacha who was destroyed by the bowstring. He would not forsake the corpse, but laid himself down by the body of his murdered master, and presently expired.

THE PERSIAN GREYHOUND

is a beautiful animal. He is more delicately framed than the English breed; the ears are also more pendulous, and feathered almost as much as those of a King Charles's spaniel. Notwithstanding, however, his apparent slenderness and delicacy, he yields not in courage, and scarcely in strength, to the British dog. There are few kennels in which he is found in which he is not the master.

In his native country, he is not only used for hunting the hare, but the antelope, the wild ass, and even the boar. The antelope is speedier than the greyhound: therefore the hawk is given to him as an ally. The antelope is no sooner started than the hawk is cast off, who, fluttering before the head of the deer, and sometimes darting his talons into his head, disconcerts him, and enables the greyhound speedily to overtake and master him. The chase, however, in which the Persians chiefly delight, and for which these greyhounds are mostly valued, is that of the *ghoo-khan*, or wild ass. This animal inhabits the mountainous districts of Persia. He is swift, ferocious, and of great endurance, which, together with the nature of the ground, renders this sport exceedingly dangerous. The hunter scarcely gives the animal a fair chance, for relays of greyhounds are placed at various distances in the surrounding country; so that, when those by which the animal is first started are tired, there are others to continue

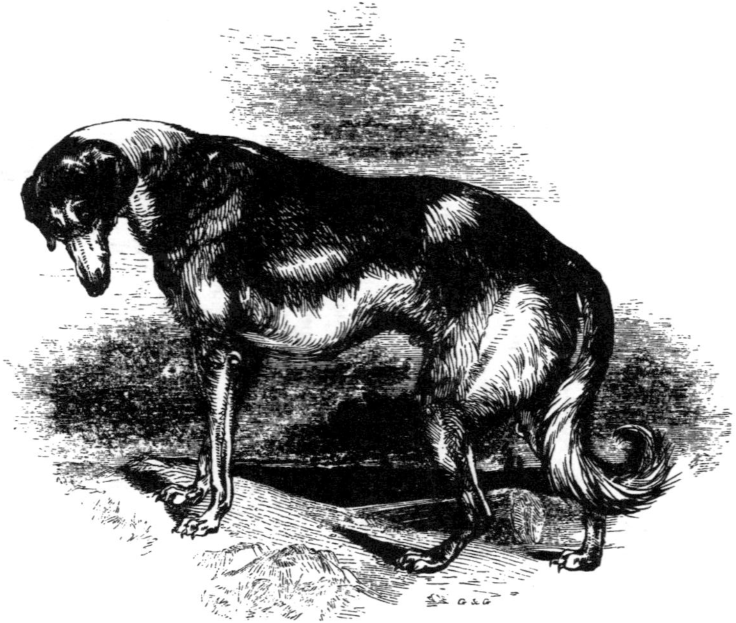

THE GRECIAN GREYHOUND.

the chase. Such, however, is the speed and endurance of the ghoo-khan, that it is seldom fairly run down by the greyhounds, its death being usually achieved by the rifle of some horseman. The Persians evince great skill and courage in this dangerous sport, galloping at full speed, rifle in hand, up and down the most precipitous hills, and across ravines and mountain streams, that might well daunt the boldest rider.[a]

The Persian greyhound, carried to Hindoostan, is not always to be depended upon; but, it is said, is apt to console itself by hunting its own master, or any one else, when the game proves too fleet or escapes into the cover.

THE ITALIAN GREYHOUND

possesses all the symmetry of the English or Persian one, on a small scale. So far as beauty can recommend it, and, generally speaking, good nature, it is deservedly a favourite in the drawing-room; but, like the large greyhound, it is inferior in intelligence. It has no strong individual attachment, but changes it with singular facility. It is not, however, seen to advantage in its petted and degraded state, but has occasionally proved a not unsuccessful courser of the rabbit and the hare, and exhibited no small share of speed and perseverance. In a country, however, the greater part of which is infested with wolves, it cannot be of much service, but exposed to unnecessary danger. It is bred along the coasts of Italy, principally for the purpose of sale to foreigners.

In order to acquire more perfect beauty of form, and more activity also, the English greyhound has received one cross from the Italian, and with decided advantage. The speed and the beauty have been evidently increased, and the courage and stoutness have not been diminished.

It has been said that Frederick the Great of Prussia was very fond of a small Italian greyhound, and used to carry it about with him under his cloak. During the seven years' war, he was pursued by a party of Austrian dragoons, and compelled to take shelter, with his favourite, under the dry arch of a bridge. Had the little animal, that was naturally ill-tempered and noisy, once barked, the monarch would have been taken prisoner, and the fate of the campaign and of Prussia decided; but it lay perfectly still, and clung close to its master, as if conscious of their mutual danger. When it died, it was buried in the gardens of the palace at Berlin, and a suitable inscription placed over its grave.

---

[a] New Sports. Mag. xiii. 124.

CHAPTER III.

THE VARIETIES OF THE DOG.

SECOND DIVISION.

The head moderately elongated, the parietals not approaching from their insertion, but rather diverging, so as to enlarge the cerebral cavities and the frontal sinuses; consequently giving to these dogs greater power of scent and intelligence. They constitute the most pleasing and valuable division of the Dog.

The Spaniel is evidently the parent of the Newfoundland dog and the setter; while the retriever, the poodle, the Bernardine, the Esquimaux, the Siberian, and the Greenland dogs, the shepherd and drover's dog, and every variety distinguished for intelligence and fidelity, have more or less of his blood in them.

THE SPANIEL

is probably of Spanish origin, and thence his name. The ears are large and pendent, the tail elevated, the fur of a different length in different parts of the body, but longest about the ears, under the neck, behind the thighs and on the tail, varying in colour, but most commonly white with brown or black patches.

There are many varieties of the spaniel. The smallest of the *land* spaniels is

THE COCKER.

It is chiefly used in flushing woodcocks and pheasants in thickets and copses into which the setter, and even the springer, can scarcely enter.

> "But, if the shady woods my cares employ,
> In quest of feathered game my spaniels beat,
> Puzzling the entangled copse, and from the brake
> Push forth the whirring pheasant."

The cocker is here very useful, although he is occasionally an exceedingly impatient animal. He is apt to whimper and babble as soon as he comes upon the scent of game, and often raises the bird before the sportsman is within reach: but when he is sufficiently broken in not to give tongue until the game rises, he is exceedingly valuable. There can scarcely be a prettier object than this little creature, full of activity, and bustling in every direction, with his tail erect; and, the moment he scents the bird, expressing his delight by the quivering of every limb, and the low eager whimpering which the best breaking cannot always subdue.

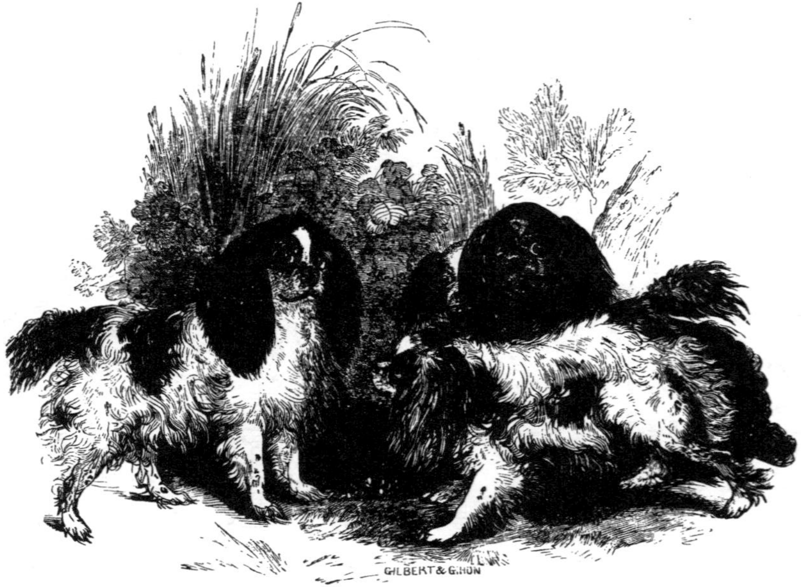

BLENHEIMS AND COCKERS.

Presently the bird springs, and then he shrieks out his ecstasy, startling even the sportsman with his sharp, shrill, and strangely expressive bark.

The most serious objection to the use of the cocker is the difficulty of teaching him to distinguish his game, and confine himself within bounds; for he will too often flush everything that comes within his reach. It is often the practice to attach bells to his collar, that the sportsman may know where he is; but there is an inconvenience connected with this, that the noise of the bells will often disturb and spring the game before the dog comes fairly upon it.

Patience and perseverance, with a due mixture of kindness and correction, will, however, accomplish a great deal in the tuition of the well-bred spaniel. He may at first hunt about after every bird that presents itself, or chase the interdicted game; but, if he is immediately called in and rated, or perhaps corrected, but not too severely, he will learn his proper lesson, and will recognise the game, to which alone his attention must be directed. The grand secret in breaking in these dogs is mildness, mingled with perseverance, the lessons being enforced, and practically illustrated by the example of an old and steady dog.

These spaniels will sometimes vie with almost every other species of dog in intelligence, and will not yield to one of them in fidelity. A gentleman in Sussex had an old cocker, that was his constant companion, both in the house and the field. If the morning was rainy, the dog was perfectly quiet; if it was fine, he became restless, and, at the usual time for his master to go out, he would take him by the flap of his coat, and gently pull at it. If the door was opened, he ran immediately to the keeper's lodge, which was at a considerable distance from the house. This was a signal for the other dogs to be brought up, and then he trotted back to announce their approach.

[This beautiful and interesting dog, so called from his peculiar suitableness for woodcock shooting, is but little known among us except as a boudoir companion for our ladies. He is, nevertheless, extensively used in England by sportsmen for finding and flushing this bird, as also the pheasant; and no doubt, if introduced into our country, would prove equally, if not more serviceable, in putting up game concealed in the thickets and marshy hollows of our uncleared grounds. Having extremely fine scenting powers, they are also employed in greyhound coursing, to give warning of the proximity of a hare, which they seldom fail to accomplish.

This active little animal hunts with great spirit, and soon becomes attached to the sport; in fact the only difficulty to be overcome in breaking him, is the effort it requires to make him suppress his natural ardour and withhold his exclamations of delight till the bird is actually on the wing. The tutelage of the cocker intended for the field should commence as early as possible, and is not, as many suppose, attended with great difficulty. His first lessons should be confined to the art of bringing and carrying, which he soon, in common with all the other members of the spaniel tribe, learns. The next thing to be inculcated is implicit obedience to our wishes; then, at the age of four months or so, he may be carried to the field, where his natural fondness for hunting will soon be developed by his chasing every bird within his reach. When this impulse is fully exhibited, and the dog expresses gratification in the amusement, he should be then instructed to give chase, or not, at his master's pleasure. When this desirable end has been accomplished, he may be introduced to the particular kinds of game which it is proposed to hunt him on, and by slow degrees teach him to confine his attentions to those varieties alone. It is absolutely necessary that the dog be forced to hunt as near to the sportsman as possible, otherwise the game will be flushed at such a distance that it will be impossible to get at it. The cocker spaniel is much smaller than the springer; his ears are long, pendulous, and silky; his body round and compact; his legs short and tufted; his coat variable; his nose black; tail bushy and feathered, and, when hunting, is kept in constant motion.

Some are black and white, others liver colour and yellow: the latter variety we have most usually seen in this country, and some of them have been represented to us as well-broken and serviceable dogs.—L.]

THE KING CHARLES'S SPANIEL,

so called from the fondness of Charles II. for it—who usually had some of them following him, wherever he went—belongs likewise to the cockers. Its form and character are well preserved in one of the paintings of the unfortunate parent of that monarch and his family. The ears deeply fringed and sweeping the ground, the rounder form of the forehead, the larger and moister eye, the longer and silken coat, and the clearness of the tan, and white and black colour, sufficiently distinguish this variety. His beauty and diminutive size have consigned him to the drawing-room or parlour.

Charles the First had a breed of spaniels, very small, with the hair black and curly. The spaniel of the second Charles was of the black and tan breed.

The King Charles's breed of the present day is materially altered for the worse. The muzzle is almost as short, and the forehead as ugly and prominent, as the veriest bull-dog. The eye is increased to double its former size, and has an expression of stupidity with which the character of the dog too accurately corresponds Still there is the long ear, and the silky coat, and the beautiful colour of the hair, and for these the dealers do not scruple to ask twenty, thirty, and even fifty guineas.

[This breed of dog was cultivated with such jealous care by the late Duke of Norfolk, that no solicitation or entreaty could induce this nobleman to part with one of these favourites, except under certain peculiar stipulations and injunctions, as detailed in the following interview of Mr. Blain with the late Duchess of York. "On one occasion, when we were accompanying Her Royal Highness to her menagerie, with almost a kennel of canine favourites behind her, after drawing our attention to a jet black pug pup she had just received from Germany, she remarked that she was going to show me what she considered a present of much greater rarity, which was a true King Charles's breed sent to her by the Duke of Norfolk. 'But,' she observed, 'would you believe he could be so ungallant as to write word that he must have a positive promise not from myself, but from the Duke of York, that I should not breed from it in the direct line?'" Notwithstanding these selfish restrictions on the part of this noble patron of the spaniel, this breed of dog has become quite common in England, and not a few have found their way to this country.—L.]

THE SPRINGER.

This dog is slower and steadier in its range than the cocker; but it is a much safer dog for the shooter, and can better stand a hard day's work. The largest and best breed of springers is said to be in Sussex, and is much esteemed in the Wealds of that county.

From a cross with the terrier a black and tan variety was procured, which was cultivated by the late Duke of Norfolk, and thence called the Norfolk Spaniel. It is larger than the common springer, and stancher, and stouter. It often forms a strong individual attachment, and is unhappy and pines away when separated from its master. It is more ill-tempered than the common springer, and, if not well broken in, is often exceedingly obstinate.

[Mr. Skinner informs us that this breed, in its greatest purity, may be found in the Carrollton family, as also in the possession of Mr. Keyworth of Washington city.—L.]

THE BLACK AND TAN SPANIEL,

the cross of the terrier being nearly or quite got rid of, is often a beautiful animal, and is much valued, although it is frequently considered a somewhat stupid animal. The cocker and the springer are sometimes used as finders in coursing.

THE BLENHEIM SPANIEL,

a breed cultivated by one of the Dukes of Marlborough, belongs to this division. From its beauty, and occasional gaiety, it is oftener an inhabitant of the drawing-room than the field; but it occasionally breaks out, and shows what nature designed it for. Some of these carpeted pets acquit themselves nobly in the covert. There they ought oftener to be; for they have not much individuality of attachment to recommend them, and, like other spoiled animals, both quadruped and biped, misbehave. The breed has degenerated of late, and is not always to be had pure, even in the neighbourhood of Blenheim. This spaniel may be distinguished by the length and silkiness of the coat, the deep fringe about the ear, the arch and deep-feathering of the tail, the full and moist eye, and the blackness of the palate.

THE WATER-SPANIEL.

Of this breed there are two varieties, a larger and smaller, both useful according to the degree of range or the work required; the smaller, however, being ordinarily preferable. Whatever be his general size, strength and compactness of form are requisite. His head is long, his face smooth, and his limbs, more developed than those of the springer, should be muscular, his carcase round, and his hair long and closely curled. Good breaking is more necessary here than even with the land-spaniel, and, fortunately, it is more easily accomplished; for, the water-spaniel, although a stouter, is a more docile animal than the land one.

Docility and affection are stamped on his countenance, and he rivals every other breed in his attachment to his master. His work is double; first to find, when ordered so to do, and to back behind the sportsman when the game will be more advantageously trodden up. In both he must be taught to be perfectly obedient to the voice, that he may be kept within range, and not unnecessarily disturb the birds. A more important part of his duty, however, is to find and bring the game that has dropped. To teach him to find is easy enough, for a young water-spaniel will as readily take to the water as a pointer puppy will stop; but to bring his game without tearing is a more difficult lesson, and the most difficult of all is to make him suspend the pursuit of the wounded game while the sportsman re-loads.

The water-spaniel was originally from Spain; but the pure breed has been lost, and the present dog is probably descended from the large water-dog and the English setter.

The water and land spaniels differ materially from each other. The water-spaniel, although when at his work being all that his

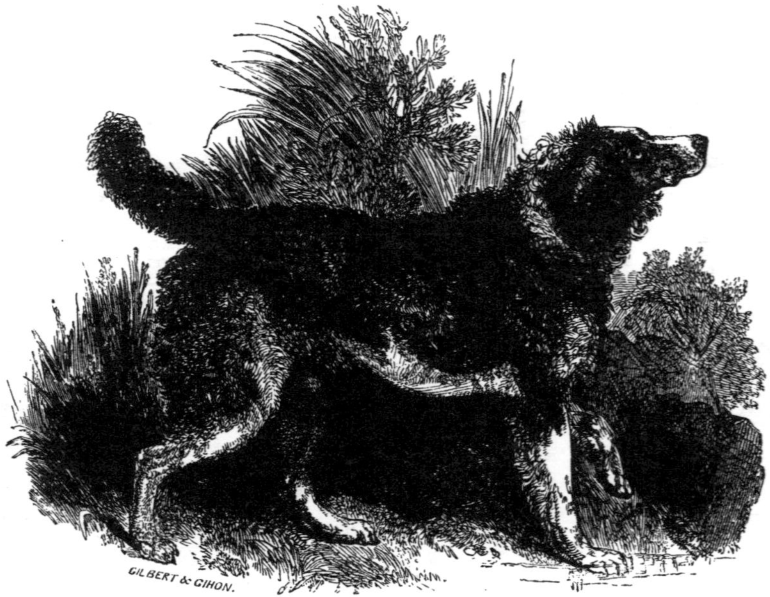

THE WATER SPANIEL.

master can desire, is, when unemployed, comparatively a slow and inactive dog; but under this sobriety of demeanor is concealed a strength and fidelity of attachment to which the more lively land-spaniel cannot always lay just claim. The writer of this work once saved a young water-spaniel from the persecution of a crowd of people who had driven it into a passage, and were pelting it with stones. The animal had the character of being, contrary to what his species usually are, exceedingly savage; and he suffered himself to be taken up by me and carried from his foes with a kind of sullenness; but when, being out of the reach of danger, he was put down, he gazed on his deliverer, and then crouched at his feet.

From that moment he attached himself to his new master with an intensity of affection scarcely conceivable—never expressed by any boisterous caresses, but by endeavouring to be in some manner in contact with him; resting his head upon his foot; lying upon some portion of his apparel, his eye intently fixed upon him; endeavouring to understand every expression of his countenance. He would follow one gentleman, and one only, to the river-side, and behave gallantly and nobly there; but the moment he was dismissed he would scamper home, gaze upon his master, and lay himself down at his feet. In one of these excursions he was shot. He crawled home, reached his master's feet, and expired in the act of licking his hand.

Perhaps the author may be permitted to relate one story more of the water-spaniel: he pledges himself for its perfect truth. The owner of the dog is telling this tale. "I was once on the sea-coast, when a small, badly-formed, and leaky fishing-boat was cast on shore, on a fearful reef of rocks. Three men and a boy of ten years old constituted the crew. The men swam on shore, but they were so bruised against the rocks, that they could not render any assistance to the poor boy, and no person could be found to venture out in any way. I heard the noise and went to the spot with my dog. I spoke to him, and in he went, more like a seal than a dog, and after several fruitless attempts to mount the wreck, he succeeded, and laid hold of the boy, who clung to the ropes, screaming in the most fearful way at being thus dragged into the water. The waves dashed frightfully on the rocks. In the anxiety and responsibility of the moment I thought that the dog had missed him, and I stripped off my clothes, resolved to render what assistance I could. I was just in the act of springing from the shore, having selected the moment when the receding waves gave me the best chance of rendering any assistance, when I saw old 'Bagsman,' for that was the name of my dog, with the struggling boy in his mouth, and the head uppermost. I rushed to the place where he must land, and the waves bore the boy and the dog into my arms.

"Some time after that I was shooting wild-fowl. I and my dog had been working hard, and I left him behind me while I went to a neighbouring town to purchase gunpowder. A man, in a drunken frolic, had pushed off in a boat with a girl in it; the tide going out carried the boat quickly away, and the man becoming frightened, and unable to swim, jumped overboard. Bagsman, who was on the spot, hearing the splash, jumped in, swam out to the man, caught hold of him, and brought him twenty yards towards the shore, when the drunken fellow clasped the dog tight round the body, and they both went down together. The girl was saved by a boat going to her assistance. The body of the man was recovered about an hour afterwards, with that of the dog clasped tight in his arms, thus dragging him to the bottom. 'Poor Bagsman! thy worth deserves to be thus chronicled.'"

THE POODLE.

The particular cross from which this dog descended is unknown, but the variety produced has been carefully preserved. It is, probably, of continental origin, and is known by its thick curly hair concealing almost every part of the face, and giving it the appearance of a short, thick, unintelligent head. When, however, that hair is removed, there is still the large head; but there is also the cerebral cavity more capacious than in any other dog, and the frontal sinuses fully developed, and exhibiting every indication of the intellectual class to which it belongs.

It was originally a water-dog, as its long and curly hair, and its propensities in its domesticated state, prove; but, from its peculiar sagacity, it is capable of being trained to almost any useful purpose, and its strong individual attachment renders it more the companion of man than a mere sporting dog: indeed, its qualities as a sporting dog are seldom recognised by its owner.

These dogs have far more courage than the water-spaniel, all the sagacity of the Newfoundland, more general talent, if the expression may be used, and more individual attachment than either of them, and without the fawning of the one, or the submissiveness of the other. The poodle seems conscious of his worth, and there is often a quiet dignity accompanying his demonstrations of friendship.

This dog, however, possesses a very peculiar kind of intelligence. It will almost perform the common offices of a servant: it will ring the bell and open the door. Mr. Wilkie, of Ladythorn in Northumberland, had a poodle which he had instructed to go through all the apparent agonies of dying. He would fall on one side, stretch himself out, and move his hind legs as if he were in

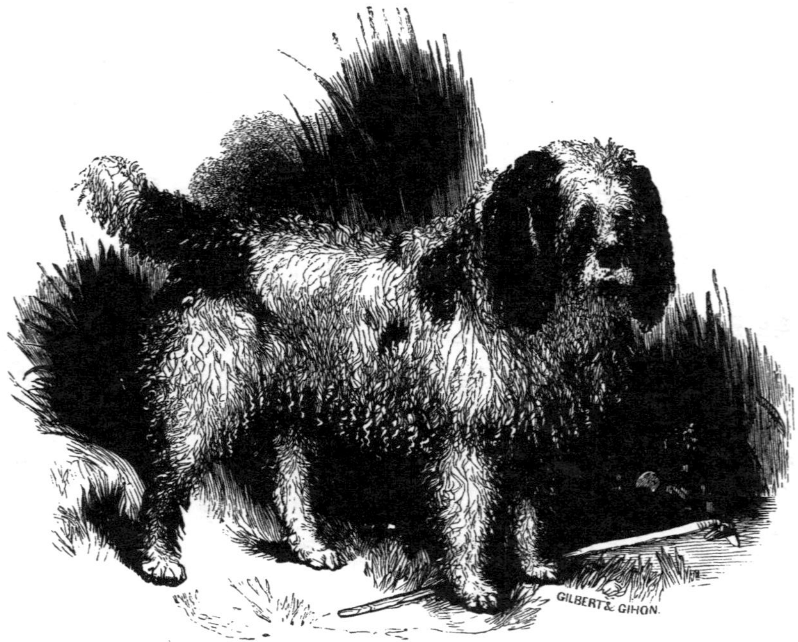

THE POODLE.

great pain; he would next simulate the convulsive throbs of departing life, and then stretch out his limbs and thus seem as if he had expired. In this situation he would remain motionless, until he had his master's command to rise.

The portrait of Sancho, a poodle, that was with difficulty forced from the grave of his master, after the battle of Salamanca, is familiar to many of our readers. Enticed from his post he could not be, nor was he at length taken away until weakened by grief and starvation. He by degrees attached himself to his new master, the Marquis of Worcester, but not with the natural ardour of a poodle. He was attentive to every command, and could perform many little domestic offices. Sometimes he would exhibit considerable buoyancy of spirit; but there oftener seemed to be about him the recollection of older and closer friendship.

Another poodle occupies an interesting place in the history of the Peninsular war. He too belonged to a French officer, who was killed at the battle of Castella. The French were compelled to retreat before they could bury their dead, and the soldiers wished to carry with them this regimental favourite; but he would not be forced from the corpse of his master. Some soldiers afterwards traversing the field of battle, one of them discovered the cross of the Legion of Honour on the breast of the fallen officer, and stooped to take it away, when the dog flew savagely at him, and would not quit his hold, until the bayonet of another soldier laid him lifeless.

A veterinary surgeon, who, before any other animal than the horse was acknowledged to be the legitimate object of medical care, did not disdain to attend to the diseases of the dog, used to say that there were two breeds which he never wished to see in his infirmary, namely, the poodle and the Norfolk spaniel; for, although not always difficult to manage, he could never attach them to him, but they annoyed him by their pitiful and imploring gaze during the day, and their mournful howling at night.

Custom has determined that the natural coat of this animal shall be taken from him. It may be a relief to the poodle for a part of his coat to be stripped off in hot weather, and the curly hair which is left on his chest, contrasted with his smooth and well-rounded loins and quarters, may make it look pretty enough; but it should be remembered that he was not designed by nature to be thus exposed to the cold of winter, and that there are no dogs so liable to rheumatism, and that rheumatism degenerating into palsy, as the well-trimmed poodle.

THE BARBET

is a small poodle, the production of some unknown and disadvantageous cross with the true poodle. It has all the sagacity of the poodle, and will perform even more than his tricks. It is always in action; always fidgety; generally incapable of much affection, but inheriting much self-love and occasional ill temper; unmanageable by any one but its owner; eaten up with red mange; and frequently a nuisance to its master and a torment to every one else.

We must not, however, do it injustice; it is very intelligent, and truly attached to its owner.

The barbet possesses more sagacity than most other dogs, but it is sagacity of a particular kind, and frequently connected with various amusing tricks. Mr. Jesse, in his Gleanings in Natural History, gives a singular illustration of this. A friend of his had a barbet that was not always under proper command. In order to keep him in better order, he purchased a small whip, with which he corrected him once or twice during a walk. On his return the whip was put on a table in the hall, but on the next morning it was missing. It was soon afterwards found concealed in an outbuilding, and again made use of in correcting the dog. Once more it would have been lost, but, on watching the dog, who was suspected of having stolen it, he was seen to take it from the hall table in order to hide it once more.

THE MALTESE DOG

can be traced back to an early period. Strabo says that "there is a town in Sicily called Melita, whence are exported many beautiful dogs called *Canes Melitæi.* They were the peculiar favourites of the women; but now (A. D. 25) there is less account made of these animals, which are not bigger than common ferrets or weasels, yet they are not small in understanding nor unstable in their love." They are also found in Malta and in other islands of the Mediterranean, and they maintain the same character of being devotedly affectionate to their owners, while, it is added,— and they are not loved the less for that, — they are ill-tempered to strangers.

THE LION DOG

is a diminutive likeness of the noble animal whose name it bears. Its head, neck, shoulders, and fore-legs down to the very feet, are covered with long, wavy, silky hairs. On the other parts of the dog it is so short as scarcely to be grasped, except that on the tail there is a small bush of hair. The origin of this breed is not known; it is, perhaps, an intermediate one between the Maltese and the Turkish dog.

THE TURKISH DOG,

as it is improperly called, is a native of hot climates. The supposition of Buffon is not an improbable one, that, being taken

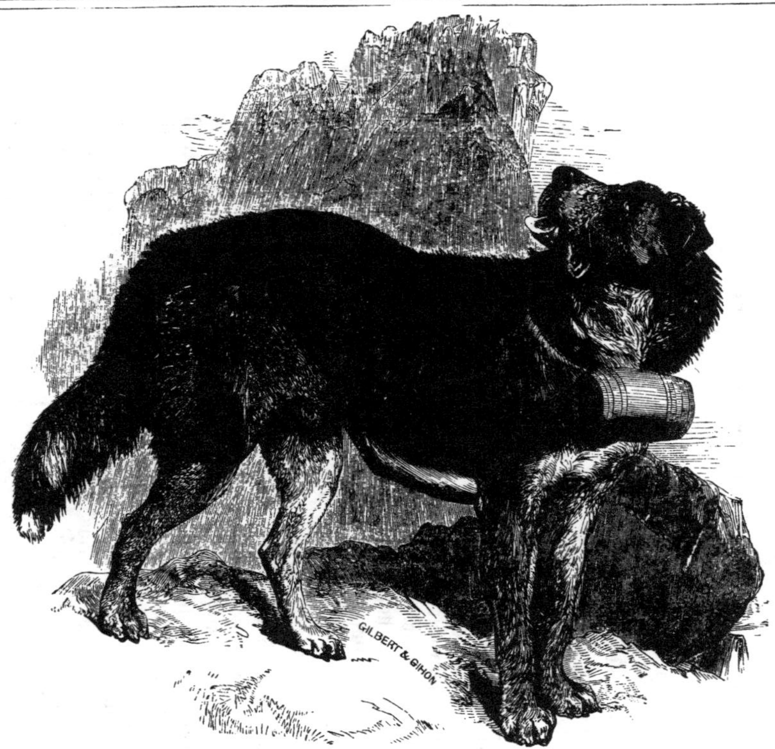

THE ALPINE SPANIEL, OR BERNARDINE DOG.

from some temperate country to one considerable hotter, the European dog probably acquired some cutaneous disease. This is no uncommon occurrence in Guinea, the East Indies, and South America. Some of these animals afterwards found their way into Europe, and, from their singularity, care was taken to multiply the breed. Aldrovandus states that the first two of them made their appearance in Europe in his time, but the breed was not continued, on account, as it was supposed, of the climate being too cold for them.

The few that are occasionally seen in England bear about them every mark of a degenerated race. They have no activity, and they show little intelligence or affection. One singular circumstance appertains to all that the author of this work has had the opportunity of seeing,—their teeth become very early diseased, and drop from the gums. That eminent zoologist, Mr. Yarrell, examining, with the author of this work, one that had died, certainly not more than five years old, found that it had neither incisors nor canine teeth, and that the molars were reduced to one on each side, the large tubercular tooth being the only one that was remaining. At the scientific meeting of the Zoological Society, the same gentleman stated, that he had examined the mouths of two individuals of the same variety, then alive at the gardens, in both of which the teeth were remarkably deficient. In neither of them were there any false molars, and the incisors in both were deficient in number. Before the age of four years the tongue is usually disgustingly hanging from the mouths of these animals.

THE ALPINE SPANIEL, OR BERNARDINE DOG,

is a breed almost peculiar to the Alps, and to the district between Switzerland and Savoy. The passes over these mountains are exceedingly dangerous from their steepness and narrowness. A precipice of many hundred feet is often found on one side, and perpendicular rocks on the other, while the path is glazed with frozen snow or ice. In many places the path is overhung with huge masses of frozen snow, which occasionally loosen and fall, when the dreadful storms peculiar to these regions suddenly come on, and form an insurmountable barrier, or sweep away or bury the unfortunate traveller. Should he escape these dangers, the path is now become trackless, and he wanders amid the dreary solitudes until night overtakes him; and then, when he pauses from fatigue or uncertainty with regard to the path he should pursue, his limbs are speedily benumbed. Fatal slumbers, which he cannot shake off, steal upon him, and he crouches under some ledge, and sleeps, to wake no more. The snow drifts on. It is almost continually falling, and he is soon concealed from all human help.

On the top of Mount St. Bernard, and near one of the most dangerous of these passes, is a convent, in which is preserved a breed of large dogs trained to search for the benighted and frozen wanderer. Every night, and particularly when the wind blows tempestuously, some of these dogs are sent out. They traverse every path about the mountains, and their scent is so exquisite that they can discover the traveller, although he may lie many feet deep in the snow. Having found him, they set to work and endeavour to scrape away the snow, uttering a deep bark that reverberates from rock to rock, and tells those who are watching in the convent that some poor wretch is in peril. Generally, a little flask of spirits is tied round the neck of the animal, by drinking which the benighted traveller may recruit his strength, until more effectual rescue arrive. The monks hasten in the direction of the sound, and often succeed in rekindling the vital spark before it is quite extinguished. Very many travellers have been thus rescued from death by these benevolent men and their intelligent and interesting quadruped servants.

One of these Bernardine dogs, named Barry, had a medal tied round his neck as a badge of honourable distinction, for he had saved the lives of forty persons. He at length died nobly in his vocation. A Piedmontese courier arrived at St. Bernard on a very stormy day, labouring to make his way to the little village of St. Pierre, in the valley beneath the mountain, where his wife and children lived. It was in vain that the monks attempted to check his resolution to reach his family. They at last gave him two guides, each of whom was accompanied by a dog, one of which was the remarkable creature whose services had been so valuable. Descending from the convent, they were overwhelmed by two avalanches or heaps of falling snow, and the same destruction awaited the family of the poor courier, who were travelling up the mountain in the hope of obtaining some news of the husband and father.

A beautiful engraving has been made of this noble dog. It represents him as saving a child which he had found in the Glacier of Balsore, and cherished, and warmed, and induced to climb upon his shoulders, and thus preserved from, otherwise, certain destruction.

THE NEWFOUNDLAND DOG.

The Newfoundland is a spaniel of large size. He is a native of the island of which he bears the name; but his history is disgraceful to the owners of so valuable an animal. The employment of the lower classes of the inhabitants of St. John, in Newfoundland, is divided between the cutting of wood, and the drawing of it and other merchandise in the winter, and fishing in the summer.

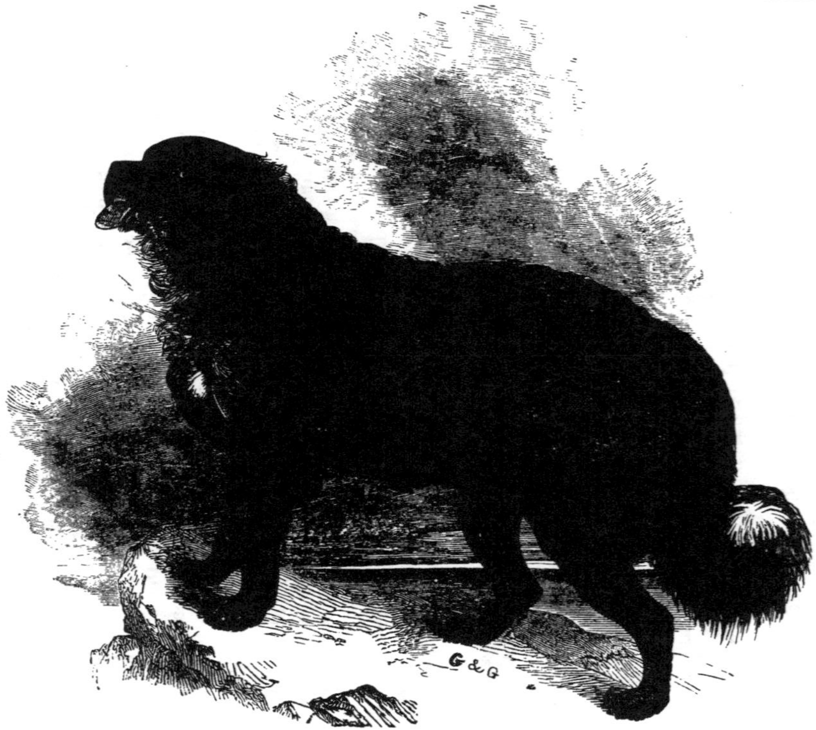

THE NEWFOUNDLAND DOG.

The carts used in the winter work are drawn by these dogs, who are almost invariably urged and goaded on beyond their strength, fed only with putrid salt-fish, and an inadequate quantity even of that. A great many of them are worn out and die before the winter is over; and, when the summer approaches, and the fishing season commences, many of them are quite abandoned, and, uniting with their companions, prowl about preying on the neighbouring flocks, or absolutely starving.

Mr. Macgregor, however, states that "in almost every other part of British America they are valuable and useful. They are remarkably docile and obedient to their masters, serviceable in all the fishing countries, and yoked in pairs to draw the winter's fuel home. They are faithful, good-natured, and ever friendly to man. They will defend their master and their master's property, and suffer no person to injure either the one or the other; and, however extreme may be the danger, they will not leave them for a minute. They seem only to want the faculty of speech, in order to make their good wishes and feelings understood, and they are capable of being trained for all the purposes for which every other variety of the canine species is used."[a]

That which most recommends the Newfoundland dog is his fearlessness of water, and particularly as connected with the preservation of human life. The writer of the present work knows one of these animals that has preserved from drowning four human beings.

[This breed of dog, though much esteemed both in England and other portions of the world, as well for his majestic appearance as for many useful and winning traits of character, has but few sportsmen as patrons with us. He is not only used in England as a water-dog for the pursuit of wild fowl, but has been trained by many sportsmen to hunt on partridges, woodcocks, and pheasants, and is represented by Captain Hawker and others as surpassing all others of the canine race, in finding wounded game of every description.

Mr. Blain remarks that, "as a retriever, the Newfoundland dog is easily brought to do almost anything that is required of him, and he is so tractable, likewise, that, with the least possible trouble, he may be safely taken among pointers to the field, with whose province he will not interfere, but will be overjoyed to be allowed to look up the wounded game, which he will do with a perseverance that no speed and no distance can slacken, nor any hedgerow baulk. In cover he is very useful; some, indeed, shoot woodcocks to a Newfoundland, and he never shines more than when he is returning with a woodcock, pheasant, or hare, in his mouth,

[a] Historical and Descriptive Sketches of British America, by J. Macgregor

which he yields up, or even puts into your hand unmutilated." Notwithstanding the high commendations of these gentlemen, we cannot look upon the Newfoundland in any other light than that of a dog, whose powers of sagacity are destined for display in the water.

In contending with this element, either in the preservation of human life, or in search of wounded fowl, he has no equal, and volumes might be filled with accounts of his various daring achievements in this particular branch, not only in England, but on the rivers of our own country. Mr. Blain mentions two varieties of these dogs as being common in England, the Labrador and St. John. The former is very large, rough-haired, and carries his tail very high; the latter is smaller, more docile, and sagacious in the extreme, and withal much more manageable. We were not aware of these varieties, and more particularly as regards the difference in docility and sagacity, but are convinced, from subsequent observations, that such is the case even in our own country, for we have often noticed a great dissimilarity in the size and appearance of these dogs and attributed it to the effects of the climate and cross breeding with inferior animals. We are indebted to Mr. Skinner for bringing before the public a faithful and minute account of two of these animals imported into this country by Mr. Law, of Baltimore, and may be pardoned for giving again publicity to this gentleman's letter in relation to these two sagacious brutes.

BALTIMORE, MARYLAND,
January 7th, 1845.

"MY DEAR SIR:—In the fall of 1807 I was on board of the ship Canton, belonging to my uncle, the late Hugh Thompson, of Baltimore, when we fell in, at sea, near the termination of a very heavy equinoctial gale, with an English brig in a sinking condition, and took off the crew. The brig was loaded with codfish, and was bound to Poole, in England, from Newfoundland. I boarded her, in command of a boat from the Canton, which was sent to take off the English crew, the brig's own boats having been all swept away, and her crew in a state of intoxication. I found on board of her two Newfoundland pups, male and female, which I saved, and, subsequently, on our landing the English crew at Norfolk, our own destination being Baltimore, I purchased these two pups of the English captain for a guinea a-piece. Being bound again to sea, I gave the dog-pup, which was called Sailor, to Mr. John Mercer, of West River; and the slut-pup, which was called Canton, to Doctor James Stewart, of Sparrow's Point. The history which the English captain gave me of these pups was, that the owner of his brig was extensively engaged in the Newfoundland trade, and had directed his correspondent to select and send him a pair of pups of the most approved Newfoundland breed, but of different families, and that the pair I purchased of him were selected under this order. The dog was of a dingy red colour, and the slut black. They were not large; their hair was short, but very thick coated; they had dew claws. Both attained great reputation as water-dogs. They were most sagacious in everything, particularly so in all duties connected with duck-shooting. Governor Lloyd exchanged a Mexican ram for the dog at the time of the merino fever, when such rams were selling for many hundred dollars, and took him over to his estate on the eastern shore of Maryland, where his progeny were well known for many years after, and may still be known there, and on the western shore, as the Sailor breed. The slut remained at Sparrow's Point till her death, and her progeny were, and are still, well known through Patapsco Neck, on the Gunpowder, and up the bay, amongst the duck-shooters, as unsurpassed for their purposes. I have heard both Doctor Stewart and Mr. Mercer relate most extraordinary instances of the sagacity and performances of both dog and slut, and would refer you to their friends for such particulars as I am unable, at this distance of time, to recollect with sufficient accuracy to repeat.

Yours, in haste,
GEORGE LAW."

These dogs are represented as being of fine carriage, broad-chested, compact figure, and in every respect built for strength and activity.

Their patience and endurance were very great when pursuing wounded ducks through the floating ice, and when fatigued from extraordinary exertions were known to rest themselves upon broken portions of ice till sufficiently recovered again to commence the chase. We have seen some of the descendants of these sagacious animals on the Chesapeake, engaged, not only in bringing the ducks from the water when shot, but also toling them into shore within range of the murderous batteries concealed behind the blind.

This may not be an inappropriate place to speak of this wonderful mode of decoying ducks, termed toling, so extensively practised upon the Chesapeake bay and its tributaries, where the canvass-back and red-heads resort in such numerous quantities every fall. A species of mongrel water-dog, or often any common cur, is taught to run backwards and forwards after stones, sticks, or other missiles thrown from one side to the other. In his activity and industry in this simple branch of education, within the comprehension of any dog, consists the almost incredible art ol toling the canvass-back.

With a dog of this character, the shooting party, consisting of several persons all prepared with heavy double-barrelled duck-guns, esconce themselves at break of day behind some one of the numerous blinds temporarily erected along the shore contiguous to the feeding-grounds of these ducks. Everything being arranged, and the morning mists cleared off, the ducks will be seen securely feeding on the shallows not less than several hundreds of yards from the shore. The dog is now put in motion by throwing stones from one side of the blind to the other. This will soon be perceived by the ducks, who, stimulated by an extreme degree of curiosity, and feeling anxious to inform themselves as to this sudden and singular phenomenon, raise their heads high in the water and commence swimming for the shore. The dog being kept in motion, the ducks will not arrest their progress until within a few feet of the water's edge, and oftentimes will stand on the shore staring, as it were, in mute and silly astonishment at the playful motions of the dog.

If well trained the dog takes no notice whatever of the duck. but continues his fascination until the quick report of the battery announces to him that his services are now wanted in another quarter, and he immediately rushes into the water to arrest the flight of the maimed and wounded, who, struggling on every side, dye the water with their rich blood.

The discovery of this mode of decoying ducks was quite an accident, being attributed to a circumstance noticed by a sportsman, who, concealed behind a blind patiently awaiting the near approach of the canvass-back, observed that they suddenly lifted up their heads and moved towards the shore. Wondering at this singular and unusual procedure on the part of this wray bird, he naturally looked round to discover the cause, and observed a young fox sporting upon the river bank, and the ducks, all eagerness to gaze upon him, were steering their course directly for the shore.

These ducks will not only be decoyed by the dog, but will often come in by waving a fancy coloured handkerchief attached to the ramrod. We have seen a dog fail to attract their attention till bound around the loins with a white handkerchief, and then succeed perfectly well. The toling season continues about three weeks from the first appearance of the ducks, often a much shorter time, as these birds become more cautious, and are no longer deceived in this way.

The canvass-back toles better than any other duck; in fact, it is asserted by many sportsmen, that this particular variety alone can be decoyed in this mode. There are always numbers of other ducks feeding with the canvass-back, particularly the red-heads and black-necks, who partake of the top of the grass that the canvass-back discards after eating off the root, which is a kind of celery. These ducks, though they come in with the canvass-back when toled, do not seem to take any notice whatever of the dog, but continue to swim along, carelessly feeding, as if entrusting themselves entirely to the guidance of the other ducks.

As far as we have been able to judge, we are inclined to this opinion also, and do not recollect ever having succeeded in toling any other species of duck, unaccompanied by the canvass-back, although we have made the effort many times. These ducks are a very singular bird, and although very cunning under ordinary circumstances, seem perfectly bewildered upon this subject, as we were one of a party several years since, who actually succeeded in decoying the same batch of ducks three successive times in the course of an hour, and slaying at each fire a large number, as we counted out over forty at the conclusion of the sport.

Although the toling of ducks is so simple in its process, there are few dogs that have sufficient industry and perseverance to arrive at any degree of perfection in the art. The dog, if not possessed of some sagacity and considerable training, is very apt to tire and stop running when the ducks have got near to the shore, but too far off to be reached by the guns, which spoils all, as the birds are very apt to swim or fly off if the motion of the animal is arrested for a few moments.—L.]

A native of Germany was travelling one evening on foot through Holland, accompanied by a large dog. Walking on a high bank which formed one side of a dyke, his foot slipped, and he was precipitated into the water; and, being unable to swim, soon became senseless. When he recovered his recollection, he found himself in a cottage on the contrary side of the dyke, surrounded by peasants, who had been using the means for the recovery of drowned persons. The account given by one of them was, that, returning home from his labour, he observed at a considerable distance a large dog in the water, swimming and dragging, and sometimes pushing along something that he seemed to have great difficulty in supporting, but which he at length succeeded in getting into a small creek on the opposite side. When the animal had pulled what he had hitherto supported as far out of the water as he was able, the peasant discovered that it was the body of a man, whose face and hands the dog was industriously licking. The peasant hastened to a bridge across the dyke, and, having obtained assistance, the body was conveyed to a neighbouring house, where proper means soon restored the drowned man to life. Two very considerable bruises, with the marks of teeth, appeared, one on his shoulder and the other on his poll; hence it was presumed that the faithful beast had first seized his master by the shoulder, and swam with him in this manner for some time, but that his sagacity had prompted him to quit this hold, and to shift it to the nape of the neck, by which he had been enabled to support the head out of water; and in this way he had conveyed him nearly a quarter of a mile before he had brought him to the creek, where the banks were low and accessible.

Dr. Beattie relates an instance of a gentleman attempting to cross the river Dee, then frozen over, near Aberdeen. The ice gave way about the middle of the river: but, having a gun in his hand, he supported himself by placing it across the opening. His dog then ran to a neighbouring village, where, with the most significant gestures, he pulled a man by the coat, and prevailed on him to follow him. They arrived at the spot just in time to save the drowning man's life.

Of the noble disposition of the Newfoundland dog, Dr. Abel, in one of his lectures on Phrenology, relates a singular instance. "When this dog left his master's house, he was often assailed by a number of little noisy dogs in the street. He usually passed them with apparent unconcern, as if they were beneath his notice; but one little cur was particularly troublesome, and at length carried his impudence so far as to bite the Newfoundland dog in the leg. This was a degree of wanton insult beyond what he could patiently endure; and he instantly turned round, ran after the offender, and seized him by the skin of the back. In this way he carried him in his mouth to the quay, and, holding him some time over the water, at length dropped him into it. He did not, however, seem to design that the culprit should be punished capitally. He waited a little while, until the poor animal, who was unused to that element, was not only well ducked, but nearly sinking, and then plunged in, and brought him safe to land."

"It would be difficult," says Dr. Hancock, in his Essay on Instinct, "to conceive any punishment more aptly contrived, or more completely in character. Indeed, if it were fully analyzed, an ample commentary might be written in order to show what a variety of comparisons and motives and generous feelings entered into the composition of this act."

No one ever drew more legitimate consequences from certain existing premises.

One other story should not be omitted of this noble breed of water-dogs. A vessel was driven on the beach of Lydd, in Kent. The surf was rolling furiously. Eight poor fellows were crying for help, but not a boat could be got off to their assistance. At length a gentleman came on the beach accompanied by his Newfoundland dog: he directed the attention of the animal to the vessel, and put a short stick into his mouth. The intelligent and courageous fellow at once understood his meaning, sprung into the sea, and fought his way through the waves. He could not, however, get close enough to the vessel to deliver that with which he was charged; but the crew understood what was meant, and they made fast a rope to another piece of wood, and threw it towards him. The noble beast dropped his own piece of wood and immediately seized that which had been cast to him, and then, with a degree of strength and determination scarcely credible,—for he was again and again lost under the waves,—he dragged it through the surge and delivered it to his master. A line of communication was thus formed, and every man on board was rescued.

There is, however, a more remarkable fact recorded in the Penny Magazine. "During a heavy gale a ship had struck on a rock near the land. The only chance of escape for the shipwrecked was to get a rope ashore; for it was impossible for any boat to live in the sea as it was then running. There were two Newfoundland dogs and a bull-dog on board. One of the Newfoundland dogs was thrown overboard, with a rope thrown round him, and perished in the waves. The second shared a similar fate: but the bull-dog fought his way through that terrible sea, and, arriving safe on shore, rope and all, became the saviour of the crew."

Some of the true Newfoundland dogs have been brought to Europe and have been used as retrievers. They are principally valuable for the fearless manner in which they will penetrate the thickest cover. They are comparatively small, but muscular, strong, and generally black. A larger variety has been bred, and is now perfectly established. He is seldom used as a sporting dog, or for draught, but is admired on account of his stature and beauty, and the different colours with which he is often marked. Perhaps he is not quite so good-natured and manageable as the smaller variety, and yet it is not often that much fault can be found with him on this account.

A noble animal of this kind was presented to the Zoological Society by His Royal Highness Prince Albert. He is a great ornament to the gardens; but he had been somewhat unmanageable, and had done some mischief before he was sent thither.

A portion of Lord Byron's beautiful epitaph on the death of his Newfoundland dog will properly close our account of this animal:—

> "The poor dog! in life the firmest friend,
> The first to welcome, foremost to defend;
> Whose honest heart is still his master's own;
> Who labours, fights, lives, breathes for him alone."

[Notwithstanding the many excellent qualities so conspicuous in this noble breed of dog, he is said to possess one most ungenerous trait of character, "a peculiar antipathy to sheep," and if not early trained to endure their presence, will take every opportunity to destroy these innocent animals.—L.]

THE ESQUIMAUX DOG

is a beast of burden and of draught, usefully employed by the inhabitants of the extreme parts of North America and the neighbouring islands. When the Esquimaux Indian goes in pursuit of the seal, the rein-deer, or the bear, his dogs carry the materials of his temporary hut, and the few necessaries of his simple life; or, yoked to the sledge, often draw him and his family full sixty miles a-day over the frozen plains of these inhospitable regions. At other times they assist in the chase, and run down and destroy the bear and the rein-deer on land, and the seal on the coast.

These dogs are very early trained to the work which they are destined to follow, and even at the tender age of four or five months are harnessed together or in company with older animals, and are compelled, either by persuasion or brutal chastisement, to draw heavy weights, and thus soon become accustomed to the trammels of the rude gearing, and familiar with the service that they afterwards perform with so much sagacity and alacrity.

Capt. Lyon states that they are very similar in appearance to the shepherd dog of England, but more muscular and broad chested, owing to severe work; ears pointed, of a savage appearance; the finer dogs are equal to the Newfoundland breed in point of height and general symmetry.

It is also somewhat curious to be informed that these dogs have no particular season of œstrum, but bear young indiscriminately at all times of the year, cold or warm, having very little or no effect upon their reproductive powers, being often seen in heat during the month of December when the thermometer was forty degrees below zero.

Their journeys are often without any certain object; but, if the dogs scent the deer or the bear, they gallop away in that direction until their prey is within reach of the driver, or they are enabled to assist in destroying their foe. Captain Parry, in his Journal of a Second Voyage for the Discovery of a North-West Passage, gives an amusing account of these expeditions. "A number of dogs, varying from six to twelve, are attached to each sledge by means of a single trace, but with no reins. An old and tried dog is placed as the leader, who, in their simple journeys, and when the chase is the object, steadily obeys the voice of the driver sitting in front of the sledge, with a whip long enough to reach the leader. This whip, however, is used as seldom as possible; for these dogs, although tractable, are ferocious, and will endure little correction. When the whip is applied with severity on one, he falls upon and worries his neighbour, and he, in his turn, attacks

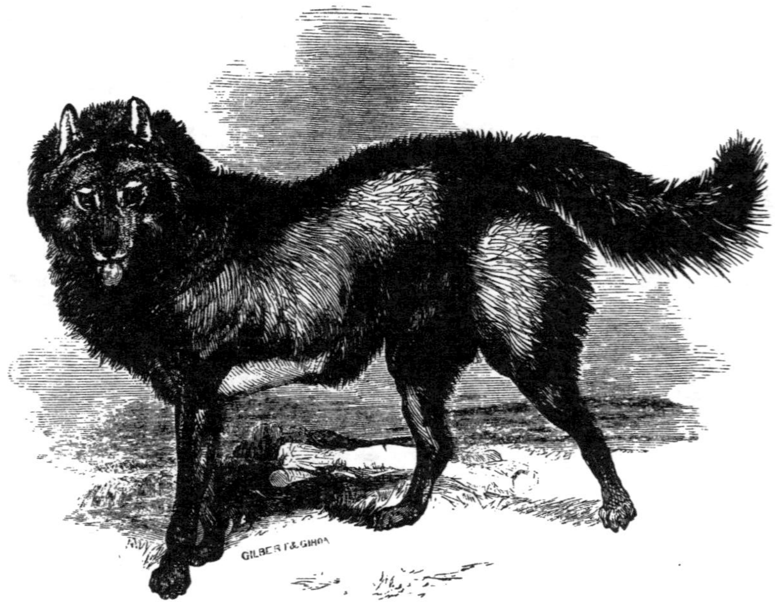

THE ESQUIMAUX DOG.

a third, and there is a scene of universal confusion, or the dogs double from side to side to avoid the whip, and the traces become entangled, and the safety of the sledge endangered. The carriage must then be stopped, each dog put into his proper place, and the traces re-adjusted. This frequently happens several times in the course of the day. The driver therefore depends principally on the docility of the leader, who, with admirable precision, quickens or slackens his pace, and starts off or stops, or turns to the right or left, at the summons of his master. When they are journeying homeward, or travelling to some spot to which the leader has been accustomed to go, he is generally suffered to pursue his own course; for, although every trace of the road is lost in the drifting snow, he scents it out, and follows it with undeviating accuracy. Even the leader, however, is not always under the control of his master. If the journey lies homeward, he will go his own pace, and that is usually at the top of his speed; or, if any game starts, or he scents it at a distance, no command of his driver will restrain him. Neither the dog nor his master is half civilized or subdued."

Each of these dogs will draw a weight of 120 lb. over the snow, at the rate of seven or eight miles an hour.

[It is extraordinary to consider the powers and wonderful speed of these animals, almost equalling that of many horses.

Captain Lyon informs us that three dogs drew a sledge weighing 100 lbs. and himself, one mile in six minutes; his leader dog, which is generally more powerful than the others, drew 196 lb. the same distance in eight minutes; seven dogs ran one mile in four minutes and thirty seconds, with a heavy sledge full of men attached to them; ten dogs ran one mile in five minutes; nine dogs drew 1611 lb. the same distance in nine minutes.—*Lyon's Journal*, p. 243.—L.]

In summer, many of these dogs are used as beasts of burden, and each carries from thirty to fifty pounds. They are then much better kept than in the winter; for they have the remains of the whale and sea-calf, which their masters disdain to eat. The majority, however, are sent adrift in the summer, and they live on the produce of the chase or of their constant thievery. The exactness with which, the summer being past, each returns to his master, is an admirable proof of sagacity, and frequently of attachment.

In some parts of Siberia, on the borders of the Oby, there are established relays of dogs, like the post-horses in other countries. Four of these are attached to a very light vehicle; but, when much haste is required, or any very heavy goods are to be conveyed, more than treble or quadruple that number are harnessed to the vehicle. M. de Lesseps[a] gives an almost incredible account

[a] Journal Historique du Voyage de M. de Lesseps. Paris, 1790. 2 vols.—tome 1

of this. He is speaking of the voracity of these poor beasts, in the midst of the snowy desert, with little or no food. "We had unharnessed our dogs, in order to bring them closer together, in the ordinary way; but, the moment they were brought up to the pole, they seized their harness, constructed of the thickest and toughest leather, and tore it to pieces, and devoured it. It was in vain that we attempted every means of restraint. A great number of them escaped into the wilds around, others wandered here and there, and seized everything that came within their reach, and which their teeth could destroy. Almost every minute some one of them fell exhausted, and immediately became the prey of the others. Every one that could get within reach struggled for his share. Every limb was disputed, and torn away by a troop of rivals, who attacked all within their reach. As soon as one fell by exhaustion or accident, he was seized by a dozen others, and destroyed in the space of a few minutes. In order to defend ourselves from this crowd of famished beasts, we were compelled to have recourse to our bludgeons and our swords. To this horrible scene of mutual destruction succeeded, on the following day, the sad appearance of those that surrounded the sledge, to which we had retreated for safety and for warmth. They were thin, and starved, and miserable; they could scarcely move; their plaintive and continual howlings seemed to claim our succour: but there was no possibility of relieving them in the slightest degree, except that some of them crept to the opening in our carriage through which the smoke escapes; and the more they felt the warmth the closer they crept, and then, through mere feebleness, losing their equilibrium, they rolled into the fire before our eyes."

These dogs are not so high as the common pointer, but much larger and stouter, although their thick hair, three or four inches long in the winter, gives them an appearance of more stoutness than they possess. Under this hair is a coating of fine close soft wool, which begins to grow in the early part of winter, and drops off in the spring. Their muzzles are sharp and generally black, and their ears erect.

The Greenland, and Siberian, and Kamtschatdale are varieties of the Esquimaux or Arctic dogs, but enlarged in form, and better subdued. The docility of some of these is equal to that of any European breed.

A person of the name of Chabert, who was afterwards better known by the title of "Fire King," had a beautiful Siberian dog, who would draw him in a light carriage 20 miles a-day. He asked £200 for him, and sold him for a considerable portion of that sum; for he was a most beautiful animal of his kind, and as docile as he was beautiful. Between the sale and the delivery, the dog fell and broke his leg. Chabert, to whom the price agreed on was of immense consequence, was in despair. He took the dog at night to a veterinary surgeon. He formally introduced them to each other. He talked to the dog, pointed to his leg, limped around the room, then requested the surgeon to apply some bandages around the leg, and he seemed to walk sound and well. He patted the dog on the head, who was looking alternately at him and the surgeon, desired the surgeon to pat him, and to offer him his hand to lick, and then, holding up his finger to the dog, and gently shaking his head, quitted the room and the house. The dog immediately laid himself down, and submitted to a reduction of the fracture, and the bandaging of the limb, without a motion, except once or twice licking the hand of the operator. He was quite submissive, and in a manner motionless, day after day, until, at the expiration of a month, the limb was sound. Not a trace of the fracture was to be detected, and the purchaser, who is now living, knew nothing about it.

The employment of the Esquimaux dogs is nearly the same as those from Newfoundland, and most valuable they are to the traveller who has to find his way over the wild and trackless regions of the north. The manner, however, in which they are generally treated seems ill calculated to cause any strong or lasting attachment. During their period of labour, they, like their brethren in Newfoundland, are fed sparingly on putrid fish, and in summer they are turned loose to shift for themselves until the return of the severe season renders it necessary to their masters' interest that they should again be sought for, and once more reduced to their state of toil and slavery.

They have been known for several successive days to travel more than 60 miles. They seldom miss their road, although they may be driven over one untrodden snowy plain, where they are occasionally unable to reach any place of shelter. When, however, night comes, they partake with their master of the scanty fare which the sledge will afford, and, crowding round, keep him warm and defend him from danger. If any of them fall victims to the hardships to which they are exposed, their master or their companions frequently feed on their remains, and their skins are converted into warm and comfortable dresses.

THE LAPLAND DOG.

Captain Clarke thus describes the Lapland dog:—" We had a valuable companion in a dog belonging to one of the boatmen. It was of the true Lapland breed, and in all respects similar to a wolf, excepting the tail, which was bushy and curled like those of the Pomeranian race. This dog, swimming after the boat, if his master merely waved his hand, would cross the lake as often as he pleased, carrying half his body and the whole of his head and tail out of the water. Wherever he landed, he scoured all the long grass by the side of the lake in search of wild-fowl, and came back to us, bringing wild-ducks in his mouth to the boat, and then, having delivered his prey to his master, he would instantly set off again in search of more."[a]

But we pass on to another and more valuable species of the dog—

THE SHEEP-DOG.

The origin of the sheep-dog is somewhat various; but the predominant breed is that of the intelligent and docile spaniel. Although it is now found in every civilized country in which the sheep is cultivated, it is not coeval with the domestication of that animal. When the pastures were in a manner open to the first occupant, and every shepherd had a common property in them, it was not so necessary to restrain the wandering of the sheep, and the voice of the shepherd was usually sufficient to collect and to guide them. He preceded the flock, and they "followed him whithersoever he went." In process of time, however, man availed himself of the sagacity of the dog to diminish his own labour and fatigue, and this useful servitor became the guide and defender of the flock.

The sheep-dog possesses much of the same form and character in every country. The muzzle is sharp, the ears are short and erect, and the animal is covered, particularly about the neck, with thick and shaggy hair. He has usually two dew claws on each of the hind legs; not, however, as in the one claw of other dogs, having a jointed attachment to the limb, but merely connected by the skin and some slight cellular substance. These excrescences should be cut off when the dog is young. The tail is slightly turned upwards and long, and almost as bushy as that of a fox, even in that variety whose coat is almost smooth. He is of a black colour or black prevails, mixed with gray or brown.

Professor Grognier gives the following account of this dog as he is found in France:—"The shepherd's dog, the least removed from the natural type of the dog, is of a middle size; his ears short and straight; the hair long, principally on the tail, and of a dark colour; the tail is carried horizontally or a little elevated. He is very indifferent to caresses, possessed of much intelligence and activity to discharge the duties for which he was designed In one or other of its varieties it is found in every part of France. Sometimes there is but a single breed, in others there are several varieties. It lives and maintains its proper characteristics, while other races often degenerate. Everywhere it preserves its proper distinguishing type. It is the servant of man, while other breeds

[a] Clarke's Scandinavia, vol. i. p. 432.

vary with a thousand circumstances. It has one appropriate mission, and that it discharges in the most admirable way: there is evidently a kind and wise design in this."

This account of the French sheep-dog, or of the sheep-dog everywhere, is as true as it is beautiful. One age succeeds to another, we pass from one climate to another, and everything varies and changes, but the shepherd's dog is what he ever was—the guardian of our flocks. There are, however, two or more species of this dog; the one which Professor Grognier has described, and which guards and guides the sheep in the open and level country, where wolves seldom intrude; another crossed with the mastiff, or little removed from that dog, used in the woody and mountainous countries, their guard more than their guide.[a] In Great Britain, where he has principally to guide and not to guard the flock, he is comparatively a small dog. He is so in the northern and open parts of the country, where activity is principally wanted; but, in the more enclosed districts, and where strength is often needed to turn an obstinate sheep, he is crossed with some larger dog, as the rough terrier, or sometimes the pointer, or now and then the bull-dog: in fact, almost any variety that has strength and stoutness may be employed. Thus we obtain the larger sheep-dog and the drover's dog. The sagacity, forbearance, and kindness of the sheep-dog are generally retained, but from these crosses there is occasionally a degree of ferocity from which the sheep often suffer.

In other countries, where the flock is exposed to the attack of the wolf, the sheep-dog is larger than the British drover's dog, and not far inferior in size to the mastiff. The strength and ferocity which qualify him to combat with the wolf, would occasionally be injurious or fatal to those who somewhat obstinately opposed his direction; therefore, in Denmark and in Spain, the dog is rarely employed to drive the flock. It is the office of the shepherd, to know every individual under his charge, to, as in olden times, "call them all by their names," and have always some docile and tamed wether who will take the lead, almost as subservient to his voice as is the dog himself, and whom the flock will immediately follow.

In whatever country the dog is used, partly or principally to protect the flock from the ravages of the wolf, he is as gentle as a lamb, except when opposed to his natural enemy; and it is only in England that the guardian of the sheep occasionally injures and worries them, and that many can be found bearing the mark

[a] The migratory sheep, in some parts of the south of France almost as numerous as in Spain, are attended by *a goat*, as a guide; and the intelligence and apparent pride which he displays are remarkable.

of the tooth. This may be somewhat excusable (although it is often carried to a barbarous extent) in the drover's dog; but it will admit of no apology in the shepherd's dog. It is the result of the idleness of the boy, or the mingled brutality and idleness of the shepherd, who is attempting to make the dog do his own work and that of his master too. We have admired the Prussian sheep-dog in the discharge of his duty, and have seen him pick out the marked sheep, or stop and turn the flock, as cleverly as any Highland colley, but he never bit them. He is a shorter, stronger, and more compact dog than ours. He pushes against them and forces them along. If they rebel against this mild treatment, the shepherd is at hand to enforce obedience; and the flock is as easily and perfectly managed as any English or Highland one, and a great deal more so than the majority that we have seen.

Mr. Trimmer, in his work on the Merinos, speaking of the Spanish flocks, says: "There is no driving of the flock; that is a practice entirely unknown; but the shepherd, when he wishes to remove his sheep, calls to him a tame wether accustomed to feed from his hands. The favourite, however distant, obeys his call, and the rest follow. One or more of the dogs, with large collars armed with spikes, in order to protect them from the wolves, precede the flock, others skirt it on each side, and some bring up the rear. If a sheep be ill or lame, or lag behind unobserved by the shepherds, they stay with it and defend it until some one return in search of it. With us, dogs are too often used for other and worse purposes. In open, unenclosed districts, they are indispensable; but in others I wish them, I confess, either managed, or encouraged less. If a sheep commits a fault in the sight of an intemperate shepherd, or accidentally offends him, it is *dogged* into obedience: the signal is given, the dog obeys the mandate, and the poor sheep flies round the field to escape from the fangs of him who should be his protector, until it becomes half dead with fright and exhaustion, while the trembling flock crowd together dreading the same fate, and the churl exults in this cowardly victory over a weak and defenceless animal.[a]

If the farmer will seriously calculate the number of ewes that have yeaned before their time, and of the lambs that he has lost, and the accidents that have occurred from the sheep pressing upon one another in order to escape from the dog, and if he will also take into account the continual disturbance of the sheep while grazing, by the approach of the dog, and the consequent interference with the cropping and the digestion of the food, he will attach more importance to the good temper of the dog and of the shepherd than he has been accustomed to do. There would be

[a] Trimmer on the Merinos, p. 50. See also the Society's work on Sheep.

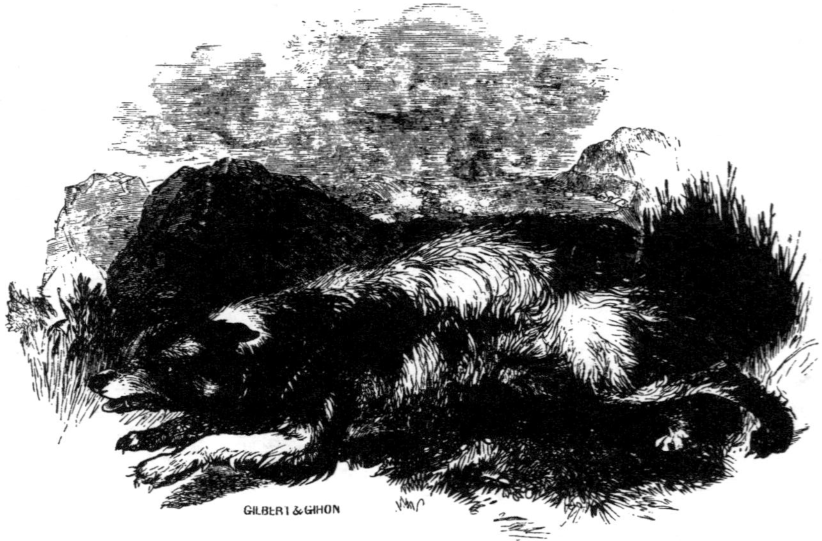

THE ENGLISH SHEEP DOG.

no injustice, or rather a great deal of propriety, in inflicting a fine for every tooth-mark that could be detected. When the sheep, instead of collecting round the dog, and placing themselves under his protection on any sudden alarm, uniformly fly from him with terror, the farmer may be assured there is something radically wrong in the management of the flock.

Instinct and education combine to fit this dog for our service. The pointer will act without any great degree of instruction, and the setter will crouch; and most certainly the sheep-dog, and especially if he has the example of an older and expert one, will, almost without the teaching of the master, become everything that can be wished, obedient to every order, even to the slightest motion of the hand. There is a natural predisposition for the office he has to discharge, which it requires little trouble or skill to develop and perfect.

It is no unpleasing employment to study the degree in which the several breeds of dogs are not only highly intelligent, but fitted by nature for the particular duty they have to perform. The pointer, the setter, the hound, the greyhound, the terrier, the spaniel, and even the bull-dog, were made, and almost perfected, by nature chiefly for one office alone, although they may be useful in many other ways. This is well illustrated in the sheep-dog. If he be but with his master, he lies content, indifferent to every surrounding object, seemingly half asleep and half awake, rarely mingling with his kind, rarely courting, and generally shrinking from, the notice of a stranger; but the moment duty calls, his sleepy, listless eye, becomes brightened; he eagerly gazes on his master, inquires and comprehends all he is to do, and, springing up, gives himself to the discharge of his duty with a sagacity, and fidelity, and devotion, too rarely equalled even by man himself.

Mr. James Hogg, the Ettrick Shepherd, living in his early days among the sheep and their quadruped attendants, and an accurate observer of nature, as well as an exquisite poet, gives some anecdotes of the colley, (the Highland term for sheep-dog,) with which the reader will not be displeased. "My dog Sirrah," says he, in a letter to the Editor of Blackwood's Edinburgh Magazine, "was, beyond all comparison, the best dog I ever saw. He had a somewhat surly and unsocial temper, disdaining all flattery, and refusing to be caressed; but his attention to my commands and interest will never again be equalled by any of the canine race. When I first saw him, a drover was leading him with a rope. He was both lean and hungry, and far from being a beautiful animal; for he was almost black, and had a grim face, striped with dark brown. I thought I perceived a sort of sullen intelligence in his countenance, notwithstanding his dejected and forlorn appearance, and I bought him. He was scarcely a year old, and knew so little of herding that he had never turned a sheep in his life; but, as soon as he discovered that it was his duty to do so, and that it obliged me, I can never forget with what anxiety and eagerness he learned his different evolutions; and when I once made him understand a direction, he never forgot or mistook it."

On one night, a large flock of lambs that were under the Ettrick Shepherd's care, frightened by something, scampered away in three different directions across the hills, in spite of all that he could do to keep them together. "Sirrah," said the shepherd, "they're a' awa!"

It was too dark for the dog and his master to see each other at any considerable distance, but Sirrah understood him, and set off after the fugitives. The night passed on, and Hogg and his assistant traversed every neighbouring hill in anxious but fruitless search for the lambs; but he could hear nothing of them nor of the dog, and he was returning to his master with the doleful intelligence that he had lost all his lambs. "On our way home, however," says he, "we discovered a lot of lambs at the bottom of a deep ravine called the Flesh Cleuch, and the indefatigable Sirrah standing in front of them, looking round for some relief, but still true to his charge. We concluded that it was one of the divisions which Sirrah had been unable to manage, until he came to that commanding situation. But what was our astonishment when we discovered that not one lamb of the flock was missing! How he had got all the divisions collected in the dark, is beyond my comprehension. The charge was left entirely to himself from midnight until the rising sun; and, if all the shepherds in the forest had been there to have assisted him, they could not have effected it with greater promptitude. All that I can say is, that I never felt so grateful to any creature under the sun as I did to my honest Sirrah that morning."

A shepherd, in one of his excursions over the Grampian Hills to collect his scattered flock, took with him (as is a frequent practice, to initiate them in their future business) one of his children about four years old. After traversing his pastures for a while, attended by his dog, he was compelled to ascend a summit at some distance. As the ascent was too great for the child, he left him at the bottom, with strict injunctions not to move from the place. Scarcely, however, had he gained the height, when one of the Scotch mists, of frequent occurrence, suddenly came on, and almost changed the day to night. He returned to seek his child, but was unable to find him, and concluded a long and fruitless search by coming distracted to his cottage. His poor dog also was missing in the general confusion. On the next morning by daylight he renewed his search, but again he came back without his child. He found, however, that during his absence his dog

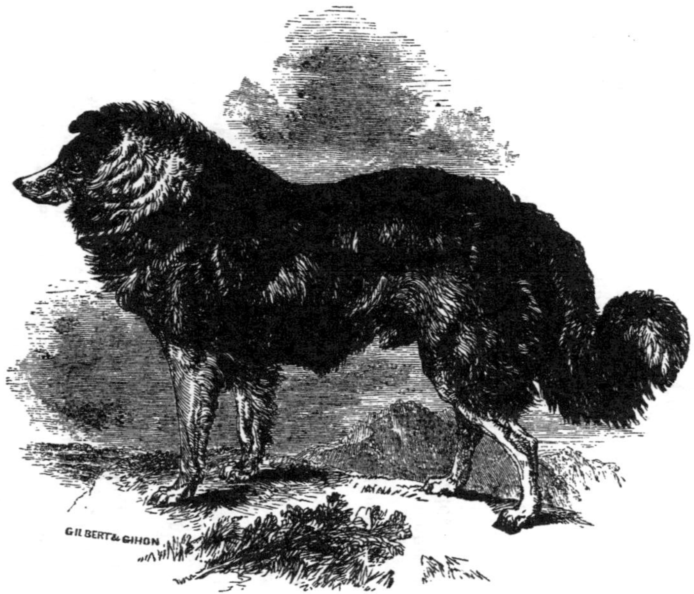

THE SCOTCH SHEEP DOG.

had been home, and, on receiving his allowance of food, instantly departed. For four successive days the shepherd continued his search with the same bad fortune, the dog as readily coming for his meal and departing. Struck by this singular circumstance, he determined to follow the dog, who departed as usual with his piece of cake. The animal led the way to a cataract at some distance from the spot where the child had been left. It was a rugged and almost perpendicular descent which the dog took, and he disappeared in a cave, the mouth of which was almost on a level with the torrent. The shepherd with difficulty followed; but, on entering the cavern, what were his emotions when he beheld the infant eating the cake which the dog had just brought to him, while the faithful animal stood by, eyeing his young charge with the utmost complacency! From the situation in which the child was found, it appeared that he had wandered to the brink of the precipice, and then either fallen or scrambled down, the torrent preventing his re-ascent. The dog by means of his scent had traced him to the spot, and afterwards prevented him from starving by giving up a part, or, perhaps, the whole of his own daily allowance. He appears never to have quitted the child night or day, except for food, as he was seen running at full speed to and from the cottage.[a]

Mr. Hogg says, and very truly, that a single shepherd and his dog will accomplish more in gathering a flock of sheep from a Highland farm than twenty shepherds could do without dogs; in fact, that without this docile animal, the pastoral life would be a mere blank. It would require more hands to manage a flock of sheep, gather them from the hills, force them into houses and folds, and drive them to markets, than the profits of the whole flock would be capable of maintaining. Well may the shepherd feel an interest in his dog; he it is indeed that earns the family bread, of which he is himself content with the smallest morsel: always grateful, and always ready to exert his utmost abilities in his master's interests. Neither hunger, fatigue, nor the worst treatment will drive him from his side, and he will follow him through every hardship without murmur or repining. If one of them is obliged to change masters, it is sometimes long before he will acknowledge the new owner, or condescend to work for him with the willingness that he did for his former lord; but, if he once acknowledges him, he continues attached to him until death.[b]

We will add another story of the colley, and proceed. It illus-

---

[a] Annals of Sporting, vol. viii. p. 83.

[b] "The Ettrick Shepherd has probably spoken somewhat too enthusiastically of his dog; but accounts of the sagacity and almost superhuman fidelity of this dog crowd so rapidly upon us that we are compelled to admire and to love him."—Hogg's Shepherd's Calendar, vol. ii. p. 308.

trates the memory of the dog. A shepherd was employed in bringing up some mountain sheep from Westmoreland, and took with him a young sheep-dog who had never made the journey before. From his assistant being ignorant of the ground, he experienced great difficulty in having the flock stopped at the various roads and lanes he passed in their way to the neighbourhood of London.

In the next year the same shepherd, accompanied by the same dog, brought up another flock for the gentlemen who had had the former one. On being questioned how he had got on, he said much better than the year before, as his dog now knew the road, and had kept the sheep from going up any of the lanes or turnings that had given the shepherd so much trouble on his former journey. The distance could not have been less than 400 miles.[a]

Buffon gives an eloquent and faithful account of the sheep-dog. —"This animal, faithful to man, will always preserve a portion of his empire and a degree of superiority over other beings. He reigns at the head of his flock, and makes himself better understood than the voice of the shepherd. Safety, order, and discipline are the fruits of his vigilance and activity. They are a people submitted to his management, whom he conducts and protects, and against whom he never employs force but for the preservation of good order." "If we consider that this animal, notwithstanding his ugliness and his wild and melancholy look, is superior in instinct to all others; that he has a decided character in which education has comparatively little share; that he is the only animal born perfectly trained for the service of others; that, guided by natural powers alone, he applies himself to the care of our flocks, a duty which he executes with singular assiduity, vigilance, and fidelity; that he conducts them with an admirable intelligence which is a part and portion of himself; that his sagacity astonishes at the same time that it gives repose to his master, while it requires great time and trouble to instruct other dogs for the purposes to which they are destined:—if we reflect on these facts we shall be confirmed in the opinion that the shepherd's dog is the true dog of nature, the stock and model of the whole species."[b]

[After reading the above history of this truly valuable dog, it is almost superfluous for us to attempt to add anything more on this head; however, we must pause for a few moments, to call the attention of our agriculturists and others engaged in raising sheep, to the immense advantages to be derived from the introduction of this sagacious animal throughout our own country.

The increased vigour that is now given for the cultivation of sheep, to supply the necessary demands of the numerous woollen

[a] Jesse's Gleanings, vol. i. p. 93. [b] Buffon's Natural History, vol. v. p. 314.

factories springing up in every quarter, renders the services of this faithful creature absolutely indispensable, not only as a guardian of the flocks, but as a mere expedient of economy.

Many portions of our country, now lying idle, particularly the mountainous ranges, are peculiarly adapted for the grazing of sheep, and we are destined not only to supply the world with cotton, but may hope ere long to add to our national wealth the other equally valuable staple commodity, that of wool.

In the care of sheep, each dog not only supplies the place of two or three men, but, as is seen in the foregoing pages, renders such assistance as cannot be obtained from any other source.

The shepherds of Mexico lead a life not unlike the patriarchs of old, shifting about from day to day, watching their immense flocks, attended only by a few dogs, who have the entire control of the sheep, keeping them from straying away, and not only defending them from the blood-thirsty wolf, but even attacking, if necessary, the skulking savage.

These dogs of Mexico are represented as being much larger than the English variety, and no doubt are the descendants of the Spanish shepherd dog, so highly prized in protecting the Merino flocks from the wolves that infest the mountainous parts of Spain, most frequented by the herds during the summer season.

These dogs are the same breed as those engaged by the philanthropic monks of St. Bernard in hunting up the benumbed traveller when sinking from exhaustion, or already overwhelmed by the sudden rushing of an avalanche into some one of the mountain passes.

The original Spanish shepherd dog is a very powerful animal, and even those of Mexico, when armed with spiked collars, are a sufficient match for the largest wolves. Mr. Kendall mentions having met on the grand prairie with a flock of sheep numbering seventeen thousand, which immense herd was guarded by a very few men, assisted by a large number of noble dogs, which appeared gifted with the faculty of keeping them together. There was no running about, no barking or biting in their system of tactics; on the contrary, they were continually walking up and down, like faithful sentinels, on the outer side of the flock, and should any sheep chance to stray from his fellows, the dog on duty at that particular post would walk gently up, take him carefully by the ear, and lead him back to the fold. Not the least fear did the sheep manifest at the approach of these dogs, and there was no occasion for it."—Vol. I. p. 268.

This account coincides with the remarks of Mr. Trinner upon this dog in old Spain; and Mr. Skinner very justly remarks, that the Mexican sheep-dog has not his equal in any part of the world, except, perhaps, in his native country, and that the Scotch or English dog sinks into insignificance when compared with him.

A flock of a thousand sheep in Spain requires the attendance of two men and an equal number of dogs, who never for a moment quit their charge, watching them without intermission day and night. The great inferiority of the English dogs, may be attributed, perhaps, to their want of care in training and bringing up, which is considered the most essential, and actually the foundation of all their future usefulness with the Mexicans. The pups when first born, are taken from the bitch, and put to a sucking ewe, already deprived of her own lamb. For several days the ewe is confined with the pups in the shepherd's hut, and either from force, or an instinctive desire to be relieved of the contents of the udder, she soon allows the little strangers to suck, and in the course of a few days more, becomes quite reconciled to the change, and exhibits a great degree of affection for her foster children, who, knowing no other parentage, becomes thus early engrafted into the general community, and returns their early kindness by every mark of affection and fidelity hereafter; never being willing for a moment to quit their society, but remains with them night and day, expressing a peculiar attachment to this particular flock, and seeming able to distinguish each member of it from all other intruders.

In the third volume of the American Agriculturist will be found an interesting article connected with this subject, and from which we might extract much useful information, if our limits would allow of its insertion in the present volume.

Mr. Skinner states, that in 1832 he had two of these dogs, a male and female, both trained, but unfortunately lost the latter before obtaining any pups from her; he also remarks, that they can be imported via Havana and Santander, at an expense of not less than $70 or $80. We see no reason why the same dogs might not be obtained at a much less cost by the Santa Fé traders, who, no doubt, would be glad to bring them into the country as companions de voyages, provided there was any demand for them. —L.]

THE DROVER'S DOG

bears considerable resemblance to the sheep-dog, and has usually the same prevailing black or brown colour. He possesses all the docility of the sheep-dog, with more courage, and sometimes a degree of ferocity, exercised without just cause upon his charge, while he is in his turn cruelly used by a brutal master.

There is a valuable cross between the colley and the drover's dog in Westmoreland, and a larger and stronger breed is cultivated in Lincolnshire; indeed it is necessary there, where oxen as well as sheep are usually consigned to the dog's care. A good drover's dog is worth a considerable sum; but the breed is too frequently and injudiciously crossed at the fancy of the owner. Some drovers' dogs are as much like setters, lurchers, and hounds, as they are to the original breed.

Stories are told of the docility and sagacity of the drover's dog even more surprising than any that are related of the sheep-dog. The Ettrick Shepherd says, that a Mr. Steel, butcher in Peebles, had such implicit dependence on the attention of his dog to his orders, that whenever he put a lot of sheep before her, he took a pride in leaving them entirely to her, and either remained to take a glass with the farmer of whom he had made the purchase, or travelled another road to look after bargains or business. At one time, however, he chanced to commit a drove to her charge, at a place called Willenslee, without attending to her condition, which he certainly ought to have done. This farm is about five miles from Peebles, over wild hills, and there is no regularly defined path to it. Whether Mr. Steel chose another road is uncertain; but, on coming home late in the evening, he was surprised to hear that his faithful animal had not made her appearance with her flock. He and his son instantly prepared to set out by different paths in search of her; but, on going into the street, there was she with the flock, and not one of the sheep missing; she, however, was carrying a young pup in her mouth. She had been taken in travail on those hills; and how the poor beast had contrived to manage the sheep in her state of suffering is beyond human calculation, for her road lay through sheep-pastures the whole way. Her master's heart smote him when he saw what she had suffered and effected; but she was nothing daunted; and, having deposited her young one in a place of safety, she again set out at full speed to the hills, and brought another and another little one, until she had removed her whole litter one by one; the last, however, was dead.

Mr. Blaine relates as extraordinary an instance of intelligence, but not mingled, like the former, with natural affection. A butcher and cattle-dealer, who resided about nine miles from Alston, in Cumberland, bought a dog of a drover. The butcher was accustomed to purchase sheep and kine in the vicinity, which, when fattened, he drove to Alston market and sold. In these excursions he was frequently astonished at the peculiar sagacity of his dog, and at the more than common readiness and dexterity with which he managed the cattle; until at length he troubled himself very little about the matter, but, riding carelessly along, used to amuse himself with observing how adroitly the dog acquitted himself of his charge. At length, so convinced was he of his sagacity, as well as fidelity, that he laid a wager that he would intrust the dog with a number of sheep and oxen, and let him drive them alone and unattended to Alston market. It was stipulated that no one should be within sight or hearing who had the least control over the dog, nor was any spectator to interfere. This extraordinary animal, however, proceeded with his business in the most steady and dexterous manner; and, although he had frequently to drive his charge through other herds that were grazing, he did not lose one; but, conducting them to the very yard to which he was used to drive them when with his master, he significantly delivered them up to the person appointed to receive them by barking at his door. When the path which he travelled lay through grounds in which others were grazing, he would run forward, stop his own drove, and then, chasing the others away, collect his scattered charge, and proceed.

THE ITALIAN OR POMERANIAN WOLF-DOG.

The wolf-dog is no longer a native of Great Britain, because his services are not required there, but he is useful in various parts of the Continent, in the protection of the sheep from the attacks of the wolf. A pair of these dogs was brought to the Zoological Society of London in 1833, and there long remained, an ornament to the Gardens. They appeared to possess a considerable degree of strength, but to be too gentle to contend with so powerful and ferocious an animal as the wolf. They were mostly covered with white or gray, or occasionally black hair, short on the head, ears, and feet, but long and silky on the body and tail. The forehead is elevated, and the muzzle lengthened and clothed with short hair. The attachment of this dog to his master and the flock is very great, and he has not lost a particle of his sagacity, but, where wolves are common, is still used as a sheep-dog.

THE CUR

is the sheep-dog crossed with the terrier. He has long and somewhat deservedly obtained a very bad name, as a bully and a coward; and certainly his habit of barking at everything that passes, and flying at the heels of the horse, renders him often a very dangerous nuisance: he is, however, in a manner necessary to the cottager; he is a faithful defender of his humble dwelling; no bribe can seduce him from his duty; and he is likewise a useful and an effectual guard over the clothes and scanty provisions of the labourer, who may be working in some distant part of the field. All day long he will lie upon his master's clothes seemingly asleep, but giving immediate warning of the approach of a supposed marauder. He has a propensity, when at home, to fly at every horse and every strange dog; and of young game of every kind there is not a more ruthless destroyer than the village cur

Mr. Hogg draws the following curious parallel between the sheep-dog and the cur :—"An exceedingly good sheep-dog attends to nothing but the particular branch of business to which he is bred. His whole capacity is exerted and exhausted in it; and he is of little avail in miscellaneous matters; whereas a very indifferent cur bred about the house, and accustomed to assist in everything, will often put the more noble breed to disgrace in these little services. If some one calls out that the cows are in the corn or the hens in the garden, the house colley needs no other hint, but runs and turns them out. The shepherd's dog knows not what is astir, and, if he is called out in a hurry for such work, all that he will do is to run to the hill, or rear himself on his haunches to see that no sheep are running away. A well-bred sheep-dog, if coming hungry from the hills, and getting into a milk-house, would likely think of nothing else than filling his belly with the cream. Not so his initiated brother: he is bred at home to far higher principles of honour. I have known such lie night and day among from ten to twenty pails full of milk, and never once break the cream of one of them with the tip of his tongue, nor would he suffer cat, rat, or any other creature to touch it. While, therefore, the cur is a nuisance, he is very useful in his way, and we would further plead for him, that he possesses a great deal of the sagacity and all the fidelity of the choicest breed of dogs."

The dog who, according to the well-known and authentic story, watched the remains of his master for two years in the churchyard of St. Olave's, in Southwark, was a cur.

The following story is strictly authentic:—"Not long ago a young man, an acquaintance of the coachman, was walking, as he had often done, in Lord Fife's stables at Banff. Taking an opportunity, when the servants were not regarding him, he put a bridle into his pocket. A Highland cur that was generally about the stables saw him, and immediately began to bark at him, and when he got to the stable-door would not let him pass, but bit him by the leg in order to prevent him. As the servants had never seen the dog act thus before, and the same young man had been often with them, they could not imagine what could be the reason of the dog's conduct. However, when they saw the end of a valuable bridle peeping out of the young man's pocket, they were able to account for it, and, on his giving it up, the dog left the stable-door, where he had stood, and allowed him to pass."[a]

[a] Travels in Scotland, by the Rev. J. Hall, vol. ii. p. 395.

THE LURCHER.

This dog was originally a cross between the greyhound and the shepherd's dog, retaining all the speed and fondness for the chase belonging to the one, and the superior intelligence and readiness for any kind of work which the latter possessed. This breed has been crossed again with the spaniel, combining the disposition to quest for game which distinguishes the spaniel with the muteness and swiftness of the greyhound. Sometimes the greyhound is crossed with the hound. Whatever be the cross, the greyhound must predominate; but his form, although still to be traced, has lost all its beauty.

The lurcher is a dog seldom found in the possession of the honourable sportsman. The farmer may breed him for his general usefulness, for driving his cattle, and guarding his premises, and occasionally coursing the hare; but other dogs will answer the former purposes much better, while the latter qualification may render him suspected by his landlord, and sometimes be productive of serious injury. In a rabbit-warren this dog is peculiarly destructive. His scent enables him to follow them silently and swiftly. He darts unexpectedly upon them, and, being trained to bring his prey to his master, one of these dogs will often in one night supply the poacher with rabbits and other game worth more money than he could earn by two days' hard labour.

Mr. H. Faull, of Helstone, in Cornwall, lost no fewer than fifteen fine sheep, and some of them store sheep, killed by lurchers in January, 1824.[a]

We now proceed to the different species of dog belonging to the second division of Cuvier, which are classed under the name of Hound; and, first we take

THE BEAGLE.

The origin of this diminutive hound is somewhat obscure. There is evidently much of the harrier and of the old southern, connected with a considerable decrease of size and speed, the possession of an exceedingly musical voice, and very great power of scent. Beagles are rarely more than ten or twelve inches in height, and were generally so nearly of the same size and power of speed, that it was commonly said they might be covered with a sheet. This close running is, however, considered as a mark of excellence in hounds of every kind.

There are many pleasurable recollections of the period when "the good old English gentleman" used to keep his pack of beagles or little harriers, slow but sure, occasionally carried to the field in a pair of panniers on a horse's back; often an object of

[a] Annals of Sporting, vol. v. p. 137.

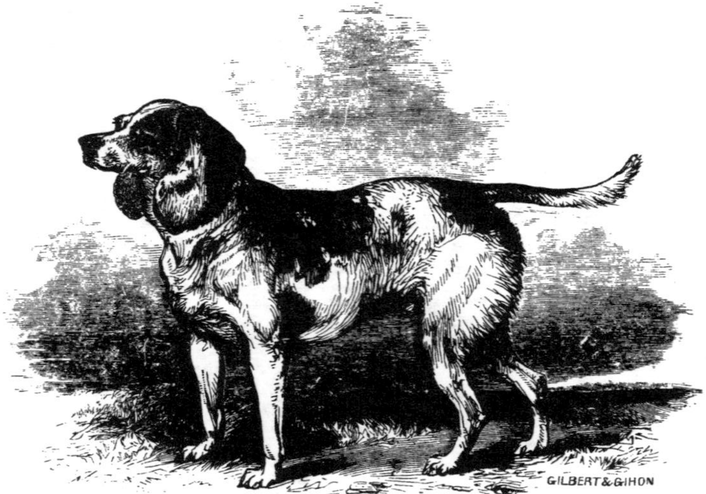

THE BEAGLE.

ridicule at an early period of the chase, but rarely failing to accomplish their object ere the day closed, "the puzzling pack unravelling wile by wile, maze within maze." It was often the work of two or three hours to accomplish this; but it was seldom, in spite of her speed, her shifts, and her doublings, that the hare did not fall a victim to her pursuers.

The slowness of their pace gradually caused them to be almost totally discontinued, until very lately, and especially in the royal park at Windsor, they have been again introduced. Generally speaking, they have all the strength and endurance which is necessary to ensure their killing their game, and are much fleeter than their diminutive size would indicate. Formerly, considerable fancy and even judgment used to be exercised in the breeding of these dogs. They were curiously distinguished by the names of "deep-flewed," or "shallow-flewed," in proportion as they had the depending upper lip of the southern, or the sharper muzzle and more contracted lip of the northern dogs. The shallow-flewed were the swiftest, and the deep-flewed the stoutest and the surest, and their music the most pleasant. The wire-haired beagle was considered as the stouter and better dog.

The form of the head in beagles has been much misunderstood. They have, or should have, large heads, decidedly round, and thick rather than long; there will then be room for the expansion of the nasal membrane, that of smell, and for the reverberation of the sound, so peculiarly pleasant in this dog.

The beagle runs very low to the ground, and therefore has a stronger impression of the scent than taller dogs. This is especially the case when the scent is more than usually low.

Among the advocates for beagles, several years ago, was Colonel Hardy. He used to send his dogs in panniers, and they had a little barn for their kennel. The door was one night broken open, and every hound, panniers and all, stolen. The thief was never discovered, nor even suspected.

The use of beagles was soon afterwards nearly abandoned by the introduction of the harrier, and by his yielding in his turn to the fox-hound; but the beagles of Colonel Thornton and Colonel Molyneux will not be soon forgotten.[a]

[a] Mr. Beckford at one time determined to try how he should like the use of beagles, and, having heard of a small pack of them, he sent his coachman, the person he could best spare, to fetch them. It was a long journey, and, although he had some assistance, yet not being used to hounds, he had some trouble in getting them along, especially as they had not been out of the kennel for several weeks before. They were consequently so riotous that they ran after everything they saw, sheep, cur dogs, birds of all sorts, as well as hares and deer. However, he lost but one hound; and, when Mr. Beckford asked him what he thought of them, he said, that they could not fail of being good hounds, for they would hunt everything.

There is, however, a practice which fair sportsmen will never resort to—the use of a beagle to start a hare in order to be run down by a brace of greyhounds, or perhaps by a lurcher. The hare is not fairly matched in this way of proceeding.

THE HARRIER

occupies an intermediate station between the beagle and the fox-hound. It is the fox-hound bred down to a diminished size, and suited to the animal he is to pursue. He retains, or did for a while retain, the long body, deep chest, large bones, somewhat heavy head, sweeping ears, and mellow voice, which the sportsman of old so enthusiastically described, with the certainty of killing, and the pleasing prolongation of the chase. With this the farmer used to be content: it did not require expensive cattle, was not attended with much hazard of neck, and did not take him far from home.

Almost every country squire used in former days to keep his little pack of harriers or beagles. He was mounted on his stout cob-horse, that served him alike for the road and the chase; and his huntsman probably had a still smaller and rougher beast, or sometimes ran afoot. He could then follow the sport, almost without going off his own land, and the farmer's boys, knowing the country and the usual doublings of the hare, could see the greater part of the chase, and were almost able to keep up with the hounds, so that they were rarely absent at the death: indeed, they saw and enjoyed far more of it than the fox-hunter or the stag-hunter now does, mounted on his fleetest horse.

The harrier was not more than 18 or 19 inches high. He was crossed with the fox-hound if he was getting too diminutive, or with the beagle if he was becoming too tall.

The principal objects the sportsman endeavoured to accomplish were to preserve stoutness, scent, and musical voice, with speed to follow the hare sufficiently close, yet not enough to run her down too quickly, or without some of those perplexities, and faults, and uncertainties which give the principal zest to the chase.

The character and speed of the hound much depend on the nature of the country. The smaller harrier will best suit a deeply enclosed country; but where there is little cover, and less doubling greater size and fleetness are requisite. The harrier, nevertheless, let him be as tall and as speedy as he may, should never be used for the fox; but every dog should be strictly confined to his own game.

Mr. Beckford, in his Thoughts upon Hunting, gives an account, unrivalled, of the chase of the hare and fox. Many sporting writers have endeavoured to tread in his steps; but they have

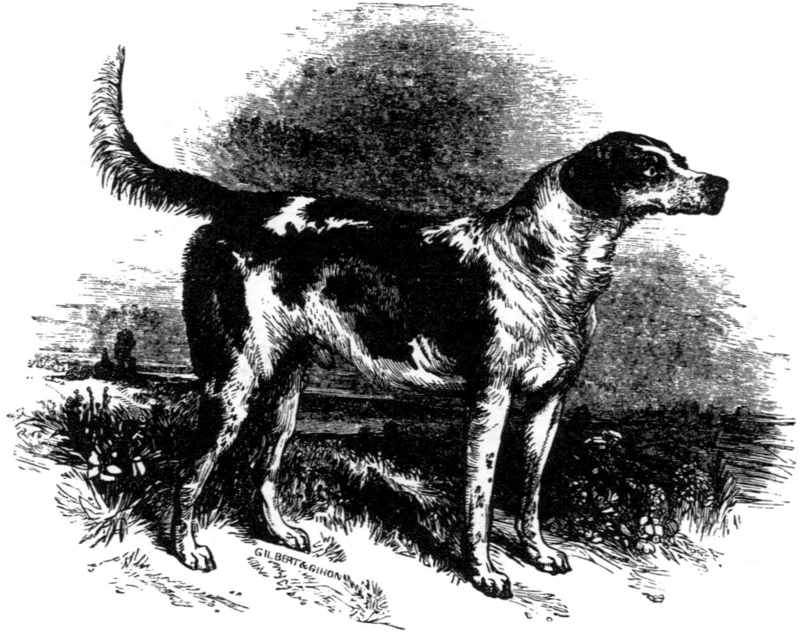

THE HARRIER.

failed in giving that graphic account of the pleasures of the field which Mr. Beckford's essay contains.

He says that the sportsman should never have more than 20 couple in the field, because it would be exceedingly difficult to get a greater number to run together, and a pack of harriers cannot be complete if they do not. A hound that runs too fast for the rest, or that lags behind them, should be immediately discarded. His hounds were between the large slow-hunting harrier and the fox-beagle. He endeavoured to get as much bone and strength in as little compass as possible. He acknowledges that this was a difficult undertaking; but he had, at last, the pleasure to see them handsome, small, yet bony, running well together, and fast enough, with all the alacrity that could be desired, and hunting the coldest scent.

He anticipates the present improvement of the chase when he lays it down as a rule never to be departed from, that hounds of every kind should be kept to their own game. They should have one scent, and one style of hunting. Harriers will run a fox in so different a style from the pursuit of a hare, that they will not readily, and often will not at all, return to their proper work. The difference in the scent, and the eagerness of pursuit, and the noise that accompanies fox-hunting, all contribute to spoil a harrier.

Mr. Beckford pleasingly expresses a sportman's consideration for the poor animal which he is hunting to death. "A hare," he says, "is a timorous little animal that we cannot help feeling some compassion for at the time that we are pursuing her destruction. We should give scope to all her little tricks, nor kill her foully nor overmatched. Instinct instructs her to make a good defence when not unfairly treated, and I will venture to say that, as far as her own safety is concerned, she has more cunning than the fox, and makes shifts to save her life far beyond all his artifice."[a]

THE FOX-HOUND

is of a middle size, between the harrier and the stag-hound; it is the old English hound, sufficiently crossed with the greyhound to give him lightness and speed without impairing his scent; and he has now been bred to a degree of speed sufficient to satisfy the man who holds his neck at the least possible price, and with which few, except thorough-bred horses, and not all of them, can live to the end of the chase. The fox-hound is lighter, or, as it is now called, more highly bred, or he retains a greater portion of his original size and heaviness, according to the nature of the country and the fancy of the master of the pack: therefore it is difficult to give an accurate description of the best variety of this dog; but

[a] Beckford on Hunting, p. 150.

there are guiding points which can never be forgotten without serious injury.

He derives from the greyhound a head somewhat smaller and longer in proportion to his size than either the stag-hound or the harrier. But considerable caution is requisite here. The beauty of the head and face, although usually accompanied by speed, must never be sacrificed to stoutness and power of scent. The object of the sportsman is to amalgamate them, or rather to possess them all in the greatest possible degree. This will generally be brought to a great degree of perfection if the sportsman regards the general excellence of the dog rather than the perfection of any particular point. The ears should not, comparatively speaking, be so large as those of the stag-hound or the harrier; but the neck should be longer and lighter, the chest deep and capacious, the fore legs straight as arrows, and the hind ones well bent at the hock.

Some extraordinary accounts have been given of the speed of the fox-hound. A match that was run over the Beacon Course at Newmarket is the best illustration of his fleetness. The distance is 4 miles 1 furlong and 132 yards. The winning dog performed it in 8 minutes and a few seconds; but of the sixty horses that started with the hounds, only twelve were able to run in with them. Flying Childers had run the same course in 7 minutes and 30 seconds.

"The size, or, as we should rather say, the height of a fox-hound, is a point on which there has been much difference of opinion. Mr. Chule's pack was three inches below the standard of Mr. Villebois', and four inches below that of Mr. Warde's. The advocates of the former assert, that they get better across a deep and strongly fenced country, while the admirers of the latter insist on their being better climbers of hills and more active in cover. As to uniformity in size, it is by no means essential to the well-doing of hounds in the field, and has been disregarded by some of our best sportsmen: Mr. Meynell never drafted a good hound on account of his being over or under sized. The proper standard of height in fox-hounds is from 21 to 22 inches for bitches, and from 23 to 24 for dog-hounds. Mr. Warde's bitches, the best of the kind that our country contained, were rather more than 23 inches. A few of his dogs were 25 inches high. The amount of hounds annually bred will depend upon the strength of the kennel. From sixty to eighty couples is the complement for a four days a-week pack, which will require the breeding of a hundred couples of puppies every year, allowing for accidents and distemper."[a]

---

[a] The Horse and the Hound, by Nimrod, p. 340.

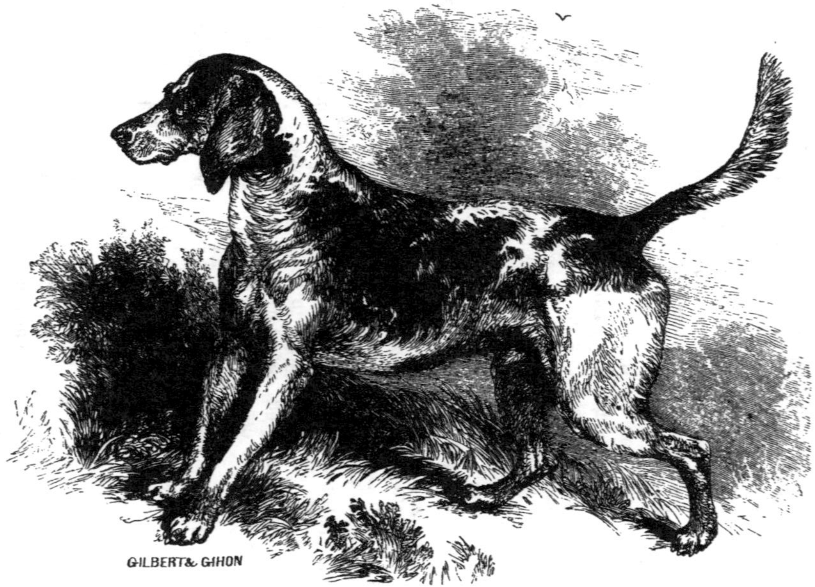

THE FOX HOUND.

Nimrod very properly observes, that "Mr. Beckford has omitted a point much thought of by the modern sportsmen, namely, *the back-ribs*, which should also be deep, as in a strong-bodied horse, of which we say, when so formed, that he has a good 'spur place;' a point highly esteemed in him. Nor is he sufficiently descriptive of the hinder legs of the hound; for there is a length of thigh discernible in first-rate hounds which, like the well-let-down hock of the horse, gives them much superiority of speed, and is also a great security against their laming themselves in leaping fences, which they are more apt to do when they become blown and consequently weak. The fore legs, 'straight as arrows,' is an admirable illustration of perfection in those parts by Beckford; for, as in a bow or bandy legged man, nothing is so disfiguring to a hound as having his elbows projecting, and which is likewise a great check to speed."[a]

Mr. Daniel gives a curious account of the prejudices of sportsmen on the subject of colour. The white dogs were curious hunters, and had a capital scent; the black, with some white spots, were obedient, good hunters, and with good constitutions; the gray-coloured had no very acute scent, but were obstinate, and indefatigable in their quest; the yellow dogs were impatient and obstinate, and taught with difficulty.[b]

The dog exhibits no criteria of age after the first two years. That period having elapsed, the whiteness and evenness of the teeth soon pass away, and the *old* dog can scarcely be mistaken. Nimrod scarcely speaks too positively when he says that an old hound cannot be mistaken, if only looked in the face. At all events, few are found in a kennel after the eighth year, and very few after the ninth.

Mr. Beckford advises the sportsman carefully to consider the size, shape, colour, constitution, and natural disposition of the dog from which he breeds, and also the fineness of the nose, the evident strength of the limb, and the good temper and devotion to his master which he displays. The faults or imperfections in one breed may be rectified in another; and, if this is properly attended to, there is no reason why improvements may not continually be made.

The separation of the sexes in the kennel and in the field is one of the latest innovations in the hunting world, and generally considered to be a good one. The eye is pleased to see a pack of hounds, nearly or quite of a size. The character of the animal is more uniformly displayed when confined to one sex. In consequence of the separation of the two, the dogs are less inclined to quarrel; and the bitches are more at their ease than when under-

---

[a] The Horse and the Hound, by Nimrod, p. 332. [b] Daniel's Fox-hound, p. 205.

going the importunate solicitations of the male. As to their performances in the field, opinions vary, and each sex has its advocates. The bitch, with a good fox before her, is decidedly more off-hand at her work; but she is less patient, and sometimes overruns the scent. Sir Bellingham Graham has been frequently heard to say, that if his kennels would have afforded it, he would never have taken a dog-hound into the field. That in the canine race the female has more of elegance and symmetry of form, consequently more of speed, than the male, is evident to a common observer; but there is nothing to lead to the conclusion that, in the natural endowments of the senses, any superiority exists.[a]

The bitch should not be allowed to engage in any long and severe chase after she has been lined. She should be kept as quiet as may be practicable, and well but not too abundantly fed; each having a kennel or place of retreat for herself. She should be carefully watched, and especially when the ninth week approaches. The huntsman and the keeper without any apparent or unnecessary intrusion, should be on the alert.

The time of pupping having arrived, as little noise or disturbance should be made as possible; but a keeper should be always at hand in case of abortion or difficult parturition. Should there be a probability of either of these occurring, he should not be in a hurry; for, as much should be left to nature as can, without evident danger, be done, and the keeper should rarely intrude unless his assistance is indispensable.

The pupping being accomplished, the mother should be carefully attended to. She should be liberally fed, and particularly should have her share of animal food, and an increased quantity of milk.

The bitch should not have whelps until she has hunted two seasons; for, before that time it will be scarcely possible to ascertain her excellences or defects. If there are any considerable faults, she should be immediately rejected.

When the time approaches for her to produce her puppies, she should be allowed a certain degree of liberty, and should choose her couch and run about a little more than usual; but, when the young ones are born, the less they are handled the better. The constitution and appearance of the mother will indicate how many should be kept. If two litters are born at or about the same time, or within two or three days of each other, we may interchange one or two of the whelps of each of them, and perhaps increase the value of both.

When the whelps are able to crawl to a certain distance, it will be time to mark them, according to their respective litters, some

---

[a] The Horse and the Hound, by Nimrod, p. 355.

on the ear and others on the lip. The dew-claws should be removed, and, usually, a small tip from the tail. Their names also should be recorded.

The whelps will begin to lap very soon after they can look about them, and should remain with the mother until they are fully able to take care of themselves. They may then be prepared to go to quarters.

Two or three doses of physic should be given to the mother, with intervals of four or five days between each: this will prepare her to return to the kennel.

There is often considerable difficulty in disposing of the whelps until they get old and stout enough to be brought into the kennel. They are mostly sent to some of the neighbouring cottages, in order to be taken care of; but they are often neglected and half starved there. In consequence of this, distemper soon appears, and many of them are lost.

Whelps *walked*, or taken care of at butchers' houses, soon grow to a considerable size; but they are apt to be heavy-shouldered and throaty, and perhaps otherwise deformed. There is some doubt whether it might not be better for the sportsman to take the management of them himself, and to have a kennel built purposely for them. It may, perhaps, be feared that the distemper will get among them: they would, however, be well fed, and far more comfortable than they now are; and, as to the distemper, it is a disease that they must have some time or other.

From twenty to thirty couples are quite as many as can be easily managed; and the principal consideration is, whether they are steady, and as nearly as possible equal of speed. When the packs are very large, the hounds are seldom sufficiently hunted to be good. Few persons choose to hunt every day, or, if they did, it is not likely that the weather would permit them. The sportsman would, therefore, be compelled to take an inconvenient number into the field, and too many must be left behind. In the first place, too many hounds in the field would frequently spoil the sport; and, on the other hand, the hounds that remained would get out of wind, or become riotous, or both. Hounds, to be useful and good, should be constantly hunted; but a great fault in many packs is their having too many old dogs among them.

Young hounds, when first taken to the kennel, should be kept separate from the rest of the pack, otherwise there will be frequent and dangerous quarrels. When these do occur, the feeder hears, and sometimes, but not so frequently as he ought, endeavours to discover the cause of the disturbance, and visits the culprits with deserved punishment; too often, however, he does not give himself time for this, but rushes among them, and flogs every hound that he can get at, guilty or not guilty. This is a shameful method of procedure. It is the cause of much undeserved punishment: it spoils the temper of the dog, and makes him careless and indifferent as long as he lives.

Mr. Beckford very properly remarks, that "Young hounds are, and must be awkward at first, and should be taken out, a few at a time, with couples not too loose. They are thus accustomed to the usual occurrences of the road, and this is most easily accomplished when a young and an old dog are coupled together."

A sheep-field is the next object, and the young hound, properly watched, soon becomes reconciled, and goes quietly along with the companion of the preceeding day. A few days afterwards the dogs are uncoupled in the field, and perhaps, at first, are not a little disposed to attack the sheep; but the cry of "Ware sheep!" in a stern tone of voice, arrests them, and often, without the aid of the whip; it being taken as a principle that this instrument should be used as seldom as possible. If, indeed, the dog is self-willed, the whip must be had recourse to, and perhaps with some severity; for, if he is once suffered to taste the blood of the sheep, it may be difficult to restrain him afterwards. A nobleman was told that it was possible to break his dogs of the habit of attacking his sheep, by introducing a large and fearless ram among them; one was accordingly procured and turned into the kennel. The men with their whips and voices, and the ram with his horns, soon threw the whole kennel into confusion. The hounds and the ram were left together. Meeting a friend soon afterwards, "Come," said he, "to the kennel, and see what rare sport the ram is making among the hounds." His friend asked whether he was not afraid that some of them might be spoiled. "No," said he; "they deserve it, and let them suffer." They proceeded to the kennel; all was quiet. The kennel-door was thrown open, and the remains of the ram were found scattered about: the hounds, having filled their bellies, had retired to rest.

The time of entering young hounds must vary in different countries. In a corn country, it should not be until the wheat is carried; in grass countries, somewhat sooner; and, in woodlands, as soon as we please. Frequent hallooing may be of use with young hounds; it makes them more eager; but, generally speaking, there is a time when it may be of use, a time when it does harm, and a time when it is perfectly indifferent.

The following remarks of Mr. Beckford are worthy of their author: — "Hounds at their first entering cannot be encouraged too much. When they begin to know what is right, it will be soon enough to chastise them for doing wrong, and, in such case, one rather severe beating will save a great deal of trouble. The voice should be used as well as the whip; and the smack of the whip will often be of as much avail as the lash to him who has felt it."

Flogging hounds in the kennel, the frequent practice of too many huntsmen, should be held in utter abhorrence, and, if carried to a considerable excess, is a disgrace to humanity. Generally speaking, none but the sportsman can form an adequate conception of the perfect obedience of the hound both in the kennel and the field. At feeding-time, each dog, although hungry enough, will go through the gate in the precise order in which he is called by the feeder; and, in a well-broken pack, to chop at, or to follow a hare, or to give tongue on a false scent, or even to break cover alone, although the fox is in view, are faults that are rarely witnessed.

Let not this obedience, however, be purchased by the infliction of a degree of cruelty that disgraces both the master and the menial. A young fox-hound may, possibly, mistake the scent of a hare for that of a fox, and give tongue. In too many hunts he will be unmercifully flogged for this, and some have almost died under the lash. Mercy is a word totally unknown to a great proportion of whippers-in, and even to many who call themselves gentlemen. There can be no occasion or excuse for barbarity: a little trouble, and moderate punishment, and the example of his fellows, will gradually teach the wildest hound his duty.

That the huntsman, and not the hound, may occasionally be in fault, the following anecdote will furnish sufficient proof. In drawing a strong cover, a young bitch gave tongue very freely, while none of the other hounds challenged. The whipper-in railed to no purpose; the huntsman insisted that she was wrong, and the whip was applied with great severity. In doing this, the lash accidentally struck one of her eyes out of its socket.

Notwithstanding the dreadful pain that must have ensued, she again took up the scent, and proved herself right; for the fox had stolen away, and she had broken cover after him, unheeded and alone. After much delay and cold hunting, the pack hit off the same scent.

At some distance a farmer informed the sportsmen, that they were a long way behind the fox, for he had seen a single hound, very bloody about the head, running breast-high, so that there was but little chance of their getting up with her. The pack, from her coming to a check, did at length overtake her.

The same bitch once more hit off the scent, and the fox was killed, after a long and severe run. The eye of the poor animal, that had hung pendent through the chase, was then taken off with a pair of scissors.

THE COMMENCEMENT OF THE SEASON.

During the beginning of autumn, the hounds should be daily exercised when the weather will permit. They should often be called over in the kennel to habituate them to their names, and walked out among the sheep and deer, in order that they may be accustomed perfectly to disregard them.

A few stout hounds being added to the young ones, some young foxes may occasionally be turned out. If they hunt improper game, they must be sternly checked. Implicit obedience is required until they have been sufficiently taught as to the game which they are to pursue. No obstinate deviation from it must ever be pardoned. The hounds should be, as much as possible, taken out into the country which they are afterwards to hunt, and some young foxes are probably turned out for them to pursue. At length they are suffered to hunt their game in thorough earnest, and to taste of its blood.

After this they are sent to more distant covers, and more old hounds are added, and so they continue until they are taken into the pack, which usually happens in September. The young hounds continue to be added, two or three couple at a time, until all have hunted. They are then divided into two packs, to be taken out alternate days. Properly speaking, the sport cannot be said to begin until October, but the two preceding months are important and busy ones.[a]

"It would appear, then," says Nimrod, "that the breeding of a pack of fox-hounds, bordering on perfection, is a task of no ordinary difficulty. The best proof of it is to be found in the few sportsmen that have succeeded in it. Not only is every good quality obtained if possible, but every imperfection or fault is avoided. The highest virtue in a fox-hound is his being true to the line his game has gone, and a stout runner at the end of the chase. He must also be a patient hunter when there is a cold scent and the pack is at fault."

While there is no country in the world that can produce a breed of horses to equal the English thorough-bred in his present improved state, there are no dogs like the English fox-hound for speed, scent, and continuance. It would seem as if there were something in the climate favourable and necessary to the perfection of the hound. Packs of them have been sent to other countries, neighbouring and remote; but they have usually become more or less valueless.

As regards the employment of the voice and the horn when out with hounds, too much caution cannot be used. A hound should

---

[a] Beckford's Thoughts on Hunting, p. 95.

never be cheered unless we are perfectly convinced that he is right, nor rated unless we are sure that he is wrong. When we are not sure of what is going on we should sit still and be silent. A few moments will possibly put us in possession of all that we wish to know.[a]

The horn should only be used on particular occasions, and a huntsman should speak by his horn as much as by his voice. Particular notes should mean certain things, and the hounds and the field should understand the language. We have heard some persons blowing the horn all the day long, and the hounds have become so careless as to render it of no use. When a hound first speaks in cover to a fox, you may, if you think it necessary, use *one single* and prolonged note to get the pack together. The same note will do at any time to call up a lost or loitering hound; but, when the fox breaks cover, then let your horn be marked in its notes: let it sound as if you said through it, "Gone away! gone away! gone away! away! away! away!" dwelling with full emphasis on the last syllable. Every hound will fly from the cover the moment he hears this, and the sportsmen and the field will know that the fox is away.

It is the perfection of the horse, and the perfection of the hound, and the disregard of trifling expense, that has given to Englishmen a partiality for field-sports, unequalled in any other country. Mr. Ware's pack of fox-hounds cost 2000 guineas, and the late Lord Middleton gave the same to Mr. Osbaldeston for ten couples of his hounds.

HUNTING-KENNELS.

It is time, however, to speak of the kennel, whether we regard the sporting architecture of Mr. G. Tattersall, or the scientific inquiries of Mr. Vyner, or a sketch of the noble buildings at Goodwood.

The lodging-rooms should be ceiled, but not plastered, with ventilators above and a large airy window on either side. The floors should be laid with flags or paved with bricks. Cement may be used instead of mortar, and the kennels will then be found

---

[a] Mr. Beckford gives the following excellent account of what a huntsman should be:—"A huntsman should be attached to the sport, and indefatigable, young, strong, active, bold, and enterprising in the pursuit of it. He should be sensible, good-tempered, sober, exact, and cleanly—a good groom and an excellent horseman. His voice should be strong and clear, with an eye so quick as to perceive which of his hounds carries the scent when all are running, and an ear so excellent as to distinguish the leading hounds when he does not see them. He should be quiet, patient, and without conceit. Such are the qualities which constitute perfection in a huntsman. He should not, however, be too fond of displaying them until called forth by necessity; it being a peculiar and distinguishing trait in his character to let his hounds alone while they thus hunt, and have genius to sssist them when they cannot."—Beckford on Hunting, Letter ix.

wholesome and dry. The doorways of the lodging-houses will generally be four feet and a half wide in the clear. The posts are rounded, to prevent the hounds from being injured when they rush out. The benches may be made of cast-iron or wood; those composed of iron being most durable, but the hounds are more frequently lamed in getting to them. The wooden benches must be bound with iron, or the hounds will gnaw or destroy them. A question has arisen, whether the benches should be placed round the kennel, or be in the centre of it, allowing a free passage by the side. There is least danger of the latter being affected by the damp. The walls should be wainscoted to the height of three feet at least. This will tend very considerably to their comfort.

The floors of all the courts should be arranged in nearly the same way; the partition walls being closed at the bottom, but with some iron work above. The doorways should also be so contrived, that the huntsman may be able to enter whenever he pleases. The boiling-house should be at as great a distance from the hunting-kennel as can be managed, continuing to give warmth to the infirmary for distempered puppies, and at the same time being out of the way of the other courts.

Mr. Vyner gives an interesting account of the young hounds' kennel: "This building," he says, "should be as far from the other lodging-rooms as the arrangements of the structure will allow. There is also an additional court, or grass-yard, an indispensable requisite in the puppies' kennel. The size must be regulated according to the waste land at the end of the building; but the longer it is, the better. At the farther end of the grass-court is a hospital for such young hounds as are distempered, so contrived as to be remote from the other kennels, and, at the same time, within an easy distance of the boiling-house, whence it is apparently approached by an outside door, through which the feeder can constantly pass to attend to the sick hounds without disturbing the healthy lots. Although this lodging-room is warmed by the chimneys of the boiling-house, it must also be well ventilated by two windows, to which shutters must be attached; ventilation and good air being quite as necessary to the cure of distemper as warmth."

KENNEL LAMENESS.

We now proceed to a most important and ill-understood subject —the nature and treatment of *kennel lameness.* It is a subject that nearly concerns the sportsman, and on which there are several and the most contrary opinions.

This is a kind of lameness connected with, or attributable to, the kennel. According to the early opinion of Mr. Asheton Smith, who is a good authority, it was referable to some peculiarity in the breed or management of the hounds; but, agreeably to a later opinion, it is dependent on situation and subsoil, and may be aggravated or increased by circumstances over which we have no control. Some kennels are in low and damp situations, yet the hounds are free from all complaint; and others, with the stanchest dogs and under the best management, are continually sinking under kennel lameness.

Mr. R. T. Vyner was one of the first who scientifically treated on this point, and taught us that *clay is not by any means an objectionable soil to build a kennel upon,* although so many pseudo-sportsmen are frightened by the very name of it.

He enters at once into his subject. "I am thoroughly convinced," says he, "from my own experience, and, I may add, my own suffering, that the disease of kennel lameness arises only from one cause, and that is an injudicious and unfortunate selection of the spot for building. The kennel is generally built on a sand-bed, or on a sandstone rock, while the healthiest grounds in England are on a stiff clay, and they are the healthiest because they are the least porous. Although this may be contrary to the opinion and prejudice of the majority of sportsmen, it is a fact that cannot be contradicted.

"Through a light and friable soil, such as sand and sandstone, a vapour, more or less dense, is continually exhaling and causing a perpetual damp, which produces that fearful rheumatism which goes by the name of kennel lameness, while the kennels that are built on a clay soil, a soil of an impervious nature, are invariably healthy.

"I could," he adds, "enumerate twenty kennels to prove the effect—the invariable effect—of the existence of the disease on the one part, and of the healthiness of the situation on the other. I turn particularly to her Majesty's kennel at Ascot, the arches of which were laid under the very foundation stones, and yet little or no amendment has ever taken place in the healthiness and comfort of the dogs. It is necessary to select a sound and healthy situation when about to erect a kennel, and that sound and healthy situation can be met with alone on a strong impervious clay soil. We must have no fluid oozing through the walls or the floor of the kennel, and producing damp and unhealthy vapours, such as we find in the sandbed." With regard to this there can be no error.

Nimrod, in his excellent treatise on Kennel Lameness, asks, whether it does not appear that this disease is on the increase. He asks, "How is it that neither Beckford nor Somerville says one word that clearly applies to the disease; and no one, however learned he might be in canine pathology, has been able clearly to define the disease, much less to discover a remedy for it?"

All that Mr. Blaine says on the matter amounts only to this:—

"The healthiness of the situation on which any kennel is to be built, is an important consideration. It is essential that it should be both dry and airy, and it should also be warm. A damp kennel produces rheumatism in dogs, which shows itself sometimes by weakness in the loins, but more frequently by lameness in the shoulders, known under the name of kennel lameness."

Mr. Blaine illustrates this by reference to his own experience. ' There is no disease, with the exception of distemper and mange, to which dogs are so liable as to a rheumatic affection of some part of the body. It presents almost as many varieties in the dog as it does in man; and it has some peculiarities observable in the dog only. Rheumatism never exists in a dog without affecting the bowels. There will be inflammation or painful torpor through the whole of the intestinal canal. It is only in some peculiar districts that this occurs; it pervades certain kennels only; and but until lately there has been little or almost no explanation of the cause of the evil."[a]

Nimrod took a most important view of the matter, and to him the sporting world is much indebted. "How is it," he asks, "that, in our younger days, we never heard of kennel lameness, or, indeed, of hounds being lame at all, unless from accident, or becoming shaken and infirm from not having been composed of that iron-bound material which the labours of a greyhound or a hound require? How is it, that, in our younger days, masters of hounds began the season with 50 or 60 couples, and, bating the casualties, left off at the end of it equally strong in their kennels, and able, perhaps, to make a valuable draft; whereas we now hear of one-half of the dogs in certain localities being disabled by disease, and some masters of hounds compelled to be stopped in their work until their kennels are replenished."

Washing hounds when they come home after work must be injurious to them, although it has almost become the fashion of modern times. If they are not washed at all, and we believe it to be unnecessary, yet the kennels in which lameness has appeared should be strictly avoided. It should be on the day following and not in the evening of a hunting-day that washing should take place.

Mr. Hodgson told Nimrod, that the Quorn Pack never had a case of kennel lameness until his late huntsman took to washing his hounds after hunting, and then he often had four or five couples ill from this cause. He deprecated even their access to water in the evening after hunting, and we believe that he was quite right in so doing.

The tongue of the dog, with the aid of clean straw, is his best

---

[a] Blaine on the Diseases of the Dog, p. 140.

and safest instrument in cleansing his person; and, if he can be brought to his kennel with tolerably clean feet, as Mr. Foljambe enables him to be brought, he will never be long before he is comfortable in his bed, after his belly is filled.

There is another mode, as a preventive of kennel lameness, which we have the best authority for saying deserves particular attention, and that is, the frequently turning hounds off their benches during the day, even if it were to the extent of every two hours throughout the entire day. We do not mean to deny the existence of a disease, which, being produced in the kennel, is properly termed kennel lameness. Some kennels are, no doubt, more unhealthy and prone to engender rheumatic affections than others; but, by proper management, and avoiding as much as possible all exciting causes, their effects may, at least, be very much lessened, if not entirely obviated.

LORD FITZHARDINGE'S MANAGEMENT.

Lord Fitzhardinge's opinion of the situation of the kennel and the management of the hounds, as given in the New Sporting Magazine, is somewhat different from that which has been just given. The following is the substance of it:[b]

He states that the kennel should be built on a dry and warm situation. Of this there can be no doubt: the comfort and almost the existence of the dog depend upon it. To this he adds that it must not be placed on a gravelly or porous soil, over which vapours more or less dense are frequently or continually travelling, and thus causing a destructive exhalation over the whole of the building. There must be no fluid oozing through the walls or the floor of the kennel, and producing damp and unhealthy vapours. When we have not a deep supersoil of clay, one or two layers of bricks or of stone may line the floor, and then, not even the most subtile vapour can penetrate through the floor. A clean bed of straw should be allowed every second day, or oftener when the weather is wet. The lodging-houses should be ceiled, and there should be shutters to the windows. A thatched roof is preferable to tiles, being warmer in winter and cooler in summer.

Stoves in the kennels are not necessary: probably they are best avoided; for, if dogs are accustomed to any considerable degree of artificial heat, they are more easily chilled by a long exposure to cold. Their teeth and the setting-up of their backs will confirm this.

Hounds, when they feel cold, naturally seek each other for warmth, and they may be seen lying upon the straw and licking

[a] See Hints to Young Masters of Fox-Hounds—New Sport. Mag., vol. viii. p. 174—290.

each other; and that is by far the most wholesome way of procuring comfort and warmth.

On returning from hunting, their feet should be washed with some warm fluid, and especially the eyes should be examined, and their food got ready for them as soon as possible. The feeding in the morning should be an hour, or an hour and a half, before they start for the field.

It is truly observed by the noble writer to whom we have referred, that there is no part of an establishment of this kind that merits more attention than the boiling and feeding house. The hounds cannot perform their work well unless judiciously fed. Each hound requires particular and constitutional care. No more than five of them should be let in to feed together, and often not more than one or two. The feeder should have each hound under his immediate observation, or they may get too much or too little of the food.

Some hounds cannot run if they carry much flesh; others are all the better for having plenty about them. The boilers should be of iron, two in number,—one for meal and the smaller one for flesh. The large boiler should render it necessary to be used not more than once in four days or a week. The food should be stirred for two hours, then transferred to flat coolers, until sufficiently gelatinous to be cut with a kind of spade. By the admixture of some portion of soups it may be brought to any thickness requisite. The flesh to be mixed with it should be cut very small, that the greedy hounds may not be able to obtain more than their share. Four bushels and a half of genuine old oatmeal should be boiled with a hundred gallons of water. The flesh should be boiled every second or third day. Too great a proportion of soup would render the mixture of a heating nature.

Mr. Delmé Radcliffe very truly observes that the feeding of hounds, as regards their condition, is one of the most essential proofs of a huntsman's skill in the management of the kennel. To preserve that even state of condition throughout the pack which is so desirable, he must be well acquainted with the appetite of every hound; for some will feed with a voracity scarcely credible, and others will require every kind of enticement to induce them to feed.

Mr. Meynell found that the use of dry unboiled oatmeal succeeded better than any other thing he had tried with delicate hounds. When once induced to take it, they would eat it greedily, and it seemed to be far more heartening than most kinds of aliment. Other hounds of delicate constitution might be tempted with a little additional flesh, and with the thickest and best of the trough, but they required to be watched, and often to be coaxed to eat.

The dog possesses the power of struggling against want of food for an almost incredible period. One of these animals, six years old, was missing three-and-twenty days; at length some children wandering in a distant wood thought that they frequently heard the baying of a dog. The master was told of it, and at the bottom of an old quarry, sixty feet deep, and the mouth of which he had almost closed by his vain attempts to escape, the voice of the poor fellow was recognised. With much difficulty he was extricated, and found in a state of emaciation; his body cold as ice and his thirst inextinguishable, and he scarcely able to move. They gave him at intervals small portions of bread soaked in milk and water. Two days afterwards he was able to follow his master a short distance.

This occurrence is mentioned by M. Pinguin as a proof that neither hunger nor thirst could produce rabies. Messrs. Majendie and F. Cousins have carried their observations to the extent of forty days,—a disgraceful period.[a]

MANAGEMENT OF THE PACK.

Sixty-five couple of hounds in full work will consume the carcases of three horses in one week, or five in a fortnight. The annual consumption of meal will be somewhat more than two tons per month.

In feeding, the light eaters should be let in first, and a little extra flesh distributed on the surface of the food, in order to coax those that are most shy. Some hounds cannot be kept to their work unless fed two or three times a day; while others must not be allowed more than six or seven laps, or they would get too much.

In summer an extra cow or two will be of advantage in the dairy; for the milk, after it has been skimmed, may be used instead of flesh. There must always be a little flesh in hand for the sick, for bitches with their whelps, and for the entry of young hounds.[b] About Christmas is the time to arrange the breeding establishment. The number of puppies produced is usually from five to eight or nine; but, in one strange case, eighteen of them made their appearance. The constitution and other appearances in the dam, will decide the number to be preserved. When the whelps are sufficiently grown to run about, they should be placed in a warm situation, with plenty of fresh grass, and a sufficient quantity of clean, but not too stimulating, food. They should then be marked according to their respective letters, that they may be always recognised. When the time comes, the ears of the dog

[a] Traité de la Folie des Animaux, tom. ii. 39.

[b] Mr. D. Radcliffe.

should be rounded; the size of the ear and of the head guiding the rounding-iron.

This being passed, the master of the pack takes care that his treatment shall be joyous and playful; encouragement is always with him the word. The dog should be taught the nature of the fault before he is corrected: no animal is more grateful for kindness than a hound; the peculiarities of his temper will soon be learned, and when he begins to love his master, he will mind, from his natural and acquired affection, a word or a frown from him more than the blows of all the whips that were ever put into the hands of the keepers.

The distemper having passed, and the young hounds being in good health, they should be walked out every day, and taught to follow the horse, with a keeper who is selected as a kind and quiet person, and will bear their occasionally entangling themselves in their couples. They are then taken to the public roads, and there exercised, and checked from riot, but with as little severity as possible; a frequent and free use of the whip never being allowed. No animals take their character from their master so much as the hounds do from theirs. If he is wild, or noisy, or nervous, so will his hounds be; if he is steady and quick, the pack will be the same. The whip should never be applied but for some immediate and decided fault. A rate given at an improper time does more harm than good: it disgusts the honest hound, it shies and prevents from hunting the timid one, and it is treated with contempt by those of another character who may at some future time deserve it. It formerly was the custom, and still is too much so, when a hound *has hung on a hare*, to catch him when he comes up, and flog him. The consequence of this is, that he takes good care the next time he indulges in a fault not to come out of cover at all.

We will conclude this part of our subject by a short account of the splendid kennel at Goodwood, for which we are indebted to Lord W. Lennox, with the kind permission of the Duke of Richmond. It is described as one of the most complete establishments of the kind in England. The original establishment of this building, although a little faulty, possesses considerable interest from its errors being corrected by the third Duke of Richmond, a man who is acknowledged to have been one of the most popular public characters of the day, and who in more private life extended his patronage to all that was truly honourable. It was to the Duke's support of native talent that we may trace the origin of the present Royal Academy. In 1758, the Duke of Richmond displayed, at his residence in Whitehall, a large collection of original plaster casts, taken from the finest statues and busts of the ancient sculptors. Every artist was freely admitted to this exhibition and, for the further encouragement of talent, he bestowed two medals annually on such as had exhibited the best models.

We have thus digressed in order to give a slight sketch of the nobleman by whom this kennel was built, and we do not think that we can do better than lay before our readers the original account of it.

Early in life the Duke built what was not then common, a tennis-court, and what was more uncommon, a dog-kennel, which cost him above 6000*l*. The Duke was his own architect, assisted by, and under the guidance of, Mr. Wyatt; he dug his own flints, burnt his own lime, and conducted the wood-work in his own shops. The result of his labours was the noble building of which a plan is here given.

The dog-kennel is a grand object when viewed from Goodwood. The front is handsome, the ground well raised about it, and the general effect good; the open court in the centre adds materially to the noble appearance of the building.

The entrance to the kennel is delineated in the centre with a flight of stairs leading above. The huntsman's rooms, four in number, first present themselves, and are marked in the plan before us by the letter C; each of them is fifteen feet four inches, by fourteen feet six inches.

At each end of the side towards the court is one of the feeding-rooms, twenty-nine feet by fourteen feet four inches, and nobly constructed rooms they are; they are designated by the letters B. At the back of the feeding-rooms, are one set of the lodging-rooms, from thirty-five feet six inches, to fourteen feet four inches, and marked by the letters A, and at either extremity is another lodging-room, thirty-two feet six inches in length, and fourteen feet six inches in width: this is also marked by the letter A.

Coming into the court we find the store-room twenty-four feet by fourteen and a half, marked by the letter D, and the stable, of the same dimensions, by the letter E.

At the top of the buildings are openings for the admission of cold air, and stoves to warm the air when too cold. There are plentiful supplies of water from tanks holding 10,000 gallons; so that there is no inconvenience from the smell, and the whole can at any time be drained, and not be rendered altogether useless.

Round the whole building is a pavement five feet wide; airy yards and places for breeding, &c., making part of each wing. For the huntsman and whipper-in there are sleeping-rooms, and a neat parlour or kitchen.

Soon after the kennel was erected, it would contain two packs of hounds.

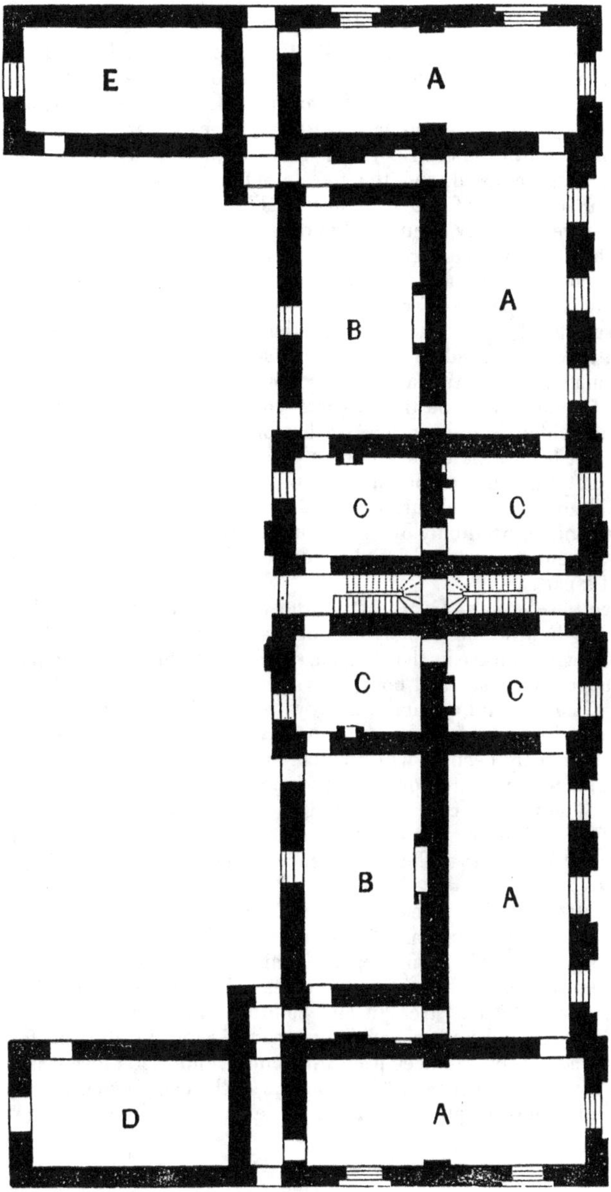

THE KENNEL AT GOODWOOD.

THE STAG-HOUND.

The largest of the English hounds that has been lately used, is devoted, as his name implies, to the chase of the deer. He is taller than the fox-hound, and with far more delicate scent, but he is not so speedy. He answers better than any other to the description given of the old English hound, so much valued when the country, less enclosed, and the forests, numerous and extensive, were the harbours of the wild deer. The deer-hound and the harrier were for many centuries the only hunting-dogs. The fox-hound has been much more recently bred.

The most tyrannic and cruel laws were enforced for the preservation of this species of game, and the life of the deer, except when sacrificed in the chase, and by those who were privileged to join in it, was guarded with even more strictness than the life of the human being. When, however, the country became more generally cultivated, and the stag was confined to enclosed parks, and was seldom sought in his lair, but brought into the field, and turned out before the dogs, so much interest was taken from the affair, that this species of hunting grew out of fashion, and was confined to the neighbourhood of the scattered forests that remained, and enjoyed only by royalty and a few noblemen, of whose establishment a kennel of deer-hounds had, from time immemorial, formed a part.

Since the death of George III., who was much attached to this sport, stag-hunting has rapidly declined, and the principal pleasure seems now to consist in the concourse of people brought together to an appointed place and hour, to witness the turning out of the deer. There is still maintained a royal establishment for the continuance of this noble sport; but, unless better supported than it has of late years been, it will gradually decline.

The stag-hounds are now a part of the regular Crown establishment. The royal kennel is situated upon Ascot Heath, about six miles from Windsor. At the distance of a mile from the kennel is Swinley Lodge, the official residence of the Master of the Stag-hounds.

The stag-hound is a beautiful animal. He is distinguished from the fox-hound by the apparent broadness and shortness of his head, his longer cheek, his straighter hock, his wider thigh and deeper chest, and better feathered and more beautifully arched tail. His appearance indicates strength and stoutness, in which indeed he is unequalled, and he has sufficient speed to render it difficult for the best horses long to keep pace with him; while, as is necessary, when the distance between the footmarks of the deer is considered, his scent is most exquisite. He is far seldomer at fault than any other hound except the blood-hound, and rarely fails of running down his game.

Of the stoutness of this dog, the following anecdotes will be a sufficient illustration. A deer, in the spring of 1822, was turned out before the Earl of Derby's hounds at Hayes Common. The chase was continued nearly four hours without a check, when, being almost run down, the animal took refuge in some outhouses near Speldhurst in Kent, more than forty miles across the country, and having actually run more than fifty miles. Nearly twenty horses died in the field, or in consequence of the severity of the chase.

A stag was turned out at Wingfield Park, in Northumberland. The whole pack, with the exception of two hounds, was, after a long run, thrown out. The stag returned to his accustomed haunt, and, as his last effort, leaped the wall of the park, and lay down and died. One of the hounds, unable to clear the wall, fell and expired, and the other was found dead at a little distance. They had run about forty miles.

When the stag first hears the cry of the hounds, he runs with the swiftness of the wind, and continues to run as long as any sound of his pursuers can be distinguished. That having ceased, he pauses and looks carefully around him; but before he can determine what course to pursue, the cry of the pack again forces itself upon his attention. Once more he darts away, and after a while again pauses. His strength perhaps begins to fail, and he has recourse to stratagem in order to escape. He practises the doubling and the crossing of the fox or the hare. This being useless, he attempts to escape by plunging into some lake or river that happens to lie in his way, and when, at last, every attempt to escape proves abortive, he boldly faces his pursuers, and attacks the first dog or man who approaches him.[a]

---

[a] The late Lord Orford reduced four stags to so perfect a degree of submission, that, in his short excursions, he used to drive them in a phaeton made for the purpose. He was one day exercising his singular and beautiful steeds in the neighbourhood of Newmarket, when their ears were saluted with the unwelcome cry of a pack of hounds, which, crossing the road in their rear, had caught the scent, and leaving their original object of pursuit, were now in rapid chase of the frightened stags. In vain his grooms exerted themselves to the utmost, the terrified animals bounded away with the swiftness of lightning, and entered Newmarket at full speed. They made immediately for the Ram Inn, to which his lordship was in the habit of driving, and, having fortunately entered the yard without any accident, the stable-keepers huddled his lordship, the phaeton, and the deer into a large barn, just in time to save them from the hounds, who came into the yard in full cry a few seconds afterwards. —Annals of Sporting, vol. iii. 1823.

THE SOUTHERN HOUND.

There used to be in the south of Devon a pack or cry of the genuine old English or southern hounds. There is some reason to believe that this was the original stock of the island, or of this part of the island, and that this hound was used by the ancient Britons in the chase of the larger kinds of game with which the country formerly abounded. Its distinguishing characters are its size and general heavy appearance; its great length of body, deep chest, and ears remarkably large and pendulous. The tones of its voice were peculiarly deep. It answered the description of Shakspeare,—

> "So flewed, so sanded; and their heads are hung
> With ears that sweep away the morning dew;
> Crook-knee'd, and dew-lapp'd, like Thessalian bulls;
> Slow in pursuit, but match'd in mouth like bells,
> Each under each."

It was the slowness of the breed which occasioned its disuse. Several of them, however, remained not long ago at a village called Aveton Gifford, in Devonshire, in the neighbourhood of which some of the most opulent of the farmers used to keep two or three dogs each. When fox-hunting had assumed somewhat of its modern form, the chase was followed by a slow heavy hound, whose excellent olfactory organs enabled him to carry on the scent a considerable time after the fox-hound passed, and also over grassy fallows, and hard roads, and other places, where the modern high-bred fox-hound would not be able to recognise it. Hence the chase continued for double the duration which it does at present, and hence may be seen the reason why the old English hunter, so celebrated in former days and so great a favourite among sportsmen of the old school, was enabled to perform those feats which were exultingly bruited in his praise. The fact is, that the hounds and the horse were well matched. If the latter possessed not the speed of the Meltonian hunter, the hounds were equally slow and stanch.

THE BLOOD-HOUND.

This dog does not materially differ in appearance from the old deer-hound of a larger size, trained to hunt the human being instead of the quadruped. If once put on the track of a supposed robber, he would unerringly follow him to his retreat, although at the distance of many a mile. Such a breed was necessary when neither the private individual nor the government had other means to detect the offender. Generally speaking, however, the blood-hound of former days would not injure the culprit that did not attempt to escape, but would lie down quietly and give notice by a loud and peculiar howl what kind of prey he had found. Some, however, of a savage disposition, or trained to unnatural ferocity, would tear to pieces the hunted wretch, if timely rescue did not arrive.

Hounds of every kind, both great and small, may be broken in to follow any particular scent, and especially when they are feelingly convinced that they are not to hunt any other. This is the case with the blood-hound. He is destined to one particular object of pursuit, and a total stranger with regard to every other.

In the border country between England and Scotland, and until the union of the two kingdoms, these dogs were absolutely necessary for the preservation of property, and the detection of robbery and murder. A tax was levied on the inhabitants for the maintenance of a certain number of blood-hounds. When, however, the civic government had sufficient power to detect and punish crime, this dangerous breed of hounds fell into disuse and was systematically discouraged. It, nevertheless, at the present day, is often bred by the rangers in large forests or parks to track the deer-stealer, but oftener to find the wounded deer.

The blood-hound is taller and better formed than the deer-hound. It has large and deep ears, the forehead broad and the muzzle narrow. The expression of the countenance is mild and pleasing, when the dog is not excited; but, when he is following the robber, his ferocity becomes truly alarming.

The Thrapstone Association lately trained a blood-hound for the detection of sheepstealers. In order to prove the utility of this dog, a person whom he had not seen was ordered to run as far and as fast as his strength would permit. An hour afterwards the hound was brought out. He was placed on the spot whence the man had started. He almost immediately detected the scent and broke away, and, after a chase of an hour and a half, found him concealed in a tree, fifteen miles distant.

Mr. John Lawrence says, that a servant, discharged by a sporting country gentleman, broke into his stables by night, and cut off the ears and tail of a favourite hunter. As soon as it was discovered, a blood-hound was brought into the stable, who at once detected the scent of the miscreant, and traced it more than twenty miles. He then stopped at a door, whence no power could move him. Being at length admitted, he ran to the top of the house, and, bursting open the door of a garret, found the object that he sought in bed, and would have torn him to pieces, had not the huntsman, who had followed him on a fleet horse, rushed up after him.

Somerville thus describes the use to which he was generally put, in pursuit of the robber —

"Soon the sagacious brute, his curling tail
Flourished in air, low bending, plies around
His busy nose, the steaming vapour snuffs
Inquisitive, nor leaves one turf untried,
Till, conscious of the recent stains, his heart
Beats quick. His snuffing nose, his active tail,
Attest his joy. Then, with deep opening mouth,
That makes the welkin tremble, he proclaims
Th' audacious felon. Foot by foot he marks
His winding way. Over the watery ford,
Dry sandy heaths, and stony barren hills,
Unerring he pursues, till at the cot
Arrived, and, seizing by his guilty throat
The caitiff vile, redeems the captive prey."

THE SETTER

is evidently the large spaniel improved to his peculiar size and beauty, and taught another way of marking his game, viz., by *setting* or crouching. If the form of the dog were not sufficiently satisfactory on this point, we might have recourse to history for information on it. Mr. Daniel, in his Rural Sports, has preserved a document, dated in the year 1685, in which a yeoman binds himself for the sum of ten shillings, fully and effectually to teach a spaniel to *sit* partridges and pheasants.

[As this old document may prove interesting to the curious, we take the liberty of inserting it, knowing full well, that Mr. Daniel's work is quite rare in this country, and copies of it are not easily obtained even in England.

Ribbesford, Oct. 7, 1685.

"I, John Harris, of Willdon, in the parish of Hastlebury, in the county of Worcester, yeoman, for and in consideration of ten shillings of lawful English money this day received of Henry Herbert of Ribbesford, in the said county, Esqr., and of thirty shillings more of like money by him promised to be hereafter pay'd me, do hereby covenant and promise to and with the said Henry Herbert, his exōrs and admōrs, that I will, from the day of the date hereof, untill the first day of March next, well and sufficiently mayntayne and keepe a Spanile Bitch named Quand, this day delivered into my custody by the said Henry Herbert, and will, before the first day of March next, fully and effectually traine up and teach the said Bitch to sitt Partridges, Pheasants, and other game, as well and exactly as the best sitting Doggers usually sett the same. And the said bitch, so trayned and taught, shall and will delivere to the said Henry Herbert, or whom he shall appoint to receive her, att his house in Ribbesford aforesaid, on the first day of March next. And if at anytime after the said Bitch shall, for want of use or practice, or ōrwise, forgett to sett Game as aforesaid, I will, at my costes and charges, maynetayne her for a month, or longer, as often as need shall require, to trayne up and teach her to sett Game as aforesaid, and shall and will, fully and effectually, teach her to sett Game as well and exactly as is above mentyon'd.

Witness my hand and seal the day and year first above written,

John Harris, his ⋈ mark.

Sealed and delivered in presence of

H. Payne, his ⋈ mark."

L.]

The first person, however, who systematically broke-in setting dogs, is supposed to have been Dudley Duke of Northumberland, in 1335.

A singular dog-cause was tried in Westminster, in July, 1822. At a previous trial it was determined that the mere possession of a dog, generally used for destroying game, was sufficient proof of its being actually so used. Mr. Justice Best, however, determined that a man might be a breeder of such dogs without using them as game-dogs; and Mr. Justice Bailey thought that if a game-dog was kept in a yard, chained up by day, and let loose at night, and, being so trained as to guard the premises, he was to be considered as a yard-dog, and not as a game-dog.

The setter is used for the same purpose as the pointer, and there is great difference of opinion with regard to their relative value as sporting-dogs. Setters are not so numerous; and they are dearer, and with great difficulty obtained pure. It was long the fashion to cross and mix them with the pointer, by which no benefit was obtained, but the beauty of the dog materially impaired; many Irish sportsmen, however, were exceedingly careful to preserve the breed pure. Nothing of the pointer can be traced in them, and they are useful and beautiful dogs, altogether different in appearance from either the English or Scotch setter. The Irish sportsmen are, perhaps, a little too much prejudiced with regard to particular colours. Their dogs are either very red, or red and white, or lemon-coloured, or white, patched with deep chestnut; and it was necessary for them to have a black nose, and a black roof to the mouth. This peculiar dye is supposed to be as necessary to a good and genuine Irish setter as is the palate of a Blenheim spaniel to the purity of his breed. A true Irish setter will obtain a higher price than either an English or Scotch one. Fifty guineas constituted no unusual price for a brace of them, and even two hundred guineas have been given. It is, nevertheless, doubtful whether they do in reality so much exceed the other breeds, and whether, although stout and hard-working dogs, and

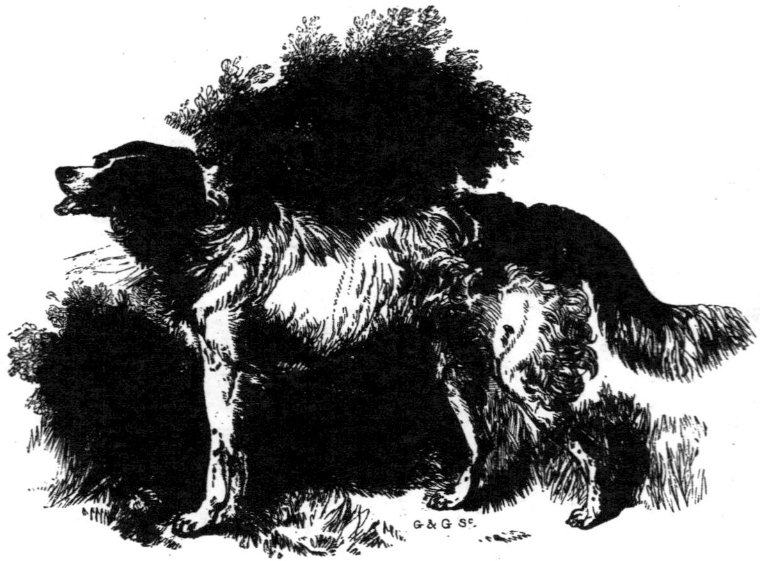

THE SETTER.

with excellent scent, they are not somewhat too headstrong and unruly.

The setter is more active than the pointer. He has greater spirit and strength. He will better stand continued hard work He will generally take the water when necessary, and, retaining the character of the breed, is more companionable and attached. He loves his master for himself, and not, like the pointer, merely for the pleasure he shares with him. His somewhat inferior scent, however, makes him a little too apt to run into his game, and he occasionally has a will of his own. He requires good breaking, and plenty of work: but that breaking must be of a peculiar character: it must not partake of the severity which too often accompanies, and unnecessarily so, the tuition of the pointer. He has more animal spirit than the pointer, but he has not so much patient courage; and the chastisement, sometimes unnecessary and cruel, but leaving the pointer perfect in his work, and eager for it too, would make the setter disgusted with it, and leave him a mere *blinker*. It is difficult, however, always to decide the claim of superiority between these dogs. He that has a good one of either breed may be content, but the lineage of that dog must be pure. The setter, with much of the pointer in him, loses something in activity and endurance; and the pointer, crossed with the setter, may have a degree of wildness and obstinacy, not a little annoying to his owner. The setter may be preferable when the ground is hard and rough; for he does not soon become foot-sore. He may even answer the purpose of a springer for pheasants and woodcocks, and may be valuable in recovering a wounded bird. His scent may frequently be superior to that of the pointer, and sufficiently accurate to distinguish, better than the pointer, when the game is sprung; but the steadiness and obedience of the pointer will generally give him the preference, especially in a fair and tolerably smooth country. At the beginning of a season, and when the weather is hot, the pointer will have a decided advantage.

[We beg leave to finish this history of the setter by referring to our essay on this dog, published in vol. xv, No. 47, of the "New York Spirit of the Times," or as lately transferred to the pages of an interesting and valuable sporting work, about being published by our esteemed friend, Wm. A. Porter, and from which we now abstract our remarks upon

THE MERITS OF THE SETTER COMPARED WITH THOSE OF THE POINTER.

It cannot for a moment be doubted that the setter has superior advantages to the pointer, for hunting over our uncleared country, although the pointer has many qualities that recommend him to the sportsman, that the setter does not possess. In the first place, the extreme hardiness and swiftness of foot, natural to the setter, enables him to get over much more ground than the pointer, in the same space of time. Their feet also, being more hard and firm, are not so liable to become sore from contact with our frozen ground. The ball pads being well protected by the spaniel toe-tufts, are less likely to be wounded by the thorns and burs with which our woods are crowded during the winter season. His natural enthusiasm for hunting, coupled with his superior physical powers, enables him to stand much more work than the pointer, and oftentimes he appears quite fresh upon a long continued hunt, when the other will be found drooping and inattentive.

The long, thick fur of the setter, enables him to wend his way through briary thickets without injury to himself, when a similar attempt on the part of a pointer, would result in his ears, tail, and body being lacerated and streaming with blood.

On the other hand, the pointer is superior to the setter in retaining his acquired powers for hunting, and not being naturally enthusiastic in pursuit of game, he is more easily broken and kept in proper subjection.

The setter frequently requires a partial rebreaking at the commencement of each season, in his younger days, owing to the natural eagerness with which he resumes the sport. The necessity of this, however, diminishes with age, as the character and habits of the dog become more settled, and then we may take them into the field, with a perfect assurance of their behaving quite as well on the first hunt of the season, as the stanchest pointer would.

The extreme caution, and mechanical powers of the pointer in the field, is a barrier to his flushing the birds, as is often witnessed in the precipitate running of the setter, who winds the game and frequently overruns it in his great anxiety to come up with it. But this occasional fault on the part of the setter, may be counterbalanced by the larger quantity of game that he usually finds in a day's hunt, owing to his enthusiasm and swiftness of foot. Setters require much more water while hunting than the pointer, owing to their thick covering of fur, encouraging a greater amount of insensible perspiration to fly off than the thin and short dress of the pointer. Consequently they are better calculated to hunt in the coldest seasons than early in our falls, which are frequently quite dry and warm.

A striking instance of this fact came under our own immediate observation this fall, when shooting in a range of country thinly settled and uncommonly dry. The day being warm and the birds scarce, the dogs suffered greatly from thirst, in so much that a very fine setter of uncommon bottom, was forced to give up entirely, completely prostrated, foaming at the mouth in the most alarming manner, breathing heavily, and vomiting from time to time a thick frothy mucus.

His prostration of both muscular and nervous powers was so great, that he could neither smell nor take the slightest notice of a bird, although placed at his nose. He could barely manage to drag one leg after the other, stopping to rest every few moments, and we were fearful that we should be obliged to shoulder and carry him to a farm-house, a considerable distance off. However, he succeeded, with much difficulty, in reaching the well, where he greedily drank several pints of water administered to him with caution.

He recovered almost immediately, gave me a look of thanks, and was off to the fields in a few moments, where he soon found a fine covey of birds.

The pointer, his associate in the day's work, and a much less hardy dog, stood the hunt remarkably well, and seemed to suffer little or no inconvenience from the want of water. The setter has natural claims upon the sportsman and man generally, in his affectionate disposition and attachment to his master, and the many winning manners he exhibits towards those by whom he is caressed.

The pointer displays but little fondness for those by whom he is surrounded, and hunts equally as well for a stranger as his master.—L.]

Of the difference between the old English setter and the setters of the present day, we confess that we are ignorant, except that the first was the pure spaniel improved, and the latter the spaniel crossed too frequently with the pointer.

It must be acknowledged, that of companionableness, and disinterested attachment and gratitude, the pointer knows comparatively little. If he is a docile and obedient servant in the field, it is all we want. The setter is unquestionably his superior in every amiable quality. Mr. Blaine says, that a large setter, ill with the distemper, had been nursed by a lady more than three weeks. At length he became so ill as to be placed in a bed, where he remained a couple of days in a dying state. After a short absence, the lady, re-entering the room, observed him to fix his eyes attentively on her, and make an effort to crawl across the bed towards her. This he accomplished, evidently for the sole purpose of licking her hand, after which he immediately expired.

[Daniel Lambert celebrated for his enormous magnitude, weighing seven hundred and thirty-nine pounds, had a very superior breed of setters, which were publicly sold, at the following prices; after his death, which forcibly illustrates the immense value placed on this dog in England; whereas, many American sportsmen considers it a great hardship to be obliged to give thirty or forty dollars for a well-bred setter in this country.

	Guineas
Peg, a black Setter Bitch	41
Punch, a Setter Dog	26
Brush, do.	17
Bob, do.	20
Bell, do.	32
Bounce, do.	22
Sam, do.	26
Charlotte, a Pointer Bitch	22
Lucy, do.	12
	218

—L.]

THE POINTER.

The pointer is evidently descended from the hound.

[We beg leave to make the following extracts from our essay on this subject, published in No. 1, vol. xvi, of the "Spirit of the Times:"

The origin of the pointer, like that of the setter, is involved in much obscurity; he is of mixed blood, and no doubt largely indebted to both hound and spaniel for his distinct existence.

Many sportsmen are under the erroneous idea that the pointer is contemporary with, if not older than, the Setter. Such, however, is not the case; and we are led to believe that the Pointer is of quite modern origin; at all events, the production of a much later date than the spaniel.

Strut, in his "Sports and Pastimes," chap. 1, sects. xv. and xvi., mentions a MS. in the Cotton Library, originally written by William Twici, or Twety, Grand Huntsman to Edward II., who ascended the throne in 1307.

This manuscript contains the earliest treatise on hunting that the English possess, and enumerates the various kinds of game and different species of dogs then in existence, as also the modes of taking the former and using the latter.

After describing, in the usual minute manner, the specific employment of each dog, he finishes by stating:—"The spaniel was for use in hawking, hys crafte is for the perdrich or partridge, and the quail; and when taught to couch, he is very serviceable to the fowler, who takes these birds with nets."

No mention is made in this treatise of the pointer, and we naturally infer that he did not exist, or he would have been noticed in connexion with the spaniel, who, it appears, even at this early

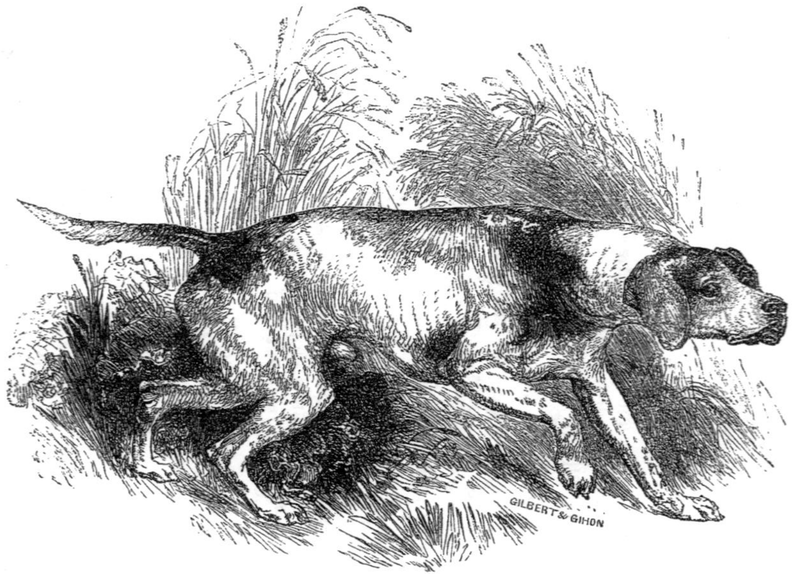

THE POINTER.

period, was taught to *couch* on and point out game to those employed in netting it.

In the early portion of the sixteenth century, we have another enumeration of dogs, *then* in use, in a book entitled—" A Jewel for Gentrie;" which, besides the dogs already descanted upon by Twici, we find added to the list, "bastards and mongrels, lemors, kenets, terrours, butchers' hounds, dung-hill dogs, trindel-tailed dogs, prychercard curs, and ladies' puppies." (Chap. 1st., Sec. XVI.—Strut.)

The pointer being the offspring of the fox-hound and spaniel, is consequently sprung from the two ancient races known as *Sagaces* and *Pugnaces* or *Bellicosi.* He certainly evinces a larger share of the *Bellicosi* blood than the setter, being ever ready for fight when assailed, while the latter generally exhibits a conciliatory disposition under the most trying circumstances.—L.]

It is the fox-hound searching for game by the scent, but more perfectly under the control of the sportsman, repressing his cry of joy when he finds his game, and his momentary pause, and gathering himself up in order to spring upon it artificially, converted into a steady and deliberate point. There still remains a strong resemblance, in countenance and in form, between the pointer and the fox-hound, except that the muzzle is shorter, and the ears smaller, and partly pendulous.

Seventy or eighty years ago, the breed of pointers was nearly white, or varied with liver-coloured spots; some, however, belonging to the Duke of Kingston, were perfectly black. This peculiarity of colour was supposed to be connected with exquisite perfection of scent. That is not the case with the present black pointers, who are not superior to any others.

Mr. Daniel relates an anecdote of one of his pointers. He had a dog that would always go round close to the hedges of a field before he would quarter his ground. He seemed to have observed that he most frequently found his game in the course of this circuit.[a]

[a] The author of the Field Book says that he saw an extremely small pointer, whose length, from the tip of the nose to the point of the tail, was only two feet and half an inch, the length of the head being six inches, and round the chest one foot and three inches. He was an exquisite miniature of the English pointer, being in all respects similar to him, except in his size. His colour was white, with dark liver-coloured patches on each side of the head, extending half down the neck. The ears, with some patches on the back, were also of the same colour, and numerous small dark-brown spots appeared over his whole body and legs.

This beautiful little animal had an exquisite sense of smell. Some of the same breed, and being the property of the Earl of Lauderdale, were broken-in and made excellent pointers, although, from their minute size, it could not be expected that they would be able to do much work. When intent upon any object, the dog assumed the same attitude as other pointers, holding up one of his feet. —The Field Book, p. 399.

Mr. Johnson gives the following characteristic sketches of the different breeds of pointer:—

THE SPANISH POINTER,

originally a native of Spain, was once considered to be a valuable dog. He stood higher on his legs, but was too large and heavy in his limbs, and had widely spread, ugly feet, exposing him to frequent lameness. His muzzle and head were large, corresponding with the acuteness of his smell. His ears were large and pendent, and his body ill-formed. He was naturally an ill-tempered dog, growling at the hand that would caress him, even although it were his master's. He stood steadily to his birds; but it was difficult to break him of chasing the hare. He was deficient in speed. His redeeming quality was his excellent scent, unequalled in any other kind of dog.

[To convince our readers of the value of this particular breed, we may mention the very singular sale of Colonel Thornton's dog Dash, who was purchased by Sir Richard Symons for one hundred and sixty pounds worth of champagne and burgundy, a hogshead of claret, and an elegant gun and another pointer, with a stipulation that if any accident befell the dog, he was to be returned to his former owner for fifty guineas. Dash unfortunately broke his leg, and in accordance with the agreement of sale was returned to the Colonel, who considered him a fortunate acquisition as a stallion to breed from. (See Blain or Daniel).—L.]

THE PORTUGUESE POINTER,

although with a slighter form than the Spanish one, is defective in the feet, often crooked in the legs, and of a quarrelsome disposition. He soon tires, and is much inclined to chase the hare. The tail is larger than that of the spaniel, and fully fringed.

THE FRENCH POINTER

is distinguished by a furrow between his nostrils, which materially interferes with the acuteness of smell. He is better formed and more active than either the Spanish or Portuguese dog, and capable of longer continued exertion; but he is apt to be quarrelsome, and is too fond of chasing the hare.

[We will close this account of the Pointer by transferring from the pages of the "Spirit of the Times" our remarks upon this particular breed.

The French variety, as described by English authors, is much smaller than either of the above breeds; and although possessed of great beauty, acute scent, and other qualifications that would render him valuable in their eyes, still is considered much inferior, not being able to cope with their dogs in hunting, owing to a want of physical power of endurance.

Youatt states, that he is distinguished by a furrow in his nose, which materially interferes with his acuteness of smell.

These accounts do not agree with the French writers, to whom, it is very true, the English should not look for any particular information respecting hunting or shooting. Nevertheless, all must admit that they are quite as capable of describing their particular breeds of animals as other nations; and, in fact, we might go farther, and say that they are much more competent to the task than English writers, judging from their extensive knowledge in comparative anatomy, and their long array of celebrated writers on natural history—the Cuviers, Buffon, &c.

Baudrillart, in his Dictionnaire des Chases, describes the Prench Pointer as having endurance and great industry, and of their being used oftentimes solely for *la grande chasse.* In the atlas of plates accompanying this interesting work, will be found two distinct and extremely correct drawings of the English Pointer, and also an engraving of the French variety, which latter, certainly, is represented as being equally, if not more muscular and hardy, than the English.

As for the furrow in the nose, as mentioned by Youatt, no reference is made to it in connection with this species, and in the engraving the nose is square. But in describing another variety, known in France as coming from Spain, *Baudrillart* states, that they are vulgarly called "*a'deux nez, parceque ce chien a les narines separées par une gouttiere.*"

As for Mr. Youatt's declaration in reference to the furrow in the nose "*materially interfering with the acuteness of smell,*" I cannot understand how, or on what principle of reasoning, this slight deviation from nature should affect the properties of the olfactory apparatus. That these furrow-nosed dogs are inferior to the English in scenting powers, as stated by Mr. Youatt, we do not question; but that their deficiency depends upon this furrow, remains to be proved.

This furrow in the nose is merely a deformity, and like many others in various breeds of animals, was solely the result of accident in the first place; and as we often see, even in the human species, the deformities and infirmities of our ancestors entailed upon their progeny, so has this '*cut in the nose*' been so extensively inherited by succeeding generations, that it has now become a distinctive mark of a whole class of dogs.

The French Pointer, as known in this country, is a beautiful, well-shaped, compact, square-nosed dog; not so long or high as the English, but extremely well built, full-chested, large head pendent ears, projecting eyes, large feet, and thickish tail.

His colour, seldom white, but generally intermingled with small spots of brown or chocolate over the body, and more particularly over the head and ears. Such a dog is in the possession of the writer, who knows nothing of his ancestry; but is convinced from those he saw in France, that they must have been imported from that country.

The English Pointer will now claim more particularly our attention. It is quite useless to go into a general description of an animal of whom we have already said much, and with whom we are all familiar; but we will endeavour to mention the most striking points of the species, which marks can be referred to as guides in the purchase of a dog.

It is a difficult matter to put on paper, in a manner satisfactory either to the reader or writer, the peculiarities of any animal, whereby he may be judged pure or mixed. However, there are, generally, some few points in each species, that can be selected as proofs of their genuineness and ability to perform certain actions peculiar to the race.

But, after all, more reliance must be placed upon the good faith of the seller, or the previous knowledge of the strain from which the purchaser selects—and what is better than either, from actual observation in the field; all of which precautions may, nevertheless, prove abortive, and our dog be worthless.

As regards the size of the English Pointer, we may say, that he averages in length about 3 feet from the tip of the muzzle to the base of the tail, and from 22 to 26 inches high. His head not bulky nor too narrow, the frontal sinuses largely developed.

The muzzle long and rather tapering, the nostrils large and well open, the ear slightly erect, not over long, and the tip triangular; if too pendent, large and rounded at the tip, there is too much of the hound present. The eyes lively, but not too prominent; the neck rather long and not over thick, the chest broad, the limbs large and muscular; the paws strong, hard and wide. The body and loins thin, rather than bulky, the hind quarters broad, and the limbs in the same proportion with the fore members; the tail long and tapering.—L.]

THE RUSSIAN POINTER

is a rough, ill-tempered animal, with too much tendency to stupidity, and often annoyed by vermin. He runs awkwardly, with his nose near the ground, and frequently springs his game. He also has the cloven or divided nose.

THE EARLY TRAINING OF THE DOG.

The education of these dogs should commence at an early period, whether conducted by the breeder or the sportsman; and the first lesson—that on which the value of the animal, and the pleasure of its owner, will much depend—is a habit of subjection on the part of the dog, and kindness on the part of the master. This is a *sine quâ non.* The dog must recognise in his owner a friend and a benefactor. This will soon establish in the mind of the quadruped a feeling of gratitude, and a desire to please. All this is natural to the dog, if he is encouraged by the master, and then the process of breaking-in may commence in good earnest.

No long time probably passes ere the dog commits some little fault. He is careless, or obstinate, or cross. The owner puts on a serious countenance, he holds up his finger, or shakes his head, or produces the whip, and threatens to use it. Perhaps the infliction of a blow, that breaks no bones, occasionally follows. In the majority of cases nothing more is required. The dog succumbs; he asks to be forgiven; or, if he has been self-willed, he may be speedily corrected without any serious punishment.

A writer, under the signature of "Soho," in The New Sporting Magazine for 1833, gives an interesting account of the schooling of the pointer or setter, thus commenced. A short abstract from it may not be unacceptable:—

"The first lesson inculcated is that of passive obedience, and this enforced by the infliction of severity as little as the case will admit. We will suppose the dog to be a setter. He is taken into the garden or into a field, and a strong cord, about eighteen or twenty yards long, is tied to his collar. The sportsman calls the dog to him, looks earnestly at him, gently presses him to the ground, and several times, with a loud, but not an angry voice, says, 'Down!' or 'Down charge!' The dog knows not the meaning of this, and struggles to get up; but, as often as he struggles, the cry of 'Down charge!' is repeated, and the pressure is continued or increased.

"This is repeated a longer or shorter time, until the dog, finding that no harm is meant, quietly submits. He is then permitted to rise; he is patted and caressed, and some food is given to him. The command to rise is also introduced by the terms 'Hie up!' A little afterwards the same process is repeated, and he struggles less, or perhaps ceases altogether to struggle.

"The person whose circumstances permit him occasionally to shoot over his little demesne, may very readily educate his dog without having recourse to keepers or professional breakers, among whom he would often be subject to imposition. Generally speaking, no dog is half so well broken as the one whose owner has taken the trouble of training him. The first and grand thing is to obtain the attachment of the dog, by frequently feeding and caressing him, and giving him little hours of liberty under his own inspection; but, every now and then, inculcating a lesson of obedience, teaching him that every gambol must be under the control of his master; frequently checking him in the midst of his riot with the order of 'Down charge!' patting him when he is instantly obedient; and rating, or castigating him, but not too severely, when there is any reluctance to obey. *Passive obedience is the first principle, and from which no deviation should be allowed.*[a]

"Much kindness and gentleness are certainly requisite when breaking-in the puppy, whether it be a pointer or a setter. There is heedlessness in the young dog which is not readily got rid of until age has given him experience. He must not, however, be too severely corrected, or he may be spoiled for life. If considerable correction is sometimes necessary, it should be followed, at a little distance of time, by some kind usage. The memory of the suffering will remain; but the feeling of attachment to the master will also remain, or rather be increased. The temper of a young dog must be almost as carefully studied as that of a human being. Timidity may be encouraged, and eagerness may be restrained, but affection must be the tie that binds him to his master, and renders him subservient to his will.

"The next portion of the lesson is more difficult to learn. He is no longer held by his master, but suffered to run over the field, seemingly at his pleasure, when, suddenly, comes the warning 'Down!' He perhaps pays no attention to it, but gambols along until seized by his master, forced on the ground, and the order of 'Down!' somewhat sternly uttered.

"After a while he is suffered again to get up. He soon forgets what has occurred, and gallops away with as much glee as ever. Again the 'Down!' is heard, and again little or no attention is paid to it. His master once more lays hold of him and forces him on the ground, and perhaps inflicts a slight blow or two, and this process continues until the dog finds that he must obey the command of 'Down charge!'

"The owner will now probably walk from him a little way backward with his hand lifted up. If the dog makes the slightest motion, he must be sharply spoken to, and the order peremptorily enforced.

"He must then be taught to 'back,' that is, to come behind his master when called. When he seems to understand all this, he is called by his master in a kindly tone, and patted and caressed. It is almost incredible how soon he will afterwards understand what he is ordered to do, and perform it.

"It will be seen by this that no one should attempt to break-in

---

[a] Another writer in the same volume gives also an interesting account of the management of the setter.

a dog who is not possessed of patience and perseverance. The sportsman must not expect to see a great deal of improvement from the early lessons. The dog will often forget that which was inculcated upon him a few hours before; but perseverance and kindness will effect much: the first lessons over, the dog, beginning to perceive a little what is meant, will cheerfully and joyfully do his duty.

"When there is much difficulty in teaching the dog his lesson, the fault lies as often with the master as with him; or they are, generally speaking, both in fault. Some dogs cannot be mastered but by means of frequent correction. The less the sportsman has to do with them the better. Others will not endure the least correction, but become either ferocious or sulky. They should be disposed of as soon as possible. The majority of dogs are exceedingly sagacious. They possess strong reasoning powers; they understand, by intuition, almost every want and wish of their master, and they deserve the kindest and best usage.

"The scholar being thus prepared, should be taken into the field, either alone, or, what is considerably better, with a well-trained, steady dog. When the old dog makes a point, the master calls out, 'Down!' or 'Soho!' and holds up his hand, and approaches steadily to the birds; and, if the young one runs in or prepares to do so, as probably he will at first, he again raises his hand and calls out, 'Soho!' If the youngster pays no attention to this, the whip must be used, and in a short time he will be steady enough at the first intimation of game.

"If he springs any birds without taking notice of them, he should be dragged to the spot from which they rose, and, 'Soho!' being cried, one or two sharp strokes with the whip should be inflicted. If he is too eager, he should be warned to 'take heed.' If he *rakes* or runs with his nose near the ground, he should be admonished to *hold up*, and, if he still persists, the *muzzle-peg* may be resorted to. Some persons fire over the dog for running at hares: but this is wrong; for, besides the danger of wounding or even killing the animal, he will for some time afterwards be frightened at the sound, or even at the very sight of a gun. The best plan to accustom dogs to the gun, is occasionally to fire one off when they are being fed.

"Some persons let their dog fetch the dead birds. This is very wrong. Except the sportsman has a double-barrelled gun, the dog should not be suffered to move until the piece is again charged. The young one, until he is thoroughly broken of it, is too apt to run in whether the bird is killed or not, and which may create much mischief by disturbing the game.

"Although excessive punishment should not be administered, yet no fault, however small, should pass without reproof: on the other hand, he should be rewarded, but not too lavishly, for every instance of good conduct.

"When the dog is grown tolerably steady, and taught to come at the call, he should also learn to range and quarter his ground. Let some clear morning, and some place where the sportsman is likely to meet with game, be selected. Station him where the wind will blow in his face; wave your hand and cry, 'Heigh on, good dog!' Then let him go off to the right, about seventy or eighty yards. After this, call him in by another wave of the hand, and let him go the same distance to the left. Walk straight forward with your eye always upon him; then, let him continue to cross from right to left, calling him in at the limit of each range.

"This is at first a somewhat difficult lesson, and requires careful teaching. The same ground is never to be twice passed over. The sportsman watches every motion, and the dog is never trusted out of sight, or allowed to break fence. When this lesson is tolerably learned, and on some good scenting morning early in the season, he may take the field, and perhaps find. Probably he will be too eager, and spring his game. Make him *down* immediately, and take him to the place where the birds rose. Chide him with 'Steady!' 'How dare you!' Use no whip; but scold him well, and be assured that he will be more cautious. If possible, kill on the next chance. The moment the bird is down, he will probably rush in and seize it. He must be met with the same rebuff, 'Down charge!' If he does not obey, he deserves to have, and will have, a stroke with the whip. The gun being again charged, the bird is sought for, and the dog is suffered to see it and play with it for a minute before it is put into the bag.

"He will now become thoroughly fond of the sport, and his fondness will increase with each bird that is killed. At every time, however, whether he kills or misses, the sportsman should make the dog 'Down charge,' and never allow him to rise until he has loaded.

"If a hare should be wounded, there will, occasionally, be considerable difficulty in preventing him from chasing her. The best broken and steadiest dog cannot always be restrained from running hares. He must be checked with '*Ware chase*,' and, if he does not attend, the sportsman must wait patiently. He will by-and-by come slinking along with his tail between his legs, conscious of his fault. It is one, however, that admits of no pardon. He must be secured, and, while the field echoes with the cry of '*Ware chase*,' he must be punished to a certain but not too great extent. The castigation must be repeated as often as he offends; or, if there is much difficulty in breaking him of the habit, he must be got rid of."

The breaking-in or subjugation of pointers and setters is a very important, and occasionally a difficult affair; the pleasure of the sportsman, however, depends upon it. The owner of any considerable property will naturally look to his keeper to furnish him with dogs on which he may depend, and he ought not to be disappointed; for those which belong to other persons, or are brought at the beginning of the season, whatever account the breaker or the keeper of them may give, will too often be found deficient.

THE OTTER HOUND

used to be of a mingled breed, between the southern hound and the rough terrier, and in size between the harrier and the fox-hound. The head should be large and broad, the shoulders and quarters thick, and the hair strong, wiry, and rough. They used to be kept in small packs, for the express purpose of hunting the otter.

Two hundred and fifty years ago, otter-hunting was a favourite amusement in several parts of Great Britain. Many of our streams then abounded with this destructive animal; but, since the population of our country has become more dense, and game-keepers are more numerous, and many contrivances are adopted to ensnare and destroy otters, few are now to be found.

THE TURNSPIT.

This dog was once a valuable auxiliary in the kitchen, by turning the spit before jacks were invented. It had a peculiar length of body, with short crooked legs, the tail curled, its ears long and pendent, and the head large in proportion to the body. It is still used in the kitchen on various parts of the Continent. There are some curious stories of the artfulness with which he often attempted to avoid the task imposed upon him.

There is a variety of this dog; the crooked-legged turnspit.

CHAPTER IV.

THE VARIETIES OF THE DOG.

THIRD DIVISION.

The muzzle more or less shortened, the frontal sinus enlarged, and the cranium elevated and diminished in capacity.

At the head of this inferior or brutal division of dogs stands

THE BULL-DOG.

The round, thick head, turned-up nose, and thick and pendulous lips of this dog are familiar to all, while his ferocity makes him in the highest degree dangerous. In general he makes a silent although ferocious attack, and the persisting powers of his teeth and jaws enable him to keep his hold against any but the greatest efforts, so that the utmost mischief is likely to ensue as well to the innocent visitor of his domicile as the ferocious intruder. The bull-dog is scarcely capable of any education, and is fitted for nothing but ferocity and combat.

The name of this dog is derived from his being too often employed, until a few years ago, in baiting the bull. It was practised by the low and dissolute in many parts of the country. Dogs were bred and trained for the purpose; and, while many of them were injured or destroyed, the head of the bull was lacerated in the most barbarous manner. Nothing can exceed the fury with which the bull-dog rushed on his foe, and the obstinacy with which he maintained his hold. He fastened upon the lip, the muzzle, or the eye, and there he hung in spite of every effort of the bull to free himself from his antagonist.

Bull-dogs are not so numerous as they were a few years ago; and every kind-hearted person will rejoice to hear that bull-baiting is now put down by legal authority in every part of the kingdom.

THE BULL-TERRIER.

This dog is a cross between the bull-dog and the terrier, and is generally superior, both in appearance and value, to either of its progenitors. A second cross considerably lessens the underhanging of the lower jaw, and a third entirely removes it, retaining the spirit and determination of the animal. It forms a steadier friendship than either of them, and the principal objection to it is its love of wanton mischief, and the dangerous irascibility which it occasionally exhibits.

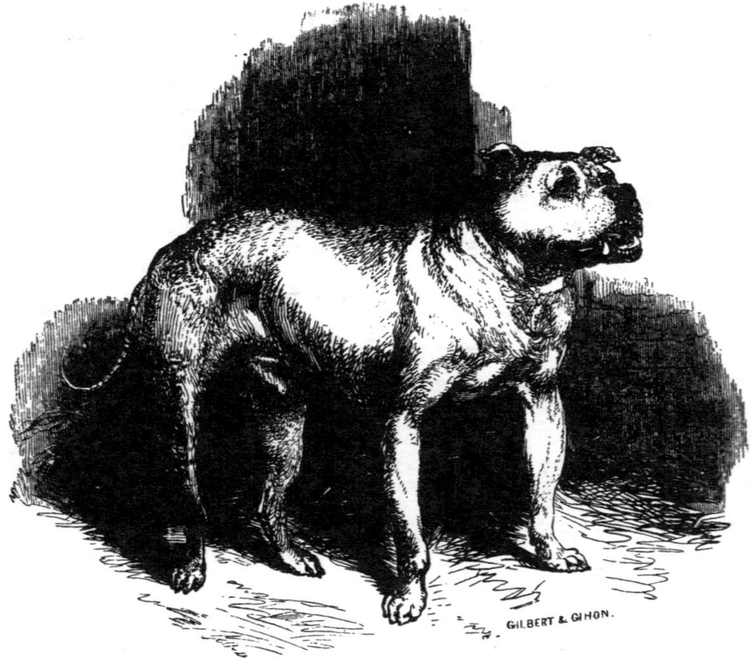

THE BULL-DOG.

Sir Walter Scott, a warm friend of dogs, and whose veracity cannot be impeached, gives an interesting account of a favourite one belonging to him. "The cleverest dog I ever had was what is called a bull-dog terrier. I taught him to understand a great many words, insomuch that I am positive the communication between the canine species and ourselves might be greatly enlarged. Camp, the name of my dog, once bit the baker when bringing bread to the family. I beat him, and explained the enormity of the offence; after which, to the last moment of his life, he never heard the least allusion to the story without creeping into the darkest corner of the room. Towards the end of his life, when he was unable to attend me while I was on horseback, he generally watched for my return, and, when the servant used to tell him, his master was coming down the hill, or through the moor, although he did not use any gesture to explain his meaning, Camp was never known to mistake him, but either went out at the front to go up the hill, or at the back to get down to the moor-side."

THE MASTIFF.

The head considerably resembles that of the bull-dog, but with the ears dependent. The upper lip falls over the lower jaw. The end of the tail is turned up, and frequently the fifth toe of the hind feet is more or less developed. The nostrils are separated one from another by a deep furrow. He has a grave and somewhat sullen countenance, and his deep-toned bark is often heard during the night. The mastiff is taller than the bull-dog, but not so deep in the chest, and his head is large compared with his general form.

It is probable that the mastiff is an original breed peculiar to the British islands.

He seems to be fully aware of the impression which his large size makes on every stranger; and, in the night especially, he watches the abode of his master with the completest vigilance; in fact, nothing would tempt him to betray the confidence which is reposed in him.

Captain Brown states that, "notwithstanding his commanding appearance and the strictness with which he guards the property of his master, he is possessed of the greatest mildness of conduct, and is as grateful for any favours bestowed upon him as is the most diminutive of the canine tribe. There is a remarkable and peculiar warmth in his attachments. He is aware of all the duties required of him, and he punctually discharges them. In the course of the night he several times examines every thing with which he is intrusted with the most scrupulous care, and, by repeated barkings, warns the household or the depredator that he is at the post of duty."[a]

The mastiff from Cuba requires some mention, and will call up some of the most painful recollections in the history of the human race. He was not a native of Cuba, but imported into the country.

The Spaniards had possessed themselves of several of the South American islands. They found them peopled with Indians, and those of a sensual, brutish, and barbarous class—continually making war with their neighbours, indulging in an irreconcilable hatred of the Spaniards, and determined to expel and destroy them. In self-defence, they were driven to some means of averting the destruction with which they were threatened. They procured some of these mastiffs, by whose assistance they penetrated into every part of the country, and destroyed the greater portion of the former inhabitants.

Las Casas, a Catholic priest, and whose life was employed in endeavouring to mitigate the sufferings of the original inhabitants, says that " it was resolved to march against the Indians, who had fled to the mountains, and they were chased like wild beasts, with the assistance of bloodhounds, who had been trained to a thirst for human blood, so that before I had left the island it had become almost entirely a desert."

THE ICELAND DOG.

The head is rounder than that of the northern dogs; the ears partly erect and partly pendent; and the fur soft and long, especially behind the fore legs and on the tail. It much resembles the Turkish dog removed to a colder climate.

This dog is exceedingly useful to the Icelanders while travelling over the snowy deserts of the north. By a kind of intuition he rarely fails in choosing the shortest and the safest course. He also is more aware than his master of the approach of the snow storms; and is a most valuable ally against the attack of the Polar bear, who, drifted on masses of ice from the neighbouring continent, often commits depredations among the cattle, and even attacks human beings. When the dog is first aware of the neighbourhood of the bear, he sets up a fearful howl, and men and dogs hasten to hunt down and destroy the depredator.

The travelling in Iceland is sometimes exceedingly dangerous at the beginning of the winter. A thin layer of snow covers and conceals some of the chasms with which that region abounds. Should the traveller fall into one of them, the dog proves a most useful animal; for he runs immediately across the snowy

[a] Brown's Biographical Sketches, p. 425.

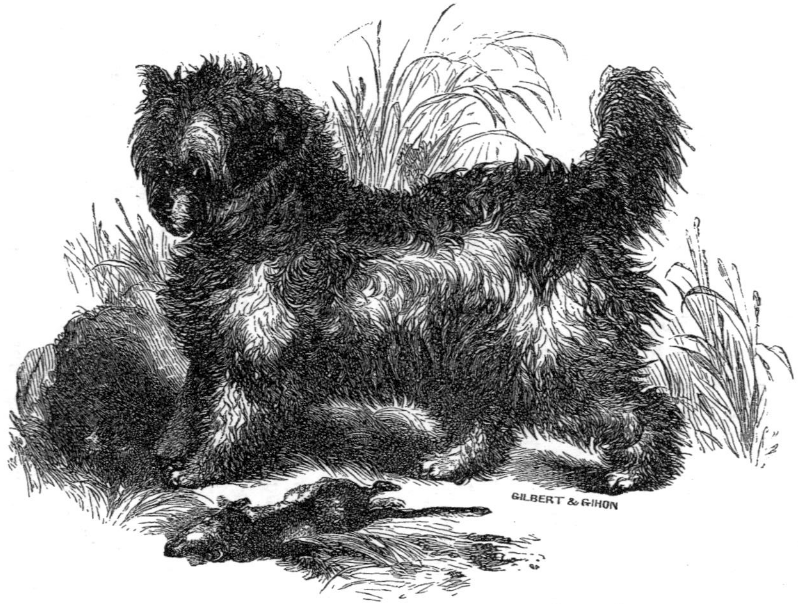

THE SCOTCH TERRIER.

waste, and, by his howling, induces the traveller's friends to hasten to his rescue.

THE TERRIER.

The forehead is convex; the eye prominent; the muzzle pointed; the tail thin and arched; the fur short; the ears of moderate size, half erect, and usually of a deep-black colour, with a yellow spot over the eyes. It is an exceedingly useful animal; but not so indispensable an accompaniment to a pack of fox-hounds as it used to be accounted. Foxes are not so often unearthed as they formerly were, yet many a day's sport would be lost without the terrier. Some sportsmen used to have two terriers accompanying in the pack, one being smaller than the other. This was a very proper provision; a large terrier might be incapable of penetrating into the earth, and a small one might permit the escape of the prey. Many terriers have lost their lives by scratching up the earth behind them, and thus depriving themselves of all means of retreat.

The coat of the terrier may be either smooth or rough; the smooth-haired ones are more delicate in appearance, and are somewhat more exposed to injury or accident; but in courage, sagacity, and strength, there is very little difference if the dogs are equally well bred. The rough terrier possibly obtained his shaggy coat from the cur, and the smooth terrier may derive his from the hound.

The terrier is seldom of much service until he is twelve months old; and then, incited by natural propensity, or the example of the older ones, or urged on by the huntsman, he begins to discharge his supposed duty.

An old terrier is brought to the mouth of the earth in which a vixen fox — a fox with her young ones — has taken up her abode, and is sent in to worry and drive her out. Some young terriers are brought to the mouth of the hover, to listen to the process that is going forward within, and to be excited to the utmost extent of which they are capable. The vixen is at length driven out, and caught at the mouth of the hole; and the young ones are suffered to rush in, and worry or destroy their first prey. They want no after-tuition to prepare them for the discharge of their duty.

This may be pardoned. It is the most ready way of training the young dog to his future business; but it is hoped that no reader of this work will be guilty of the atrocities that are often practised. An old fox, or badger, is caught, his under jaw is sawn off, and the lower teeth are forcibly extracted, or broken. A hole is then dug in the earth, or a barrel is placed large and deep enough to permit a terrier, or perhaps two of them, to enter. Into this cavity the fox or badger is thrust, and a terrier rushes after him, and drags him out again. The question to be ascertained is, how many times in a given period the dog will draw this poor tortured animal out of the barrel—an exhibition of cruelty which no one should be able to lay to the charge of any human being. It is a principle not to be departed from, that wanton and useless barbarity should never be permitted. The government, to a certain extent, has interfered, and a noble society has been established to limit, or, if possible, to prevent the infliction of useless pain.

The terrier is, however, a valuable dog, in the house and the farm. The stoat, the pole-cat, and the weazel, commit great depredations in the fields, the barn, and granary; and to a certain extent, the terrier is employed in chasing or destroying them; but it is not often that he has a fair chance to attack them. He is more frequently used in combating the rat.

The mischief effected by rats is almost incredible. It has been said that, in some cases, in the article of corn, these animals consume a quantity of food equal in value to the rent of the farm. Here the dog is usefully employed, and in his very element, especially if there is a cross of the bull-dog about him.

There are some extraordinary accounts of the dexterity, as well as courage, of the terrier in destroying rats. The feats of a dog called "Billy" will be long remembered. He was matched to destroy one hundred large rats in eight and a half minutes. The rats were brought into the ring in bags, and, as soon as the number was complete, he was put over the railing. In six minutes and thirty-five seconds they were all destroyed. In another match he destroyed the same number in six minutes and thirteen seconds. At length, when he was getting old, and had but two teeth and one eye left, a wager was laid of thirty sovereigns, by the owner of a Berkshire bitch, that she would kill fifty rats in less time than Billy. The old dog killed his fifty in five minutes and six seconds. The pit was then cleared, and the bitch let in. When she had killed thirty rats, she was completely exhausted, fell into a fit, and lay barking and yelping, utterly incapable of completing her task.

The speed of the terrier is very great. One has been known to run six miles in thirty-two minutes. He needs to be a fleet dog if, with his comparatively little bulk, he can keep up with the foxhound.

A small breed of *wry-legged* terriers was once in repute, and, to a certain degree, is retained for the purpose of hunting rabbits. It probably originated in some rickety specimens, remarkable for the slow development of their frame, except in the head, the belly, and the joints, which enlarge at the expense of the other parts.

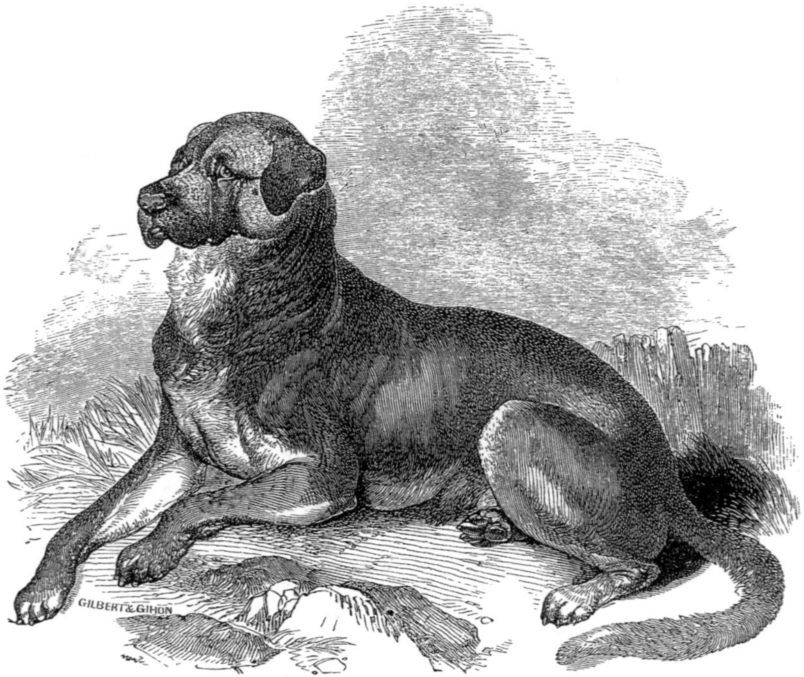

THE MASTIFF.

THE SCOTCH TERRIER.

There is reason to believe that this dog is far older than the English terrier. There are three varieties: first the common Scotch terrier, twelve or thirteen inches high; his body muscular and compact — considerable breadth across the loins — the legs shorter and stouter than those of the English terriers. The head large in proportion to the size of the body—the muzzle small and pointed—strong marks of intelligence in the countenance—warm attachment to his master, and the evident devotion of every power to the fulfilment of his wishes. The hair is long and tough, and extending over the whole of the frame. In colour, they are black or fawn: the white, yellow, or pied are always deficient in purity of blood.

Another species has nearly the same conformation, but is covered with longer, more curly, and stouter hair; the legs being apparently, but not actually, shorter. This kind of dog prevails in the greater part of the Western Islands of Scotland, and some of them, where the hair has obtained its full development, are much admired.

Her Majesty had one from Islay, a faithful and affectionate creature, yet with all the spirit and determination that belongs to his breed. The writer of this account had occasion to operate on this poor fellow, who had been bitten under somewhat suspicious circumstances. He submitted without a cry or a struggle, and seemed to be perfectly aware that we should not put him to pain without having some good purpose in view.

A third species of terrier is of a considerably larger bulk, and three or four inches taller than either of the others. Its hair is shorter than that of the other breeds, and is hard and wiry.

THE SHOCK-DOG

is traced by Buffon, but somewhat erroneously, to a mixture of the small Danish dog and the pug. The head is round, the eyes large, but somewhat concealed by its long and curly hair, the tail curved and bent forward. The muzzle resembles that of the pug. It is of small size, and is used in this country and on the Continent as a lap-dog. It is very properly described by the author of "The Field Book" as a useless little animal, seeming to possess no other quality than that of a faithful attachment to his mistress.

THE ARTOIS DOG,

with his short, flat muzzle, is a produce of the shock-dog and the pug. He has nothing peculiar to recommend him.

THE ANDALUSIAN, OR ALICANT DOG,

has the short muzzle of the pug with the long hair of the spaniel

THE EGYPTIAN AND BARBARY DOG,

according to Cuvier, has a very thick and round head, the ears erect at the base, large and movable, and carried horizontally, the skin nearly naked, and black or dark flesh-colour, with large patches of brown. A sub-variety has a kind of mane behind the head, formed of long stiff hairs.

Buffon imagines that the shepherd's dog—transported to different climates, and acquiring different habits—was the ancestor of the various species with which almost every country abounds; but whence they originally came it is impossible to say. They vary in their size, their colour, their attitude, their usual exterior, and their strangely different interior construction. Transported into various climates, they are necessarily submitted to the influence of heat and cold, and of food more or less abundant and more or less suitable to their natural organization; but the reason or the derivation of these differences of structure it is not always easy to explain.

CHAPTER V.

THE GOOD QUALITIES OF THE DOG; THE SENSE OF SMELL; INTELLIGENCE; MORAL QUALITIES; DOG-CARTS; CROPPING; TAILING; BREAKING-IN; DOG-PITS; DOG-STEALING.

In our history of the different breeds of the dog we have seen enough to induce us to admire and love him. His courage, his fidelity, and the degree in which he often devotes every power that he possesses to our service, are circumstances that we can never forget nor overlook. His very foibles occasionally attach him to us. We may select a pointer for the pureness of his blood and the perfection of his education. He transgresses in the field. We call him to us; we scold him well; perchance, we chastise him. He lies motionless and dumb at our feet. The punishment being over, he gets up, and, by some significant gesture, acknowledges his consciousness of deserving what he has suffered. The writer operated on a pointer bitch for an enlarged cancerous tumour, accompanied by much inflammation and pain in the surrounding parts. A word or two of kindness and of caution were all that were necessary, although, in order to prevent accidents, she had been bound securely. The flesh quivered as the knife pursued its course—a moan or two escaped her, but yet she did not struggle; and her first act, after all was over, was to lick the operator's hand.

From the combination of various causes, the history of no animal is more interesting than that of the dog. First, his intimate association with man, not only as a valuable protector, but as a constant and faithful companion throughout all the vicissitudes of life. Secondly, from his natural endowments, not consisting in the exquisite delicacy of one individual sense—not merely combining memory with reflection—but possessing qualities of the mind that stagger us in the contemplation of them, and which we can alone account for in the gradation existing in that wonderful system which, by different links of one vast chain, extends from the first to the last of all things, until it forms a perfect whole on the wonderful confines of the spiritual and material world.

We here quote the beautiful account of Sir Walter Scott and his dogs, as described by Henry Hallam:—

"But looking towards the grassy mound
Where calm the Douglass chieftains lie,
Who, living, quiet never found,
I straightway learnt a lesson high;

For there an old man sat serene,
And well I knew that thoughtful mien
Of him whose early lyre had thrown
O'er mouldering walls the magic of its tone.

It was a comfort, too, to see
Those dogs that from him ne'er would rove,
And always eyed him reverently,
With glances of depending love.
They know not of the eminence
Which marks him to my reasoning sense,
They know but that he is a man,
And still to them is kind, and glads them all he can.

And hence their quiet looks confiding;
Hence grateful instincts, seated deep,
By whose strong bond, were ill betiding,
They 'd lose their own, his life to keep.
What joy to watch in lower creature
Such dawning of a moral nature,
And how (the rule all things obey)
They look to a higher mind to be their law and stay !"

The subject of the intellectual and moral qualities of the inferior animals is one highly interesting and somewhat misunderstood —urged perhaps to a ridiculous extent by some persons, yet altogether neglected by others who have no feeling for any but themselves.

Anatomists have compared the relative bulk of the brain in different animals, and the result is not a little interesting. In man the weight of the brain amounts on the average to 1-30th part of the body. In the Newfoundland dog it does not amount to 1-60th part, or to 1-100th part in the poodle and barbet, and not to more than 1-300th part in the ferocious and stupid bull-dog.

When the brain is cut, it is found to be composed of two substances, essentially different in construction and function—the cortical and the medullary. The first is small in quantity, and principally concerned in the food and reproduction of the animal, and the cineritious in a great measure the register of the mind. Brute strength seems to be the character of the former, and superior intelligence of the latter. There is, comparing bulk with bulk, less of the medullary substance in the horse than in the ox —and in the dog than in the horse—and they are characterized as the sluggish ox, the intelligent horse, and the intellectual and companionable dog.

From the medullary substance proceed certain cords or prolongations, termed *nerves*, by which the animal is enabled to receive impressions from surrounding objects and to connect himself with them, and also to possess many pleasurable or painful sensations. One of them is spread over the membrane of the nose, and gives the sense of smell; another expands on the back of the eye, and the faculty of sight is gained; a third goes to the internal structure of the ear, and the animal is conscious of sound. Other nerves, proceeding to different parts, give the faculty of motion, while an equally important one bestows the power of feeling. One division, springing from a prolongation of the brain, and yet within the skull, wanders to different parts of the frame, for important purposes connected with respiration or breathing. The act of breathing is essential to life, and were it to cease, the animal would die.

There are other nerves—the sympathetic—so called from their union and sympathy with all the others, and identified with life itself. They proceed from a small ganglion or enlargement in the upper part of the neck, or from a collection of minute ganglia within the abdomen. They go to the heart, and it beats; and to the stomach, and it digests. They form a net-work round each vessel, and the frame is nourished and built up. They are destitute of sensation, and they are perfectly beyond the control of the will.

We have been accustomed, and properly, to regard the nervous system, or that portion of it which is connected with animal life—that which renders us conscious of surrounding objects and susceptible of pleasure and of pain—as the source of intellectual power and moral feeling. It is so with ourselves. All our knowledge is derived from our perception of things around us. A certain impression is made on the outward fibres of a sensitive nerve. That impression, in some mysterious way, is conveyed to the brain; and there it is received—registered—stored—and compared; there its connections are traced and its consequences appreciated; and thence a variety of interesting impressions are conveyed, and due use is made of them.

THE SENSE OF SMELL.

Our subject—the intellectual and moral feelings of brutes, and the mechanism on which they depend — may be divided into two parts, the portion that receives and conveys, and that which stores up and compares and uses the impression.

The portion that receives and conveys is far more developed in the brute than in the human being. Whatever sense we take, we clearly perceive the triumph of animal power.

The olfactory nerve in the horse, the dog, the ox, and the swine, is the largest of all the cerebral nerves, and has much greater comparative bulk in the quadruped than in the human being. The sense of smell, bearing proportion to the nerve on which it depends, is yet more acute. In man it is connected with pleasure—in the inferior animals with life. The relative size of the nerve bears an invariable proportion to the necessity of an acute sense of smell in the various animals—large in the horse compared with the olfactory nerve in the human being—larger in the ox, who is often sent into the fields to shift for himself—larger still in the swine, whose food is buried under the soil, or deeply immersed in the filth or refuse,—and still larger in the dog, the acuteness of whose scent is so connected with our pleasure.

[The disposition to hunt by scent is not peculiar to the setter or pointer, but in fact is common to all animals; developing itself in different proportions according to their various physical constructions and modes of life. The method of finding and pointing at game, now peculiar to these dogs, and engendered in their progeny through successive generations, is not the result of any special instinct, that usually governs the actions of the brute creation—but rather the effect of individual education and force of habit upon their several ancestors. This habit of life, engrafted through progressive generations into these two breeds, has become a second nature, and so entirely the property of the species, that all its members, with but little care on the part of man, will perform these same actions in the same way, and will ever continue to exhibit these propensities for hunting, provided opportunities be offered for indulging them. Nevertheless, as these peculiar predilections for "*setting or pointing*," as before said, are the effect of education and habit, the artificial impulse would very soon be entirely obliterated, if not encouraged in the young dogs of each generation. This circumstance alone, proves to us the importance of getting dogs from a well-known good strain, whose ancestors have been remarkable for their exploits in the field. This necessary precaution will insure a favourable issue to our troubles, and lessen materially our labours. In fact young puppies have been frequently known to exhibit this propensity the first time they have been taken to the field. Some of these dogs have come under the notice of the writer, who at a few months old exhibited all the peculiarities of their race; in fact were "*self-broke.*" These dogs were the progeny of a well-known imported stock, in the possession of a gentleman who selected them in England.

Although other dogs, and other animals even, have been with great difficulty and perseverance taught to find and point game, still these two breeds seem especially adapted by nature, both in their physical and intellectual construction, for the performance of this particular duty to man.

The sense of smell is differently developed in different animals; the olfactory nerve of the dog is larger than any other in the cerebrum, which peculiarity will at once account for their wonderful powers of scent.

Swine, also, have these nerves largely developed; and necessarily so, as both in a state of nature or half-civilization, the greater portion of their food is buried under the earth or mingled with the filth and mire of their sties, and would pass unheeded, if not for the acuteness of their nasal organs.

In Daniels' "Rural Sports," will be found an interesting account of a sow having been taught to find and point game of various kinds, and often having been known to stand on partridges at a distance of forty yards, which is more than can reasonably be expected of every first-rate dog. She was not only broke to find and stand game, but hunted with the dogs, and backed successfully when on a point. This extraordinary animal evinced great aptness for learning, and afterwards great enthusiasm in the sport; showing symptoms of pleasure at the sight of a gun, or when called upon to accompany a party to the field. Her hunting was not confined to any particular game, but stood equally well on partridges, pheasants, snipes, rabbits, &c. (See Blaine, part vii, chap. iii, page 792.)

Most of animals instinctively employ the organ of scent to seek out food, or avert personal danger, in preference to that of sight; but some depend more upon the latter than the former, either from instinct or the force of education.

For instance, the greyhound, though equally gifted with the sense of smell, as that of sight, has been taught to depend upon the one organ to the entire exclusion of the other, which is quite the reverse of the setter and pointer; but the wonderful speed of these dogs renders it quite unnecessary that he should employ the olfactory nerves, as no animal, however swift, can hope to escape from him in a fair race, when once near enough to be seen; though there are some that may elude his grasp by a "*ruse de guerre*" when too hardly pressed. (*Extracted from our essay in No.* 1, *vol.* xvi, *of the* "*Spirit of the Times.*")—L.]

INTELLIGENCE.

We find little mention of insanity in the domesticated animals in any of our modern authors, whether treating on agriculture, horsemanship, or veterinary medicine, and yet there are some singular and very interesting cases of aberration of intellect. The inferior animals are, to a certain extent, endowed with the same faculties as ourselves. They are even susceptible of the same moral qualities. Hatred, love, fear, hope, joy, distress, courage, timidity, jealousy, and many varied passions influence and agitate them, as they do the human being. The dog is an illustration of this — the most susceptible to every impression — approaching the nearest to man in his instincts, and in many actions that surprise the philosopher, who justly appreciates it.

What eagerness to bite is often displayed by the dog when

labouring under enteritis, and especially by him who has imbibed the poison of rabies! How singular is the less dangerous malady which induces the horse and the dog to press unconsciously forward under the influence of vertigo!—the eagerness with which, when labouring under phrenitis, he strikes at everything with his foot, or rushes upon it to seize it with his teeth! A kind of nostalgia is often recognised in that depression which nothing can dissipate, and the invincible aversion to food, by means of which many animals perish, who are prevented from returning to the place where they once lived, and the localities to which they had been accustomed.

These are circumstances proving that the dog is endowed with intelligence and with affections like ours; and, if they do not equal ours, they are of the same character.

With regard to the foundation of intellectual power, viz.: attention, memory, association, and imagination, the difference between man and animals is in degree, and not in kind. Thus stands the account,—with the quadruped as well as the biped,—the impression is made on the mind; attention fixes it there; memory recurs to it; imagination combines it, rightly or erroneously, with many other impressions; judgment determines the value of it, and the conclusions that are to be drawn from it, if not with logical precision, yet with sufficient accuracy for every practical purpose.

A bitch, naturally ill-tempered, and that would not suffer a stranger to touch her, had scirrhous enlargement on one of her teats. As she lay in the lap of her mistress, an attempt was repeatedly made to examine the tumour, in spite of many desperate attempts on her part to bite. All at once, however, something seemed to strike her mind. She whined, wagged her tail, and sprung from the lap of her mistress to the ground. It was to crouch at the feet of the surgeon, and to lay herself down and expose the tumour to his inspection. She submitted to a somewhat painful examination of it, and to a far more serious operation afterwards. Some years passed away, and whenever she saw the operator, she testified her joy and her gratitude in the most expressive and endearing manner.

A short time since, the following scene took place in a street adjoining Hanover-square. It was an exhibition of a highly interesting character, and worthy to be placed upon record. The editor of the Lancet having heard that a French gentleman (M. Léonard), who had for some time been engaged in instructing two dogs in various performances that required the exercise, not merely of the natural instincts of the animal and the power of imitation, but of a higher intellect, and a degree of reflection and judgment far greater than is commonly developed in the dog, was residing in London, obtained an introduction, and was obligingly favoured by M. Léonard with permission to hold a *conversazione* with his extraordinary pupils. He thus describes the interview :—

Two fine dogs, of the Spanish breed, were introduced by M. Léonard, with the customary French politesse, the largest by the name of M. Philax, the other as M. Brac (or spot); the former had been in training three, the latter two, years. They were in vigorous health, and, having bowed very gracefully, seated themselves on the hearth-rug side by side. M. Léonard then gave a lively description of the means he had employed to develop the cerebral system in these animals—how, from having been fond of the chase, and ambitious of possessing the best-trained dogs, he had employed the usual course of training—how the conviction had been impressed on his mind, that by gentle usage, and steady perseverance in inducing the animal to repeat again and again what was required, not only would the dog be capable of performing that specific act, but that part of the brain which was brought into activity by the mental effort would become more largely developed, and hence a permanent increase of mental power be obtained.

This reasoning is in accordance with the known laws of the physiology of the nervous system, and is fraught with the most important results. We may refer the reader interested in the subject to the masterly little work of Dr. Verity, "Changes produced in the Nervous System by Civilization."

After this introduction, M. Léonard spoke to his dogs in French, in his usual tone, and ordered one of them to walk, the other to lie down, to run, to gallop, halt, crouch, &c., which they performed as promptly and correctly as the most docile children. Then he directed them to go through the usual exercises of the *manége*, which they performed as well as the best-trained ponies at Astley's.

He next placed six cards of different colours on the floor, and, sitting with his back to the dogs, directed one to pick up the blue card, and the other the white, &c., varying his orders rapidly, and speaking in such a manner that it was impossible the dogs could have executed his commands if they had not had a perfect knowledge of the words. For instance, M. Léonard said, "Philax, take the red card and give it to Brac; and, Brac, take the white card and give it to Philax;" the dogs instantly did this, and exchanged cards with each other. He then said, "Philax, put your card on the green, and Brac, put yours on the blue;" and this was instantly performed. Pieces of bread and meat were placed on the floor, with figured cards, and a variety of directions were given to the dogs, so as to put their intelligence and obedience to a severe test. They brought the meat, bread, or cards, as com manded, but did not attempt to eat or to touch unless ordered. Philax was then ordered to bring a piece of meat and give it to Brac, and then Brac was told to give it back to Philax, who was to return it to its place. Philax was next told he might bring a piece of bread and eat it; but, before he had time to swallow it, his master forbade him, and directed him to show that he had not disobeyed, and the dog instantly protruded the crust between his lips.

While many of these feats were being performed, M. Léonard snapped a whip violently, to prove that the animals were so completely under discipline, that they would not heed any interruption.

After many other performances, M. Léonard invited a gentleman to play a game of dominos with one of them. The younger and slighter dog then seated himself on a chair at the table, and the writer and M. Léonard seated themselves opposite. Six dominos were placed on their edges in the usual manner before the dog, and a like number before the writer. The dog having a double number, took one up in his mouth, and put it in the middle of the table; the writer placed a corresponding piece on one side; the dog immediately played another correctly, and so on until all the pieces were engaged. Other six dominos were then given to each, and the writer intentionally placed a wrong number. The dog looked surprised, stared very earnestly at the writer, growled, and finally barked angrily. Finding that no notice was taken of his remonstrances, he pushed away the wrong domino with his nose, and took up a suitable one from his own pieces, and placed it in its stead. The writer then played correctly; the dog followed, and won the game. Not the slightest intimation could have been given by M. Léonard to the dog. This mode of play must have been entirely the result of his own observation and judgment. It should be added that the performances were strictly private. The owner of the dogs was a gentleman of independent fortune, and the instruction of his dogs had been taken up merely as a curious and amusing investigation.[a]

Another strange attainment of the dog is the learning to speak. The French Academicians mention one of these animals that could call in an intelligible manner for tea, coffee, chocolate, &c. The account is given by the celebrated Leibnitz, who communi-

---

[a] Plutarch relates that, at the theatre of Marcellus, a dog was exhibited before the emperor Vespasian, so well instructed as to exercise in every kind of dance. He afterwards feigned illness in a most singular manner, so as to strike the spectators with astonishment. He first exhibited various symptoms of pain; he then fell down as if dead, and, afterwards seeming to revive, as if waking from a profound sleep, and then sported about and showed various demonstrations of joy.

cated it to the Royal Academy of France. This dog was of a middling size, and was the property of a peasant in Saxony.

A little boy, a peasant's son, imagined that he perceived in the dog's voice an indistinct resemblance to certain words, and therefore took it into his head to teach him to speak. For this purpose he spared neither time nor pains with his pupil, who was about three years old when his learned education commenced, and in process of time he was able to articulate no fewer than thirty distinct words. He was, however, somewhat of a truant, and did not very willingly exert his talent, and was rather pressed than otherwise into the service of literature. It was necessary that the words should be pronounced to him each time, and then he repeated them after his preceptor. Leibnitz attests that he heard the animal talk in this way, and the French Academicians add, that unless they had received the testimony of so celebrated a person they would scarcely have dared to report the circumstance. It took place in Misnia, in Saxony.

THE MORAL QUALITIES OF THE DOG.

We pass on to another division of our subject, *the moral qualities of the dog*, strongly developed and beautifully displayed, and often putting the biped to shame.

It is truly said of the dog that he possesses

"Many a good
And useful quality, and virtue too,
Attachment never to be weaned or changed
By any change of fortune; proof alike
Against unkindness, absence, and neglect;
Fidelity, that neither bribe nor threat
Can move or warp; and gratitude, for small
And trivial favours, lasting as the life,
And glistening even in the dying eye."

It may here be noticed that, among the inferior animals with large nerves and more medullary substance, there are acuter senses; but man, excelling them in the general bulk of his brain, and more particularly in the cortical portion of it, has far superior powers of mind. These are circumstances that deserve the deepest consideration. In their wild state the brutes have no concern—no idea beyond their food and their reproduction. In their domesticated state, they are doomed to be the servants of man. Their power of mind is sufficient to qualify them for this service: but were proportionate intellectual capacity added to this—were they made conscious of their strength, and of the objects that could be effected by it—they would burst their bonds, and man would in his turn be the victim and the slave.

There is an important faculty, termed *attention*. It is that which distinguishes the promising pupil from him of whom no good hope could be formed, and the scientific man from the superficial and ignorant one. The power of keeping the mind steadily bent upon one purpose, is the great secret of individual and moral improvement. We see the habit of attention carried in the dog to a very considerable extent. The terrier eagerly watching for vermin—the sporting dog standing staunch to his point, however he may be annoyed by the blunders of his companion or the unskilfulness of his master—the foxhound, insensible to a thousand scents, and deaf to every other sound, while he anxiously and perseveringly searches out the track of his prey—these are striking illustrations of the power of attention.

Then, the impression having been received, and the mind having been employed in its examination, it is treasured up in the storehouse of the mind for future use.

This is the faculty of memory; and a most important one it is. Of the *memory* of the *dog*, and the recollection of kindness received, there are a thousand stories, from the return of Ulysses to the present day, and we have seen enough of that faithful animal to believe most of them. An officer was abroad with his regiment, during the American war. He had a fine Newfoundland dog, his constant companion, whom he left with his family. After the lapse of several years he returned. His dog met him at the door, leaped upon his neck, licked his face, and died.

Of the accuracy and retentiveness of memory in the dog, as respects the instruction he has received from his master, we have abundant proof in the pointer and the hound, and it may perhaps be with some of them, as with men, that the lesson must sometimes be repeated, and even impressed on the memory in a way not altogether pleasant.

[We know an imported Irish setter, formerly in possession of a gentleman of this city, who on many occasions, while hunting, displayed an extraordinary instinct, even sufficiently remarkable to make us believe that he possessed not only the most acute powers of observation, but that he also enjoyed the faculty of "inductive reasoning," independent of any mechanical training, many of his performances being entirely voluntary, and the result of causes dependent upon accidental circumstances alone: for instance, when lost from observation, he would noiselessly withdraw from his point, hunt up his master, and induce him, by peculiar signs, to follow him to the spot where he had previously observed the birds.

In his old days, "Smoke" was much opposed to hunting with an indifferent shot, and would leave the field perfectly disgusted, after a succession of bad shooting; seeming to argue that he no longer sought after game for amusement, but that he expected his efforts to be repaid by the death of the birds.

This dog was of a morose and dignified disposition, surly with strangers, and inclined to quarrel with any one who carried a stick or whip in their hands; never forgetting an injury, and growling whenever any person who had offended him made their appearance. He was also particularly irritable and tenacious of his rights when hunting, shunning all puppies or heedless dogs, and exhibiting a very irascible disposition if superseded in a point by another dog; and on one occasion attacked a young pointer in the field, who, in opposition to all his growling and show of irony, would persist in crawling before him, when on a point.—L.]

DOG-CARTS.

These were, and still are, in the country, connected with many an act of atrocious cruelty. We do not object to the dog as a beast of draught. He is so in the northern regions, and he is as happy as any other animal in those cold and inhospitable countries. He is so in Holland, and he is as comfortable there as any other beast that wears the collar. He is not so in Newfoundland: there he is shamefully treated. It is to the abuse of the thing, the poor and half-starved condition of the animal, the scandalous weight that he is made to draw, and the infamous usage to which he is exposed, that we object. We would put him precisely on the same footing with the horse, and then we should be able, perhaps, to afford him, not all the protection we could wish, but nearly as much as we have obtained for the horse. We would have every cart licensed, not for the sake of adding to the revenue, but of getting at the owner; and therefore the taxing need not be any great sum. We would have the cart licensed for the carrying of goods only; or a separate license taken out if it carried or drew a human being.

It is here that the cruelty principally exists. Before the dog-carts were put down in the metropolis, we then saw a man and a woman in one of these carts, drawn by a single dog, and going at full trot. Every passenger execrated them, and the trot was increased to a gallop, in order more speedily to escape the just reproaches that proceeded from every mouth. We would have the name and address of the owner, and the number of the cart, painted on some conspicuous part of the vehicle, and in letters and figures as large as on the common carts. Every passenger who witnessed any flagrant act of cruelty would then be enabled to take the number of the cart, and summon the owner; and the police should have the same power of interference which they have with regard to other vehicles.

After a plan like this had been working a little while, the nui sance would be materially abated; and, indeed, the consciousness of the ease with which the offender might be summoned, would go far to get rid of it.

CROPPING.

This is an infliction of too much torture for the gratification of a nonsensical fancy; and, after all, in the opinion of many, and of those, too, who are fondest of dogs, the animal looks far better in his natural state than when we have exercised all our cruel art upon him. Besides, the effects of this absurd amputation do not cease with the healing of the ear. The intense inflammation that we have set up, materially injures the internal structure of this organ. Deafness is occasionally produced by it in some dogs, and constantly in others. The frequent deafness of the pug is solely attributable to the outrageous as well as absurd rounding of his ears. The almost invariable deafness of the white wire-haired terrier is to be traced to this cause.

[Among the many tastes and fancies that the Americans have inherited from their ancestors, the English, may be enumerated the absurd practice of fashioning the ears of different breeds of dogs to a certain standard of beauty. Mr. Blain very justly remarks that it must be a false taste which has taught us to prefer a curtailed organ to a perfect one, without gaining any convenience by the operation. The dogs upon which this species of barbecuing are more particularly practised in this country, are the bull-dogs and terriers.

We imagine that many of our readers will be surprised when they learn that this operation, although so simple in itself, and performed by every reckless stable-boy, is attended with great suffering to the puppy, and not unfrequently with total deafness. Severe inflammation, extending to the interior of the ear, often follows this operation, more especially when awkwardly performed, as is frequently the case, by the aid of the miserable instruments within the reach of our hostlers; to say nothing of the savage fashion of using the teeth for this purpose, as is often done by ignorant fellows, who even take credit to themselves for the clever style in which they perform this outlandish operation. Mr. Blain states, that it is a barbarous custom to twist the ears off, by swinging the dog around; and we are satisfied that every sensible person will respond to this humane sentiment. We have never had the misfortune to see this latter method put into practice, and trust that such an operation is unknown among us, although, from the manner in which this gentleman condemns it, we are led to suppose that this mode is not uncommon in the old country.

As custom has sanctioned the cropping of dogs, in spite of all that can be said upon the subject, it should be done in such a manner as to cause the least possible pain to the animal. The fourth or fifth week is the proper age for this operation; if done sooner, the flap is apt to sprout and become deformed; if later, the cartilage has grown more thick and sensitive. The imaginary beauty of a terrier crop consists in the foxy appearance of the ears, which is easily produced by the clean cut of a sharp, strong pair of scissors. The first cut should commence at the posterior base of the ear, near to the head, and be carried to the extremity of the flap, taking off about the eighth of an inch or more in width. The second cut should extend from the base of the ear in front, somewhat obliquely, to intersect the other cut within a few lines of the point of the flap. These two cuts will shape the ear in such a style as to please the most fastidious eye, and will require no further trimming. The pieces taken from the first ear will answer as guides in cutting the other. The mother should not be allowed to lick the ears of the puppies, as is generally done, under the supposition that she assists in the healing process, when, in fact, she irritates them, and occasions increased inflammation. If the wounds are tardy at healing, or become mangy, they may be bathed gently with a weak solution of alum.

We regret to find that Mr. Skinner, so well known to the sporting world as the able extoller and defender of the rights of our canine friends, should recommend the cropping of terriers. We are convinced that he would change his feelings upon this subject, if he placed any confidence in the opinions of Blain, Youatt, Scott, or Daniel, all of whom condemn the practice as barbarous, and as often occasioning great suffering, and even total deafness, throughout the progeny of successive generations, as witnessed in the white wire-haired terrier and pug above mentioned.

We have had the good fortune to persuade some of our friends to desist from thus mutilating their terrier pups, all of whom, consequently, grew up with beautiful full ears and long tails, which were much admired; and to the eyes of many, the dogs seemed more sprightly and knowing with their long flaps, than when deprived of those natural appendages.—L.]

TAILING.

Then *the tail* of the dog does not suit the fancy of the owner. It must be shortened in some of these animals, and taken off altogether in others. If the sharp, strong scissors, with a ligature, were used, the operation, although still indefensible, would not be a very cruel one, for the tail may be removed almost in a moment, and the wound soon heals; but for the beastly gnawing off of the part, and the drawing out of the tendons and nerves—these are the acts of a cannibal; and he who orders or perpetrates a barbarity so nearly approaching to cannibalism, deserves to be scouted from all society.

[As a matter of necessity, we cannot sanction the too frequent and cruel practice of cutting or otherwise barbecuing different portions of the bodies of our domestic animals, and more particularly the often absurd fancy of cropping and sterning dogs. Nevertheless, we must admit the propriety of, and, in fact, recommend, the taking off a small portion of the pointer's tail, not to increase his beauty, but to save him some after suffering. A long tail is frequently lacerated in close thickets, and thus rendered sore and mangy: this is prevented by the operation, as it becomes better protected by the body, as also more thickly covered by the feather which generally forms over it.

When the pups are a month or six weeks old, this operation can be performed with little pain to the animal, by means of sharp scissors or a knife; but never allow any one to bite the tail off, as is often done by some dirty and unfeeling stable-men. Although a long tail is inconvenient, a too short one is more unsightly; care should therefore be taken not to remove too much. The quantity should be regulated by the size of the breed: for a medium breed, an inch is sufficient to be cut off at this age. Some sportsmen in England, Mr. Blain also informs us, draw out the lower tendons of the tail, which present themselves after amputation, with a pair of forceps, with a view of causing the tail to be carried higher, which adds to the style and appearance of the dog, when in the field. This practice, we agree with Mr. Youatt, is cannibal-like, and very painful; and, to say the least of it, of very doubtful propriety, as it is but seldom we find a good breed of dog carrying, while hunting, a slovenly tail.

If there should be any appearance of hemorrhage after this operation, a small piece of tape or twine may be tied around the tail, which will immediately arrest the bleeding. This ligature should not remain on longer than a few hours, as the parts included in it will be apt to slough and make a mangy ulcer, difficult to heal.—L.]

DEW-CLAWS.

Next comes the depriving the dog of his *dew-claws*—the supplementary toes a little above the foot. They are supposed to interfere with hunting by becoming entangled with the grass or underwood. This rarely happens. The truth of the matter is, they are simply illustrations of the uniformity of structure which prevails in all animals, so far as is consistent with their destiny. The *dew-claws* only make up the number of toes in other animals. If they are attached, as they are in some dogs, simply by a portion of skin, they may be removed without any very great pain, yet the man of good feeling would not meddle with them. He would not unnecessarily inflict any pain that he can avoid; and here, in several of the breeds, the toe is united by an actual joint; and if they are dissected because they are a little in the way, it is a barbarous operation, and nothing can justify it.

[Notwithstanding our author's condemnation of this practice, there are many sportsmen who think it very necessary to remove this supernumerary toe, fearing that it may interfere with the dog while hunting, as above stated.

Mr. Blain, both a practical sportsman and scientific gentleman, to whose opinions we must at all times show a due regard, considers the removal of these false appendages very necessary, stating that they often become troublesome, not only in the field, but that they frequently turn in and wound the flesh with their nails.

We have never seen any particular inconvenience arising from the presence of these dew-claws, and are not in the habit of taking them off; but, as the operation is a trifling one, and attended with little or no pain, we are disposed to recommend its general adoption, as it improves the appearance of the legs; and their presence may sometimes prove inconvenient to the animal, as stated by Mr. Blain. These claws most commonly have a ligamentous attachment only to the leg, which may be divided, a few days after birth, by a pair of sharp scissors or a knife; and if a bony union exists, it is generally of such a trifling nature that it can be severed in the same way.—L.]

The cruelties that are perpetrated on puppies during the course of their education or *breaking-in*, are sometimes infamous. Young dogs, like young people, must be to a certain degree coerced; but these animals receive from nature so great an aptitude for learning, and practising that which we require of them, and their own pleasure is so much connected with what they learn, that there is no occasion for one-tenth part of the correction that is occasionally inflicted; and the frequent consequence of the cruelty to which they are subjected, is cowardice or ferocity during life.

Not many years ago, as the author was going over one of the commons in the neighbourhood of the metropolis, now enclosed, he heard the loud sounds of the lash and the screams of a dog. He hurried on, and found two men, one holding a greyhound while another was unmercifully flogging him. He had inflicted many lashes, and was continuing the correction. The author indignantly interfered, and the dog was liberated, but with a great deal of abuse from the men; and a gentleman galloping up, and who was the owner of the dog, and a Middlesex magistrate to boot, seemed disposed to support his people in no very measured terms On being addressed, however, by name, and recognising the speaker, and his attention being directed to the *whaled* and even bloody state of the dog, he offered the best excuse that he could.

We met again some months afterwards. "That hiding," said he, "that offended you so much did Carlo good, for he has not been touched since." "No," was the reply; "you were a little ashamed of your fellows, and have altered your system, and find that your dogs do not want this unmerciful negro-whipping."

Stories are told of the *kennel-hare*—a hare kept on purpose, and which is sometimes shown to the fox or stag-hounds. The moment that any of them open, they are tied up to the whipping-post, and flogged, while the keepers at every stroke call out "Ware hare!" A sheep has also been shown to them, or still is, after which another unmerciful flogging is administered, amidst cries of "Ware sheep!" If this is not sufficient, some of the wool is dipped in train oil, and put into the dog's mouth, which is sewed up for many hours in order to cure him of sheep-biting. There was an almost similar punishment for killing poultry; and there was the *puzzle* and the *check-collar*, cruelly employed, for killing other dogs.

There is a great deal of truth, and there may occasionally be some exaggeration, in these accounts; but the sportsman who is indebted for the pleasures of the field to the intelligence and exertions of his horses and his dogs, is bound, by every principle that can influence an honourable mind, to defend them from all wanton and useless cruelty. There is a dog, and a faithful and valuable one, that powerfully demands the assistance of the humane—the yard or watch-dog. He is not only for the most part deprived of his liberty, but too often neglected and made unnecessarily to suffer. How seldom do we see him in the enjoyment of a good bed of straw, or, rather, how frequently is everything about his kennel in a most filthy and disgusting state! The following hint not only relates to him, but to every dog that is tied up out of doors. "Their cribs or their kennels, as they are called, should be constructed so as to turn, in order to prevent their inmates from being exposed to the cutting blasts of winter. Where they have no other refuge, all animals seek shelter from the weather by turning their backs to the wind; but, as the dog thus confined cannot do so, his kennel should be capable of turning, or at least should be placed so as not to face the weather more than is necessary. The premises would be in quite as great security, for the dog depends as much upon his ear and sense of smell as upon his eye, and would equally detect a stranger's presence if he were deprived of sight."

In the Zoological Gardens, an old blind dog used to be placed at the door of the dissecting-house. Few had any business there, and every one of them he, after a while, used to recognise and welcome full ten yards off, by wagging his tail; at the same distance, he would begin to growl at a stranger unless accompanied by a friend. From the author's long habit of noticing him, he used to recognise his step before it would seem possible for its sound to be heard. He followed him with his sightless eyes in whatever direction he moved, and was not satisfied until he had patted and fondled him.

DOG-PITS.

Of the demoniacal use of the dog in the *fighting-pits*, and the atrocities that were committed there, I will not now speak. These places were frequented by few others than the lowest of the low Cruelties were there inflicted that seemed to be a libel on human nature; and such was the baneful influence of the scene, that it appeared to be scarcely possible for any one to enter these pits without experiencing a greater or less degree of moral degradation

The public dog-pits have now been put down; but the system of dog-fighting, with most of its attendant atrocities, still continues. There are many more low public-houses than there used to be pits, that have roomy places behind, and out of sight, where there are regular meetings for this purpose. Those among the neighbours who cannot fail of being annoyed and disgusted by the frequent uproar, might give a clue to these dens of infamy; and the depriving of a few of the landlords of their license would go a great way towards the effectual suppression of the practice.

Would it be thought possible that certain of our young aristocracy keep fighting-dogs at the repositories of various dealers in the outskirts of the metropolis; and that these animals remain there, as it were, at livery, the owners coming at their pleasure, and making and devising what matches they think proper?

However disgraceful it may be, it is actually the fact. Here is a field for "the suppression of cruelty!"

DOG-STEALING.

The practice of stealing dogs is both directly and indirectly connected with a great deal of cruelty. There are more than twenty miscreants who are well known to subsist by picking up dogs in the street. There are generally two of them together with aprons rolled round their waists. The dog is caught up at the corner of one of the streets, concealed in a moment in the apron, and the thieves are far away before the owner suspects the loss. These dogs, that have been used to every kind of luxury, are crowded into dark and filthy cellars, where they become infected by various diseases. The young ones have distemper, and the old ones mange, and all become filled with vermin. There they remain until a sufficient reward is offered for their recovery, or they are sent far into the country, or shipped for France or some other foreign market. Little or nothing is done by punishing the inferior rogues in this traffic. The blow must be struck at those of a superior class. I will not assert that every dog-dealer is in league with, and profits by, the lower thieves; but it is true of a great many of them, and it is the principal and most lucrative part of their trade. They are likewise intimately connected with the dog-fights, and encourage them, for the sake of their trade as dealers. An attempt should be made to bring the matter home to these scoundrels.[a]

[Dog-stealing, we are more particularly informed by Col. Hawker, is reduced to a perfect system in London, and carried on by a set of fellows who, by their cunning and peculiar knack, are enabled to avoid all detection in their nefarious traffic, and thus, by extortion of rewards or sales of stolen dogs, reap a rich harvest for the whole fraternity from the well-stored pockets of the numerous dog-fanciers of the English capital.

The villains engaged in this business are known among themselves under the too often abused sobriquet of "the Fancy," and assuming the garb of different mechanics, prowl about the streets, oftentimes with the proper tools in their hands, carelessly watching the movements of every dog that passes by, ready to grab him up the first fitting opportunity. The dog is then concealed till a suitable reward is offered for him, when, through the intervention of a third person, a trusty agent of the society, he is delivered over to his rightful owner, the actual rogue never appearing in the whole transaction.

If no reward, or an insufficient one, is offered for the recovery of the dog, he is either sent off to the country, or, perhaps, cautiously exposed for sale in some distant quarter of the city, or perhaps killed for his skin alone.

These gentry, however, prefer returning dogs to their owners for a moderate compensation, as they thus know at what rate the animal is valued, and cherish the hope of soon being able to steal him again, and thus obtaining another reward.

---

[a] Mr. Bishop, of Bond-street, has assured the public, that he is able to prove that money has recently been extorted from the owners of dogs by dog-stealers and their confederates, to the amount of more than a thousand pounds. Surely this calls for the decided interposition of the legislature. A strange case of atrocity and cruelty was related by a gentleman to Mr. Bishop. "A young dog of mine," says he, "was lost in London, and, being aware that, if a noise was made about it, a great price would be asked for it, I gave out that I wanted to purchase one: I was shown my own dog. I seized it; but there were several scoundrels present who professed to belong to it, and threatened to kill the dog if I did not pay for it. I proceeded to describe it as my own, stating that it had *bad back or double teeth.* Judge of my surprise when, after great difficulty, and the dog crying greatly, its mouth was opened, and all the back teeth had been taken out! I paid two pounds for it before they would let me take it away; but, in consequence of the injuries it had received, it died a few days afterward.'

There have been instances of a lady paying, in successive rewards, a sum not less than fifteen guineas for a miserable little lap-dog not worth as many shillings.

If anything is said about the law, or threats of prosecution held out in the notice offering a reward for a "lost or stolen dog," the death of the kidnapped animal is inevitable, as the "Fancy" prefer sacrificing an occasional prize rather than run the risk of detection by some enthusiastic or stubborn dog owner. These fellows, as well as thieves generally, are said to have a method of quieting the fiercest watch-dogs by throwing them a narcotic ball, which they call "puddening the animal."

The following account, extracted from Hawker's work, will give the American reader a *perfect* insight into the manœuvering of these sharpers.

"In the month of May, 1830, Mr. Lang lost a favourite setter. He posted handbills offering two guineas reward; on hearing of which a man came and told him the reward was not enough, but that if he would make it four guineas he could find his dog, and the amount must be deposited in the hands of a landlord who would procure him a ticket-card. He should then be met to his appointment in some private field, where he would receive his dog on condition that no questions should be asked. Mr. Lang sent his shopman, about half-past ten at night, to White Conduit Fields to meet the parties, who, on receiving the ticket, delivered up the dog. But there was great hesitation in transacting this affair, in consequence of the dog having on a lock to a steel chain collar with Mr. Lang's name, and which, therefore, induced them to proceed with extreme caution, through fear, as they supposed, of detection for felony. The whole amount paid for recovering this setter was £4 17*s*., £2 10*s*. of which went to the men who had him. The rest was divided among others of the "Fancy." The same person who gave Mr. Lang the information, said that if ever he lost a dog, and applied to him, he could undertake to get him back again within thirty-six hours, provided he would make it worth his while to do so; because all dogs taken by the "Fancy" are brought to their office and regularly booked by the secretary." (*Hawker on Shooting*, p. 592.)—L.]

INTRODUCTION TO CANINE PATHOLOGY.

BY THE EDITOR.

PREDISPOSITION TO, AND CAUSES OF, DISEASES IN DOGS. — THE CLAIMS OF DOGS UPON US.

> "Unnumbered accidents and various ills
> Attend thy pack, hang hovering o'er their heads,
> And point the way that leads to death's dark cave.
> Short is their span, few at the date arrive
> Of ancient Argus, in old Homer's song
> So highly honour'd."

THE dog from early youth, in fact oftentimes at the very period of birth, is exposed to many dangerous and troublesome affections, the result of causes not less complex and multifarious than those that exert an influence over the human organization. Many diseases are the consequence of their domesticity and the hereditary defects of their progenitors, others are dependent upon accidental circumstances, bad treatment, and improper nourishment. Not a few, however, of their most mortal maladies are the production of contagion, infection, and other like causes, all exercising a general tendency to disease difficult to define and impossible to avoid.

Although every species of dog is more or less subject to certain diseases peculiar to their race, those breeds of most value and more particularly subservient to the will of man are liable to a greater number of ills and casualties than other dogs, for the reason that they are more frequently exposed to unnatural fatigue, extremes of heat and cold, as also to the various dangers dependent upon the chase of wild animals. Those diseases resulting from specific causes, either natural to the race or artificially produced by the animal itself in a state of morbid derangement, are most frequent and fatal, as witnessed in distemper, rabies, mange, &c. The intimate connexion existing between the diseases of our canine friends and those of the human race, as also the strong similarity in the action of many drugs over the two systems, render the study of one branch almost synonymous with that of the other.

A little attention, therefore, on the part of the physician will render him quite familiar with and competent to relieve the many sufferings of these our most faithful and grateful of companions, and at the same time create an interest in a study that cannot fail to be productive of pleasure as well as information.

This subject, though claiming the attention of many skilful and intelligent persons in England and other countries, has scarce been thought of among us, and the mere mention of an infirmary or hospital for the accommodation of invalid dogs, would involuntarily create a smile of incredulity or contempt upon the face of most of our countrymen. Notwithstanding this display of ignorance and positive want of humane feeling for animal suffering, or a just appreciation of canine worth, we must beg leave to inform these unbelievers that such institutions are quite numerous in many large cities of the old world; and they must also learn that these institutions are conducted by gentlemen of science upon a system not less regular and useful in this particular branch, than similar establishments appropriated for the relief of suffering humanity.

To these hospitals hundreds of valuable sick dogs are annually sent, where they receive every attention, and are often snatched from the very jaws of death, or prevented, when attacked by rabies or other frightful affections, from doing mischief or propagating infection. Medicines the most potent are administered to these interesting patients with the utmost care, either as assuagers of temporary pain, or as remedial agents in the cure of disease. Operations the most complex are performed with the greatest skill, and every attention is bestowed upon these invalids in their different wards, and no trouble is considered too great to save the life and secure the services of a valuable and faithful dog.

As we have no such establishments in this country, and but few persons upon whom we can rely for assistance in case of need, it behooves every lover of the dog to make himself familiar with, and the mode of treating the most prominent affections of these companions of our sports, and at the same time acquire a knowledge of the operations of certain medicines upon the system in a state of health or disease, so that our trusty followers may not be left to the tender mercies and physicking propensities of ignorant stablemen, or the officious intermeddling of the "*pill-directing horse doctor.*"

The necessity of resorting to the assistance of either one or the other of these worthies is equally unfortunate, as the former will most generally kill the patient by slow degrees in forcibly and largely administering the two modern specifics for all canine affections, viz.: "soap pills and flowers of sulphur." While the latter, more bold but not less ignorant than the former, and his practice is perhaps the preferable of the two evils, will murder the dog outright by the free exhibition of calomel, nux vomica and other deleterious substances, of the operation of which he has but little knowledge or conception. This latter system, as before said, is the most preferable, as its adoption secures for our favourite a speedy termination of his sufferings, and also relieves our own minds from a state of suspense that illustrates too forcibly the remark, "Hope deferred maketh the heart sick."

REMEDIAL MEANS FOR THE CURE OF DISEASES.

There are but few remedies useful for the cure of diseases in the human race that might not be employed by a skilful practitioner in overcoming the same or different ailments in the dog. There are, however, several drugs that cannot be used in the same proportions for the one as for the other, without danger of producing fatal consequences, as instanced in calomel, a medicine so often abused by those who pretend to a knowledge of its administration in the maladies of dogs.

This article, though given with impunity to mankind in doses varying from five grains to twenty grains, as also oftentimes administered to horses in quantities three or four times as great, without any appreciable effect, will not unfrequently, in minute doses of three grains to four grains, produce the most violent symptoms in the strongest dogs. We have seen severe vomiting and purging occasioned by these small doses, and we once salivated a large mastiff by the administration of two blue pills. It is thus that both the regular physician, and even the veterinary surgeon, unacquainted with this remarkable peculiarity, will make fatal mistakes; and how much oftener must such blunders take place when we intrust our canine friends to the care of stable-boys, or a "routine horse-doctor!"

Nux vomica, another medicine much used, and most important in the treatment of all nervous affections, is particularly noxious to dogs even in small quantities; a dose sufficient for a human subject under some circumstances, would almost inevitably destroy the animal under the same or analogous conditions.

A drachm of the powdered nux vomica is sufficient to destroy the largest and most powerful dog, while a few grains will sometimes produce death in a few minutes if administered to smaller animals.

We prescribed forty grains in a roll of butter for a worthless cur a short time since, which, as expected, produced great anxiety, difficulty of respiration, severe vomiting, tremors, spasmodic twitchings of the muscles, convulsions, and ultimate death in the course of half an hour. This powerful drug acts by causing a spasmodic stricture of the muscles engaged in respiration, as no signs of inflammation are observable in the stomach and other organs after death.

Spirits of turpentine, another remedy both simple and innocent in its operations upon the human economy, and so frequently prescribed for the expulsion of worms from the bowels, is a dangerous medicine for a dog, and will often in very small quantities prove fatal.

Aloes, a medicine more extensively used in canine pathology than any other in the materia medica, is also very peculiar in its operations upon these animals, they being able to bear immense doses of it, in fact quite sufficient to produce death if given to a hearty man.

Thus we might continue to enumerate other drugs which we have ascertained, from practical observation as well as the experiments of other, to exercise a peculiar action on the vital functions of the whole canine race, quite at variance with that common to both man and the other domestic animals.

In combating with the diseases of animals, the veterinary surgeon has more to contend with than the regular physician, and, in fact, should possess a knowledge and habit of observation even superior to the former; although the responsibility of his calling, in a moral sense, is much inferior to that of the other, as the importance of animal existence, under no circumstances, can be placed in comparison with that of human life: still acuteness of observation alone can direct him to the main cause of suffering in the brute creation, as the animal, though groaning under the most severe pains, cannot by any word of explanation point out to us the seat, the probable cause, or peculiar characteristics of such pain. We see that our dog is ill, he refuses his food, retires gloomily to his house, looks sullen, breathes heavy, is no longer delighted at our call. We cannot question him as to his feelings, or ask him to point out the particular region of his sufferings; we watch his motions, study his actions, and rely for our diagnosis upon general symptoms deduced from close observation.

Besides these external ocular evidences of morbid action, we have, as in the human subject, guides to direct us in forming a just opinion as to the nature of a dog's indisposition.

The state of the circulation is the first thing that should command our particular attention.

The pulse of dogs in health varies from one hundred to one hundred and twenty strokes per minute, according to the size and peculiar temperament of the animal, being more frequent in the small breeds.

The standard of the setter, pointer, hound, &c., may be stated at one hundred and five.

The action of the heart may be felt by placing the hand immediately over that organ, or applying the fingers to several points in the body and limbs where the large arteries are somewhat superficial, as on the inside of the fore-knee and the thigh of the hind-leg.

If the pulse in a state of rest exceeds the average standard in frequency, regularity, and softness, and a general feeling of uneasiness be present, together with reddened eyes, warm nose, and coated tongue, we know at once that there is an unnatural derangement of the vital functions, and that fever in some form is present. The next question to determine is, upon what does this fever depend? whether it be idiopathic, arising from morbific causes difficult to define, or whether it be sympathetic, with some organic affection yet to be discovered.

The appearance of the tongue in canine diseases will often materially assist us in forming a correct diagnosis; this organ in simple fever loses its rose-colour and becomes pale and coated, the gums and fauces also participate in this change.

If, however, the tongue be much furred, with a bright inflammatory appearance around the edges, with high arterial excitement, and disgust of food, with general anxiety and craving for water in small but frequent quantities, inflammation of the stomach or bowels may be suspected. If, on the other hand, the tongue remains brown and streaked, with less action of the pulse, variable appetite and diminution of pain, derangement of the liver may be apprehended.

If, in connection with some or all of the above symptoms, the breathing be laboured and painful, with a disposition to remain in the erect or sitting position, with great anxiety and general distress, we must look to the pulmonic viscera as the seat of the disease.

Thus, by examining each and every individual symptom of disease, the intelligent sportsman will soon be able to arrive at the proximate cause of all this unnatural state of things, and then he will be competent to administer such remedies as may seem most likely to afford relief. Without these precautions, however, he would often be groping in the dark, and, consequently, not unfrequently, apply those remedies more calculated to aggravate than cure the malady.

CHAPTER VI.

DESCRIPTION OF THE SKELETON.

DISEASES OF THE NERVOUS SYSTEM:—FITS; TURNSIDE, OR GIDDINESS EPILEPSY; CHOREA; RHEUMATISM AND PALSY.

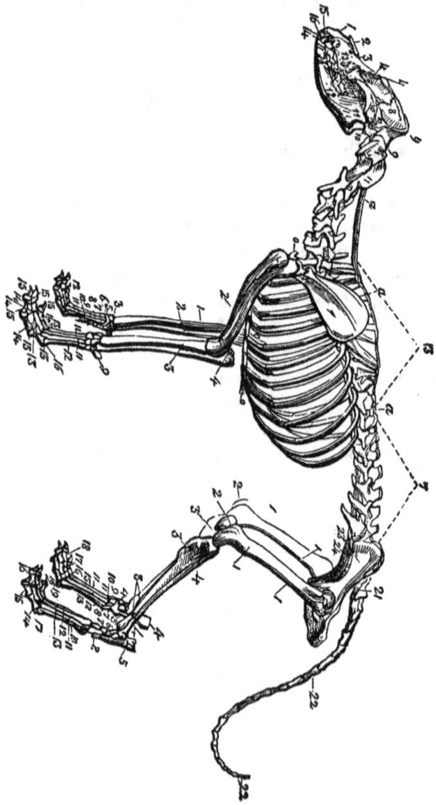

THE SKELETON OF THE DOG.

THE HEAD AND ITS FUNCTIONS.

1. The intermaxillary bone.
2. Nasal bone.
3. 3. Maxilla superior.
4. Lachrymal bone.
5. Zygomatic bone.
6. Orbit of the eye.
7. Frontal bone.
8. Summit of the head.
9. 9. Occipital bones.
10. 10. 10. Temporal bones.
11. 11. 11. Inferior maxillary or jaw bones.
12. 12. Seven inferior maxillary molar teeth.
13. 13. Six molar teeth of the superior jaw.
14. Canine teeth of the superior and inferior jaws.
15. Three incisor teeth of the superior maxillary bone.
16. The three inferior ditto.

THE TRUNK.

a. a. a. The ligamentum nuchæ.
I. II. III. IV. V. VI. VII. The seven vertebræ of the neck.
13. The thirteen dorsal vertebræ.
7. The seven lumbar vertebræ.
21. Os sacrum, or rump-bone.
22. 22. Twenty caudal vertebræ — vertebræ of the tail.
23. The left os innominatum.
24. Right ditto.
The nine true ribs, with their cartilages.
The four false ribs, with their cartilages.
o. The sternum.

THE LEFT ANTERIOR EXTREMITY.

1. The scapula, or shoulder-blade.
2. 2. Os humeri, or shoulder.
3. 3. Radius—the lesser bone of the arm.
4. 4. Ulna—the elbow.
5. Os naviculare—the navicular bone.
6. Os triquetrum, or triangulare.
7. Os pisiforme, or pisiform bone.
8. Os semilunare, or semilunar bone.
9. Os capitatum—the nail.
10. Os metacarpi digiti tertii — the third metacarpal bone.
11. Os metacarpi digiti quarti — fourth metacarpal.
12. Os metacarpi digiti quinti.
13. 13. 13. 13. The first digits of the fore-feet
14. 14. 14. 14. The second ditto.
15. The third ditto.
16. The sessamoid bone.

THE RIGHT ANTERIOR EXTREMITY.

1. 1. Radius.
2. Ulna—elbow.
3. Os triquetrum—the triangular bone.
4. Os naviculare—the navicular bone.
5. Os semilunare—the semilunar bone.
6. Os multangulum majus—the larger multangular bone.
7. Os multangulum minus—the small multangular bone.
8. Os metacarpi pollicis—the thumb.
9. Ossa metacarpi digitorum quatuor—the four bones of the metacarpi.
10. Phalanx prima pollicis—first phalange of the thumb.
11. Phalanx tertia pollicis—third phalange of ditto.
12. Digiti quatuor — fourth phalange of ditto.

THE LEFT POSTERIOR EXTREMITY.

1. 1. Os femoris—thigh-bone.
2. 2. Patella—the knee-pan.
3. 3. Tibia—the shank of the leg.
4. 4. Fibula—the small bone of ditto.
5. Calcareus—the heel.
6. Astragalus — one of the seven bones of the tarsus.
7. Os naviculare—the navicular bone.
8. Os cuboideum—or cubic bone.
9. Os cuneiforma tertium et maximum.
10. Os metatarsi digiti quarti.
11. Os metatarsi digiti tertii.
12. Os metatarsi digiti secundi.
13. Os metatarsi digiti primi.
14. Phalanges primæ digitorum pedis.
15. Phalanges secundæ.
16. Phalanges tertiæ.
17. Os sesamoideum—the sessamoid.

THE RIGHT POSTERIOR EXTREMITY.

1. Os femoris—the thigh-bone.
2. Patella—the knee-pan.
3. Tibia—the shank of the leg.
4. Calcareus—the heel.
5. Astragalus—one of the seven bones of the tarsus.
7. Os naviculare—the navicular bone.
8. Os cuneiforma primum et medium.
9. Os cuboideum, or cubic bone.
10. Os cuneiforma tertium et maximum.
11. Os cuneiforma secundum et minimum.
12. Radimentum ossis metatarsi hallucis
13. Os metatarsi digiti primi.
14. Os metatarsi digiti secundi.
15. Os metatarsi digiti tertii.
16. Phalanges primæ digitorum pedis.
17. Phalanges secundæ.
18. Phalanges tertiæ.
19. Os sesamoideum—the sessamoid.

DISEASES OF THE NERVOUS SYSTEM.

FITS.

24th Feb. 1814. — A pug was accustomed to howl frequently when his young master played on the flute. If the higher notes were sounded, he would leap on his master's lap, look in his face, and howl vehemently. To-day the young man purposely blew the shrillest sound that he could. The dog, after howling three or four times, began to run round the room, and over the tables and chairs, barking incessantly. This he continued more than an hour.

When I saw him all consciousness of surrounding objects was gone. He was still running feebly, but barking might and main.

I dashed a basin of cold water in his face, and he dropped as if he had been shot. He lay motionless nearly a minute, and then began to struggle and to bark; another cup of water was dashed in his face, and he lay quite motionless during two minutes or more. In the mean time I had got a grain each of calomel and tartar emetic, which I put on his tongue, and washed it down with a little water. He began to recover, and again began to yelp, although much softer; but, in about a quarter of an hour, sickness commenced, and he ceased his noise. He vomited three or four times, and lay frightened and quiet. A physic-ball was given him in the evening, and on the following morning.

On the next day, the young man put open the door, and sat himself down, and began to prepare the flute; the dog was out in a moment, and did not return during a couple of hours. On the following day he made his escape again, and so the matter went on; but before the expiration of the week, his master might play the flute if he pleased.

TURNSIDE, OR GIDDINESS.

This is a singular disease prevalent among cattle, but only occasionally seen in the dog. He becomes listless, dull, off his food, and scarcely recognises any surrounding object. He has no fit, but he wanders about the room for several hours at a time, generally or almost invariably in the same direction, and with his head on one side. At first he carefully avoids the objects that are in his way; but by degrees his mental faculties become impaired; his sense of vision is confused or lost, and he blunders against everything: in fact, if uninterrupted, he would continue his strange perambulation incessantly, until he was fairly worn out and died in convulsions.

I used to consider the complaint to be uniformly fatal. I have resorted to every remedial measure that the case could suggest. I have bled, and physicked and setoned, and blistered, and used the moxa; but all without avail, for not in a single case did I save my patient

No opportunity of *post-mortem* examination was lost. In some cases I have found spicula projecting from the inner plate of the skull, and pressing upon or even penetrating the dura mater. I know not why the dog should be more subject to these irregularities of cranial surface than any of our other patients; but decidedly he is so, and where they have pressed upon the brain, there has been injection of the membranes, and sometimes effusion between them.

In some cases I have found effusion without this external pressure, and, in some cases, but comparatively few, there has not been any perceptible lesion. Hydatids have been found in the different passages leading to the cranium, but they have not penetrated.

I used to recommend that the dog should be destroyed; but I met with two or three favourable cases, and, after that, I determined to try every measure that could possibly be serviceable. I bled, and physicked, and inserted setons, and tried to prevent the utter exhaustion of the animal. When he was unable longer to perform his circumvolutions, and found that he was foiled, he laid himself down, and by degrees resumed his former habits. He was sadly impatient and noisy; but in a few cases he was cured.

[We have seen but two or three cases of this disease in dogs, and are led to believe that it is quite uncommon with our domestic animals. One case in a valuable setter came on suddenly, and without any apparent cause (except perhaps over-feeding), and terminated fatally in the course of a few days.—L.]

EPILEPSY

in the dog assumes a most fatal character. It is an accompaniment, or a consequence, of almost every other disease. When the puppy is undergoing the process of dentition, the irritation produced by the pressure of the tooth, as it penetrates the gum, leads on to epilepsy. When he is going through the stages of distemper, with a very little bad treatment, or in spite of the best, fits occur. The degree of intestinal irritation which is caused by worms, is marked by an attack of epilepsy. If the usual exercise be neglected for a few days, and the dog is taken out, and suffered to range as he likes, the accumulation of excitability is expended in a fit.

The dog is, without doubt, the most intellectual animal. He is the companion and the friend of man: he exhibits, and is debased by some of his vices; but, to a greater degree than many will allow, he exhibits all the intelligence and the virtues of the biped. In proportion to his bulk, the weight of his brain far exceeds that of any other quadruped—the very smallest animals alone being excepted, in whom there must be a certain accumulation of medullary matter in order to give origin to the nerves of every system, as numerous in the minutest as in him of greatest bulk.

As it has been said of the human being that great power and exertion of the mental faculties are sometimes connected with a tendency to epilepsy, and, as violent emotions of joy or of grief have been known to be followed by it, I can readily account for its occurrence in the young dog, when frightened at the chiding of his master, or by the dread of a punishment which he was conscious that he had deserved. Then, too, I can understand that, when breaking loose from long confinement, he ranges in all the exuberance of joy; and especially when he flushes almost his first covey, and the game falls dead before him, his mental powers are quite overcome, and he falls into an epileptic fit.

The treatment of epilepsy in the dog is simple, yet often misunderstood. It is connected with distemper in its early stage. It is the produce of inflammation of the mucous passages generally, which an emetic and a purgative will probably, by their direct medicinal effect, relieve, and free the digestive passages from some source of irritation, and by their mechanical action unburthen the respiratory ones.

When it is symptomatic of a weak state of the constitution, or connected with the after stages of distemper, the emeto-purgative must be succeeded by an anodyne, or, at least, by that which will strengthen, but not irritate the patient.

A seton is an admirable auxiliary in epilepsy connected with distemper; it is a counter-irritant and a derivative, and its effects are a salutary discharge, under the influence of which inflammation elsewhere will gradually abate.

I should, however, be cautious of bleeding in distemper fits. I should be fearful of it even in an early stage, because I well know that the acute form of that general mucous inflammation soon passes over, and is succeeded by a debility, from the depression of which I cannot always rouse my patient. When the fits proceed from dentition, I lance the jaws, and give an emetic, and follow it up with cooling purgative medicine. When they are caused by irregular and excessive exercise, I open the bowels and make my exercise more regular and equable. When they arise from excitation, I expose my patient more cautiously to the influence of those things which make so much impression on his little but susceptible mind.

If the fit has resisted other means, bleeding should be resorted to. A fit in other animals is generally connected with dangerous determination of blood to the head, and bleeding is imperative.

A fit in the dog may be the consequence of sudden surprise and irritation. If I had the means I should see whether I could not break the charm; whether I could not get rid of the disturbance, by suddenly affecting the nervous system, and the system generally, in another way. I would seize him by the nape of the neck, and, with all my force, dash a little cold water in his face. The shock of this has often dispersed the epileptic agency, as it were by magic. I would give an emeto-purgative; a grain or a grain and a half of calomel and the same quantity of tartar emetic: I would soothe and coax the poor animal. Then,—and if I saw it at the beginning, I would do it early,—if the fit was more dependent upon, or was beginning to be connected with, determination of blood to the head, and not on any temporary cause of excitation or irritation, I would bleed freely from the jugular.

The folowing singular case of epilepsy is narrated by M. W. Leblanc:—

A dog of small size, three years old, was very subject to those epileptic fits that are so frequent among dogs. After a considerable period, the fits would cease, and the animal recover the appearance of perfect health; but the more he advanced in age the more frequent were the fits, which is contrary to that which usually happens.

The last fit was a very strong one, and was followed by peculiar symptoms. The animal became dispirited. The eyes lost their usual lively appearance, and the eyelids were often closed. The dog was very drowsy, and, during sleep, there were observed, from time to time, spasmodic movements, principally of the head and chest. *He always lay down on the left side.* When he walked, he had a marked propensity to turn to the left.

M. Leblanc employed purgatives, a seton to the back part of the neck, and the application of the cautery to the left side of the forehead; but nothing would stop the progress of the disease, and he died in the course of two months after the last fit. The nearer he approached his end the smaller were the circles that he took; and, in the latter part of his existence, he did little more than turn as if he were on a pivot, and, when the time arrived that he could walk no more, he used to lay himself down on the right side.

On the *post-mortem* examination, a remarkable thickness of the meninges was found on almost the whole of the left lobe of the brain. The dura mater, the two leaves of the arachnoid membrane, and the pia mater did not constitute more than one membrane of the usual thickness, and presented a somewhat yellow colouring. The cerebral substance of the left lobe appeared to be a little firmer than that of the right lobe. The fissures of the cerebral convolutions were much less deep than those of the other side

The red vessels which ran in the fissures were of smaller size, and in some places could scarcely be discovered.

[Confinement, over-feeding, blows on the head or spine, drying up of old ulcers, repelling of cutaneous affections, or, in fact, anything that is liable to derange the general health of the animal, will produce epileptic fits.

We formerly had a beagle hound of very active temperament, which we were necessarily obliged to keep much confined while in the city; and to restrain her from running too wildly when taken into the streets, we were in the habit of coupling her with a greyhound of much milder disposition. Not being willing to submit tamely to this unpleasant check upon her liberty, she was ever making fruitless attempts to escape, either by thrusting herself forwards, or obstinately pulling backwards. These efforts resulted on several occasions in fits, produced by congestion of the brain, owing to the pressure of the collar on the neck, thereby interrupting the circulation, and inducing an influx of blood to those parts. We were ultimately obliged to abandon this method of restraint, which nearly proved fatal to our much-admired beagle: she being suddenly seized with one of these fits on a hot summer's day in one of our principal thoroughfares, the crowd of ignorant bystanders concluded it to be a case of rabies, and nothing but my taking her up in my arms, and carrying her from the scene of action, saved her from falling a victim to their ignorance.

If the disease appears dependent upon plethora the result of confinement and gross living, the animal must be reduced by bleeding and purging, low diet, and exercise. If, however, the malady proceeds from weakness, as is sometimes the case in bitches while suckling a large litter, it will be necessary to relieve her of some of the pups, and supply her with the most nutritious diet, as also administer tonic balls; the following will answer.

℞ Extract of Gentian,
" Quassia, â â (each) grs. V, made into two pills, and one or two given morning and evening; or,

℞ Powdered Columbo.
Carbonate of Iron, â â, grs. V, made into two pills, and one given morning and evening, or more frequently if desirable.

A seton placed in the pole will often prevent these attacks, particularly when depending upon slight cerebral irritation, accompanying distemper and mange. Blisters and frictions to the spine are also serviceable.—L.]

CHOREA.

This is an irregular reception or distribution of nervous power —a convulsive involuntary twitching of some muscle or set of muscles. It is an occasional consequence of distemper that has been unusually severe or imperfectly treated, and sometimes it is seen even after that disease has existed in its mildest form.

[This nervous affection, more commonly known as St. Vitus' dance, is not a rare disease, and we doubt not that examples of it have been seen by most of our readers, more particularly in young dogs affected with distemper.

This malady is characterized by sudden involuntary twitchings of the different muscles of the body, the disease being sometimes confined to one limb, sometimes to two, and frequently pervades the whole system, giving the dog a distressing and painful appearance. These involuntary motions, it is very true, are generally restricted during sleep, although in old chronic cases of long standing they often continue in full activity without any remission whatever. The disease is not attended with fever, and all the functions generally remain for a considerable time unimpaired. —L.]

It first appears in one leg or shoulder, and is long, or perhaps entirely, confined to that limb. There is a singular spasmodic jerking action of the limb. It looks like a series of pulsations, and averages from forty to sixty in a minute. Oftener, perhaps, than otherwise, both legs are similarly affected. When the animal is lying down, the legs are convulsed in the way that I have described, and when he stands there is a pulsating depressing or sinking of the head and neck. In some cases, the muscles of the neck are the principal seat of the disease, or some muscle of the face; the temporal muscle beating like an artery; the masseter opening and closing the mouth, the muscles of the eyelid, and, in a few cases, those of the eye itself being affected. These convulsive movements generally, yet not uniformly, cease during sleep, but that sleep is often very much disturbed. If the case is neglected, and the dog is in a debilitated state, this spasmodic action steals over the whole frame, and he lies extended with every limb in constant and spasmodic action.

In the majority of cases, such an expenditure of nervous and muscular power slowly destroys the strength of the animal, and he dies a mere skeleton; or the disease assumes the character of epilepsy, or it quiets down into true palsy.

In the most favourable cases, no curative means having been used, the dog regains his flesh and general strength; but the chorea continues, the spasmodic action, however, being much lessened. At other times, it seems to have disappeared; but it is ready to return when the animal is excited or attacked by other disease. In a variety of instances, there is the irritable temper which accompanies chorea in the human being, and most certainly when the disease has been extensive and confirmed.

Chorea, neglected or improperly treated, or too frequently pursuing its natural course, degenerates into paralysis agitans. There is a tremulous or violent motion of almost every limb. The spasms are not relaxed, but are even increased during sleep, and when the animal awakes, he rises with agitation and alarm. There is not a limb under the perfect control of the will; there is not a moment's respite; the constitution soon sinks, and the animal dies. No person should be induced to undertake the cure of such a case: the owner should be persuaded to permit a speedy termination to a life which no skill can render comfortable.

Chorea is oftenest observed in young dogs, and especially after distemper; and it seems to depend on a certain degree of primary or sympathetic inflammatory affection of the brain.

Chorea is often very plainly a consequence of debility: either the distribution of nervous power is irregular, or the muscles have lost their power of being readily acted upon, or have acquired a state of morbid irritability. The latter is the most frequent state. Their action is irregular and spasmodic, and it resembles the struggles of expiring nature far more than the great and uniform action of health. It is not the chorea that used to be described, in which there was an irresistible impulse to excessive action, and which was best combated by complete muscular exhaustion; but the foundation of this disease is palpable debility.

[Rickets, bad feeding, cold and damp housing, worms in the alimentary canal, mange, and other chronic affections, are all forerunners of this malady.—L.]

In the treatment of chorea there must be no bleeding, no excessive purgation, but aperients or alteratives, merely sufficient to keep the fœces in a pultaceous state, so as to carry off any source of irritation to the intestinal canal, and particularly some species of worms, too frequent sources of irritation there. To these should be added nutritious food, gentle exercise, tonic medicines, and general comforts. Counter-irritants may be applied—such as blisters over the head, and setons, extending from poll to poll—the application of turpentine, or the tincture of cantharides; but all of these will frequently be of no effect, and occasionally a rapid and fearful increase of irritability will ensue: antispasmodics are in this case of no use, and narcotics are altogether powerless. As for tonics, iron and gentian have been serviceable to a certain extent, but they have never cured the complaint. The nitrate of silver will be the sheet-anchor of the practitioner, and if early used will seldom deceive him. It should be combined with ginger, and given morning and night, in doses varying from one-sixth to one-third of a grain, according to the size of the dog.

The condition and strength of the dog, and the season of the year, will be our best guides. If the patient has not lost much flesh, *and is not losing it* at the time that we have to do with him, and has few symptoms of general debility, and spring or summer are approaching, we may with tolerable confidence predict a cure; but, if he has been rapidly losing ground, and is doing so still, and staggers about and falls, there is no medicine that will restore him.

5th October, 1840.—A pointer, eighteen months old, had had the distemper, but not severely, and was apparently recovering, when he suddenly lost all voluntary power over his limbs. He was unable to get up, and his legs were in constant, rapid, and violent motion. This continued three days, during which he had refused all food, when, the dog being in the country, my advice was asked. I ordered a strong emetic to be given to him, and after that a dose of Epsom salts, the insertion of a seton, and, in addition to this, our usual tonic was to be given twice every day. His food to consist chiefly of good strong soup, which was to be forced upon him in a sufficient quantity.

In two days he was able to get up and stagger about, although frequently falling. His appetite returned. He continued to improve, and most rapidly gained strength and especially flesh. A very peculiar, high-lifting, clambering, and uncertain motion of the legs remained, with an apparent defect of sight, for he ran against almost everything.

In six weeks the seton was removed, and the dog remained in the same state until the 7th of December. The uncertain clambering motion was now increasing, and likewise the defect of sight. He ran against almost every person and every thing. The cornea was transparent, the iris contracted, there was no opacity of the lens, or pink tint of the retina, but a peculiar glassy appearance, as unconscious of everything around it. An emetic was given, and, after that, an ounce of sulphate of magnesia.

8th. He was dreadfully ill after taking the salts; perhaps they were not genuine. For two days he panted sadly, refused his food, and vomited that which was forced upon him. His muzzle was hot; he could scarcely stand; he lost flesh very rapidly. An emetic was given immediately, and a distemper-ball daily.

16th. He soon began rapidly to recover, until he was in nearly the same state as before, except that the sight was apparently more deficient. The sulphate of magnesia was given every fourth day, and another seton inserted.

21st. He continued the medicine, and evidently improved, the sight returning, and the spasms being considerably less. The distemper-ball was continued.

4th January, 1841.—The spasms were better; but the vision did not improve. In the afternoon he fell into a momentary fit. He almost immediately rose again, and proceeded as if nothing had happened. An ounce of Epsom salts was given, and then the tonic balls as before.

22*d.* The spasms were lessened, the clambering gait nearly ceased, but the vision was not improved. The seton was removed, and only an additional dose of salts given.

27*th.* The spasms suddenly and very considerably increased. The left side appeared now to be particularly affected. The left leg before and behind were most spasmed, the right scarcely at all so. The vision of the left eye was quite gone. The dog had been taken to Mr. Alexander's, the oculist, who attributed the affection of the eye and the general spasmodic disease to some pressure on the brain, and recommended the trial of copious and repeated bleeding.

28*th.* The dog was dull; the spasms appeared to have somewhat increased and decidedly to affect the left side. Fever-balls were ordered to be given.

29*th.* Considerable change took place. At three o'clock this morning I was disturbed by a noise in the hospital. The poor fellow was in a violent fit. Water was dashed in his face, and a strong emetic given; but it was not until seven o'clock that the fit had ceased; he lay until eleven o'clock, when the involuntary spasms were almost suspended. When he was placed on his feet, he immediately fell; he then gradually revived and staggered about. His master brought a physician to see him, who adopted Mr. Alexander's idea and urged bleeding. Ten ounces of blood were immediately taken; the dog refused to eat.

1*st February.*—The strength of the animal was not impaired, but the spasms were more violent, and he lay or wandered about stupid and almost unconscious. I subtracted eight ounces more of blood.

2*d.* The spasms were fully as violent, and no amendment in the vision. Eight ounces more of blood were subtracted without benefit. A fever-ball was ordered to be given.

3*d.* No amendment; but the bleeding having been carried to its full extent, I again resorted to the tonic balls, which were given morning and night. The dog was well fed and the seton replaced.

5*th.* A very considerable amendment is evident.

9*th.* The spasms rapidly subsided and almost disappeared. Vision was not perfectly restored; but the dog evidently saw with his left eye. He was taken away, and tonic-balls sent with him and ordered to be continued.

6*th March.*—The dog had improved in strength and no spasmodic affection remained; he likewise evidently saw with his left eye. The tonic-balls had been discontinued for a week, and his master hoped that all would turn out well, when suddenly, while at home, he was seized with a fit that lasted ten minutes. A strong emetic was given, which brought up a vast quantity of undigested food. A strong purging-ball was given to him in the evening.

13th. The dog had lain slightly spasmed for two or three days, when they all at once ceased, and the animal appeared as well as before. Suddenly he was taken with another fit, and again a vast quantity of food was vomited. These spasms remained two days, but on the 21st the fit returned with the same discharge of food. Courses of purgatives were then determined on. A strong dose of sulphate of magnesia was given every third day. After four doses had been given, it was impossible to force any more upon him. The syrup of buckthorn was tried, but the fourth dose of that it was impossible to give. The dog was then sent into the country; no fit occurred, but there were occasional spasms.

23d September.—He was brought back to town, and I saw him. During the last month he had had many fits. His owner at length consented that the actual cautery should be applied to his head. The searing-iron for doctoring was used, and applied red-hot to the centre of the head. It was exceedingly difficult so to confine the dog as to make the application effectual, without destroying the skin.

Under the influence of the sudden violent pain, he wandered about for more than two hours, and then the spasms returned with greater force than usual. He refused all food.

We determined to try the cautery to its full extent. We chained him up in the morning, and penetrated through the skin with the budding-iron. The spasms were dreadfully violent, and he was scarcely able to walk or to stand. This gradually subsided, and then he began to run round and round, and that increased to an extraordinary velocity: he would then lie for a while with every limb in action. The owner then yielded to all our wishes, and he was destroyed with prussic acid. No morbid appearance presented itself in the brain; but, on the inner plate of the right parietal bone, near the sagittal suture, were two projections, one-sixth of an inch in length, and armed with numerous minute spicula. There was no peculiar inflammation or vascularity of any other part of the brain.

[We once cured a case quite accidentally, by throwing a pup into a cold stream of water, and making him swim ashore; we do not recommend the plan, although we should be willing to try it again with one of our own dogs. The animal should be forced to swim till nearly exhausted, and wrapped up in blankets on coming out of the water. The intense alarm created in the pup, together with the violent struggle and coldness of the water, all act as revulsives to the disease, which, if purely nervous, may be overcome by these powerful agents.

If the dog be weak, and the stomach deranged, the following tonic balls will answer a good purpose:

℞. Carbonate of Iron.
Ground Ginger, â â, grs. X, made into two pills, one given morning and evening, or more frequently according to the age or size of the animal.—L.]

RHEUMATISM AND PALSY.

I do not know any animal so subject to *rheumatism* as the dog, nor any one in which, if it is early and properly treated, it is so manageable.

[We agree with our author, that the canine family are exceedingly liable to inflammation of the fibrous and muscular structures of the body, and there is no disease from which they suffer more, both in their youth and old age, than rheumatism. No particular species of dogs are more subject to its attacks than others, all being alike victims to its ravages. Mr. Blaine remarks, that the bowels always sympathize with other parts of the body suffering under this disease, and that inflammation will always be found existing in the abdominal viscera, if rheumatism be present, and the lower bowels will be attended with a painful torpor, which he designates as rheumatic colic. We ourselves noticed, that old setters particularly, when suffering from this disease, are frequently attacked with an acute diarrhœa, or suffer from obstinate constipation attended by griping pains, but did not know that this state of things was so uniform an accompaniment to the other affection. There are two varieties of rheumatism, the *acute* and *chronic*, both of which are attended with either general fever or local inflammation. The attacks usually come on rather suddenly, the joints swell, the pulse becomes full and tense, the parts tender, and the eyes blood-shot, the stomach deranged, and the bowels costive. Severe lancinating pain runs through the articulation, and along the course of the larger muscles, the tongue is coated, the muzzle hot and dry, and the poor animal howls with agony. The breathing becomes laboured, all food is rejected, and if you attempt to move the sufferer he sends forth piteous cries of distress. *The causes* of this serious affection are very numerous among the most usual and active agents may be enumerated, exposure to atmospherical vicissitudes, remaining wet and idle after coming from the water, damp kennels, suppressed perspiration, metastasis of eruptive diseases, luxurious living, laziness and overfeeding. These and many other causes are all busy in the production of this disease. Duck dogs on the Chesapeake, we have

17

noticed as often suffering from this affection, owing no doubt to the great exposure they are obliged to endure; but few of them arrive at old age without being martyrs to the chronic form. *Chronic rheumatism*, generally the result of the other form of disease, is most usually met with in old dogs: it is attended with little fever, although the local inflammation and swelling is sometimes considerable. The pain is often stationary in one shoulder or loin, at other times shifts about suddenly to other portions of the body. The muscles are tender and the joints stiff, the animal seems lame till he becomes heated, and limber when all appearance of the disease vanishes. In old cases the limbs become so much enlarged, and the joints so swollen, that the dog is rendered perfectly useless, and consequently increases his sufferings by idleness. *This form of the disease is known as gout.*

Treatment of *acute rheumatism*.—bleeding largely is very important in this affection, and if followed up with two or three purges of aloes, gamboge, colocynth and calomel will arrest the progress of this disease.

℞.	Extract of Colocynth	℈i.
	Calomel	grs. x.
	Powdered Gamboge	grs. ii.
	Socet. Aloes	grs. x.

Made into four pills, two to be given at night, and the other the following morning. If these medicines should not be handy, give a large purging ball of aloes, to be followed by a full dose of salts. When the inflammatory action is not sufficiently high to demand depletion, warm bathing, friction and keeping the dog wrapped up in blankets before a fire will generally afford relief. If the pain appear very severe, it will be necessary to repeat the baths at short intervals: great attention must be paid to the state of the bowels: if a diarrhœa supervenes, it must not be checked too suddenly, by the use of astringent medicines, but rather corrected by small doses of oil and magnesia. If constipation attended with colic be the character of the affection, small quantities of oil and turpentine in connexion with warm enemata will be the proper remedies. If paralysis should occur, it will be found very difficult to overcome, but must be treated, after the reduction of inflammation, upon principles laid down under the head of this latter affection. Blisters to the spine, setons, electricity, acupuncturation, &c.

Treatment of chronic rheumatism—warm baths are useful, and warm housing absolutely necessary, attention to diet, and an occasional purge of blue mass and aloes, together with electricity, acupuncture, rubefacient applications to the spine, &c.—L.]

A warm bath—perchance a bleeding—a dose or two of the castor-oil mixture, and an embrocation composed of spirit of turpentine, hartshorn, camphorated spirit, and laudanum, will usually remove it in two or three days, unless it is complicated with muscular sprains, or other lesions, such as the *chest-founder* of kennels.

This chest-founder is a singular complaint, and often a pest in kennels that are built in low situations, and where bad management prevails. Where the huntsman or whippers-in are too often in a hurry to get home, and turn their dogs into the kennel panting and hot; where the beds are not far enough from the floor, or the building, if it should be in a sufficiently elevated situation, has yet a northern aspect and is unsheltered from the blast, chest-founder prevails; and I have known half the pack affected by it after a severe run, the scent breast-high, and the morning unusually cold. It even occasionally passes on into palsy.

The veterinary surgeon will be sometimes consulted respecting this provoking muscular affection. His advice will comprise—dryness, attention to the bowels, attention to the exercise-ground, and perhaps, occasionally, setons—not where the huntsman generally places them, on the withers above, but on the brisket below, and defended from the teeth of the dog by a roller of a very simple construction, passing round the chest between the fore legs and over the front of the shoulders on either side.

The pointer, somewhat too heavy before, and hardly worked, becomes what is called chest-foundered. From his very make it is evident that, in long-continued and considerable exertion, the subscapular muscles will be liable to sprain and inflammation. There will be inflammation of the fasciæ, induration, loss of power, loss of nervous influence and palsy. Cattle, driven far and fast to the market, suffer from the same causes.

[By palsy, we mean a partial or complete loss of the powers of motion or sensation in some portion of the muscular system: this affection is very common to the canine race, and very few of them reach an advanced age without having at some time in their life experienced an attack of this malady.

The loins and hind legs suffer oftener than other parts, in fact we do not recollect ever meeting with paralysis of the fore limbs alone. Although the limbs become perfectly powerless, and are only dragged after the animal by the combined efforts of the fore legs and back, it is seldom that they lose their sensibility.—L.]

Palsy is frequent, as in the dog. However easy it may be to subdue a rheumatic affection, in its early stage, by prompt attention, yet if it is neglected, it very soon simulates, or becomes essentially connected with, or converted into, palsy.

No animal presents a more striking illustration of the connexion between intestinal irritation and palsy than the dog. He rarely or never has enteritis, even in its mildest form, without some loss of power over the hinder extremities. This may at first arise from the participation of the lumbar muscles with the intestinal irritation; but, if the disease of the bowels continues long, it will be evident enough that it is not pain alone that produces the constrained and incomplete action of the muscles of the hind extremities, but that there is an actual loss of nervous power. A dog is often brought to the veterinary surgeon, with no apparent disease about him except a staggering walk from weakness of the hind limbs. He eats well and is cheerful, and his muzzle is moist and cool; but his belly is tucked up, and there are two longitudinal cords, running parallel to each other, which will scarcely yield to pressure. The surgeon orders the castor-oil mixture twice or thrice daily, until the bowels are well acted upon, and, as soon as that is accomplished, the dog is as strong and as well as ever. Perhaps his hind limbs are dragged behind him; a warm bath is ordered, he is dosed well with the castor-oil mixture, and, if it is a recent case, the animal is well in a few days. In more confirmed palsy, the charge, or plaster on the loins, is added to the action of the aperient on the bowels. The process may be somewhat slow, but it is seldom that the dog does not ultimately and perfectly recover.

It is easy to explain this connexion, although we should have scarcely supposed that it would have been so intimate, had not frequent experience forced it on our observation. The rectum passes through the pelvis. Whatever may be said of that intestine, considering its vertical position in the human being, it is always charged with fæces in the quadruped. It therefore shares more in the effect, whatever that may be, which is produced by the retention of fæces in the intestinal canal, and it shares also in the inflammatory affection of other parts of the canal. Almost in contact with this viscus, or at least passing through the pelvis, are the crural nerves from the lumbar vertebræ, the obtusator running round the rim of the pelvis, the glutal nerve occupying its back, and the sciatic hastening to escape from it. It is not difficult to imagine that these, to a certain degree, will sympathize with the healthy and also the morbid state of the rectum; and that, when it is inert, or asleep, or diseased, they also may be powerless too. Here is something like fact to establish a very important theory, and which should be deeply considered by the sportsman and the surgeon.

[Loss of the contractile power of the sphincters of the bladder and rectum, sometimes attends this disease, and involuntary evacuations are constantly taking place, or costiveness and retention are the consequences.—L.]

Mr. Dupuy has given a valuable account of the knowledge we

possess of the diseases of the spinal marrow in our domestic quadrupeds.

He has proved—

1. That in our domestic animals the spinal marrow is scarcely ever affected through the whole of its course.

2. That the dorsal and lumbar regions are the parts oftenest affected.

3. That inflammation of the spinal marrow of these regions always produces palsy, more or less complete, of the abdominal members.

4. That, in some cases, this inflammation is limited to the inferior or superior parts of the spinal marrow, and that there is loss only of feeling or of motion.

5. That sometimes animals die of palsy without any organic lesion.

[Blows on the head, producing effusion on the brain, poisoning by lead, inflammation of the spinal marrow, affections of the nerves, caries of the spine, costiveness and affections of the bowels, are all productive of palsy. If the disease proceeds from rheumatism, or other inflammatory affections, independent of any organic lesion, the disease, if taken early, is not difficult to overcome in the young subject. Warm baths, bleeding, purging, and stimulating applications to the parts and along the spine, will answer. Castor oil and turpentine is a good purge: where the malady depends upon costiveness, purges of aloes should be administered in connexion with warm enemata, stimulating frictions along the spine, and hot baths. Croton oil dropped on the tongue will also be of great benefit: if there should be effusion or compression from fracture of the bones of the cranium, nothing but trephining will be of any service, as we can hardly hope for the absorption of the matter, and the removal of the spicula of bone can alone afford relief to the patient. Paralysis arising from poisoning should be treated as described under the head of mineral poisons. Chronic cases of paralysis arising from want of tone of the nerves and spinal marrow, repeated blistering, introduction of the seton along the spine, electricity, &c., have all been tried with some success.

Strychnia, from its peculiar effects upon the animal economy, and its almost exclusive direction to the nerves of motion, makes it a medicine particularly applicable to the treatment of this disease. It may be given in all stages of the malady, but is most serviceable after the reduction of inflammatory action, and when we are convinced that the disease depends upon want of tone in the motor muscles.

Great care should be had in its administration, as it is a powerful poison in too large doses, to a large dog; commence with a quarter of a grain in pill, three times daily, and gradually increase to a half grain or more if the animal seems to bear it well. But it should be discontinued immediately on the appearance of any constitutional symptoms, such as spasmodic twitchings of the eye-lids or muzzle.—L.]

PALSY—MANGE.

11th February, 1835.—A Persian bitch, at the Zoological Gardens, who was well yesterday, now staggers as she walks, and has nearly lost the use of her hind legs. Gave a good dose of the castor-oil mixture. *18th.* She is materially worse and drags her hind legs after her. I would fain put on a charge, but the keeper does not like that her beautiful coat should be spoiled, and wishes to try what gentle exercise will do. She certainly, after she has been coaxed a great deal, will get on her legs and stagger on fifty yards or more. Gave the castor-oil mixture daily. *19th.* She is a little stronger, and walks a little better. Continue the mixture. Embrocate well with the rheumatic mixture—sp. tereb., sp. camph., liq. ammon., et tinct. opii—and give gentle exercise.

2d March. — She does improve, although slowly; the charge is therefore postponed. Continue treatment. *30th.* She is considerably better. Continue the mixture, and use the embrocation every second day.

10th April.—She has mange in the bend of her arm, and on her chest. Use the sulphur ointment and alterative balls, and omit the embrocation and mixture. In less than a week she nearly recovered from her lameness, and ran about almost as well as ever. *30th.* She runs about very fairly, but the mange has assumed that character of scurvy which I do not know how to grapple with. Continue the alterative balls, and the ointment.

18th May.—The mange has disappeared, but the palsy is returning; she staggers slightly, and droops behind. Give the castor-oil mixture and use the embrocation.

14th June.—Mange quite gone, but palsy continues to a very considerable degree. I want to use the plaster; but the keeper pleads for a little delay. Continue the treatment.

1st July.—I have at length determined to have recourse to the charge. A piece of thick sheep's leather was fitted to her loins and haunches. *18th.* She appears to be improving, but it is very slowly. *31st.* Very little change. The plaster keeps on well: she has no power over her hind limbs; but she eats and drinks as well as ever.

23d August.—No change. Give her half a grain of strychnia, morning and night. *26th.* That singular secretion of milk, to which the bitch is subject nine weeks after œstrum, is now appearing. Her mammæ are enlarged, and I can squeeze a considerable quantity of milk out of the teats. Give an aloetic pill, and continue the strychnia. 31*st*. The secretion of milk continues. There is slight enlargement and some heat of the mammæ; but she feeds as well as ever. Increase the dose of strychnia to three-quarters of a grain.

On the following day she was found dead. In making the usual longitudinal incision through the integuments of the abdomen, a considerable quantity of milky fluid, mingled with blood, followed the knife. There was very slight enlargement of the teats, but intense inflammation of the whole of the mammary substance. The omentum, and particularly the portion opposite to the external disease, was also inflamed. Besides this there was not a vestige of disease.

This is an interesting case and deserves record. I fear that justice was not done to the animal at the commencement of the paralytic affection. In nineteen cases out of twenty in the dog, the constant but mild stimulus of a charge over the lumbar and sacral regions removes the deeper-seated inflammation of the spinal cord or its membranes, when the palsy is confined to the hind extremities, and has not been sufficiently long established to produce serious change of structure. The charge should have been applied at first. The almost total disappearance of the palsy during the cutaneous disease, which was attended with more than usual inflammation of the integument, is an instructive illustration of the power of counter-irritation, and of what might possibly have been effected in the first case; for much time was lost before the application of the charge, and when at length it was applied, it and the strychnia were powerless.

I consider the following case as exceedingly valuable, at least with reference to the power of strychnia in removing palsy:—

19*th August*, 1836.—A fine Alpine dog was suddenly attacked with a strange nervous affection. He was continually staggering about and falling. His head was forcibly bent backward and a little on one side, almost to his shoulder. A pound of blood was abstracted, a seton inserted from ear to ear, and eight grains of calomel administered. 21*st*. He has perfectly lost the use of every limb. He has also amaurosis, perfect blindness, which had not appeared the day before. He hears perfectly, and he eats, and with appetite, when the food is put into his mouth. Gave him two large spoonfuls of the castor-oil mixture daily; this consists of three parts of castor-oil, two of syrup of buck-thorn, and one of syrup of white poppies. 23*d*. A little better; can lift his head and throw it upon his side, and will still eat when fed. Continue the mixture, and give half a grain of strychnia daily. 24*th*. Little change. 27*th*. No change, except that he is rapidly losing flesh. Continue the treatment. 31*st*. The strychnia increased to three-fourths of a grain morning and night. The castor-oil mixture continued in its full quantity. He was fed well, but there was a sunken, vacant expression of countenance.

2d September. — He can move his head a little, and has some slight motion in his limbs. *4th.* He can almost get up. He recognises me for the first time. His appetite, which was never much impaired, has returned: this is to be attributed to strychnia, or the seton, or the daily aperient mixture. They have all, perhaps, been serviceable, but I attribute most to the strychnia; for I have rarely, indeed, seen any dog recover from such an attack. Continue the treatment. *6th.* Fast recovering. Medicine as before. *14th.* Improving, but not so fast as before. Still continue the treatment. *28th.* Going on slowly, but satisfactorily. Remove the seton, but continue the other treatment.

13th October.—Quite well.

CHAPTER VII.

RABIES.

We are now arrived at one of the most important subjects in veterinary pathology. In other cases the comfort and the existence of our quadruped patients are alone or chiefly involved, but here the lives of our employers, and our own too, are at stake, and may be easily, and too often are, compromised. Here also, however other portions of the chain may be overlooked or denied, we have the link which most of all connects the veterinary surgeon with the practitioner of human medicine; or, rather, here is the circumscribed but valued spot where the veterinary surgeon has the vantage-ground.

In describing the nature, and cause and treatment of rabies, it will be most natural to take the animal in which it oftenest appears, by which it is most frequently propagated; the time at which the danger commences, and the usual period before the death of the patient.

Some years ago a dog, naturally ferocious, bit a child at Lisson Grove. The child, to all appearance previously well, died on the third day, and an inquest was to be held on the body in the evening. The Coroner ordered the dog to be sent to me for examination. The animal was, contrary to his usual habit, perfectly tractable. This will appear to be of some importance hereafter. I examined him carefully. No suspicious circumstance could be found about him. There was no appearance of rabies. In the mean time the inquest took place, and the corpse of the child was carefully examined. One medical gentleman thought that there were some suspicious appearances about the stomach, and another believed that there was congestion of the brain.

The owner of the dog begged that the animal might not be taken from him, but might accompany him home. He took him home and destroyed him that no experiments might be made.

With great difficulty we procured the carcass, and from some inflammatory appearances about the tongue and the stomach, and the presence of a small portion of indigestible matter in the stomach, we were unanimously of opinion that the dog was rabid.

I do not mean to say that the child died hydrophobous, or that its death was accelerated by the nascent disease existing in the dog. There was probably some nervous affection that hastened the death of the infant, and the dog bit the child at the very period when the malady first began to develop itself. On the following day there were morbid lesions enough to prove beyond doubt that he was rabid.

This case is introduced because I used afterwards to accompany every examination of supposed or doubtful rabies with greater caution than I probably had previously used.

It is occasionally very difficult to detect the existence of rabies in its nascent state. In the year 1813, a child attempted to rob a dog of its morning food, and the animal resisting the theft, the child was slightly scratched by its teeth. No one dreamed of danger. *Eight days afterwards* symptoms of rabies appeared in the dog, the malady ran its course, and the animal died. A few days afterwards the child sickened — undoubted characteristics of rabies were observed — they ran their course and the infant was lost.

There are other cases—fortunately not numerous—in the records of human surgery, resembling this. A person has been bitten by a dog, he has paid little or no attention to it, and no application of the caustic has been made. Some weeks, or even months, have passed, he has nearly or quite forgotten the affair, when he becomes languid and feverish, and full of fearful apprehensions, and this appearing perhaps during several days, or more than a week. The empoisonment has then ceased to be a local affair, the virus has entered into the circulation, and its impression is made on the constitution generally. Fortunately the disposition to bite rarely develops itself until the full establishment of the disease, otherwise we might sometimes inquire whether it were not our duty to exterminate the whole race of dogs.

The following case deserves to be recorded. On the 21st of October, 1813, a dog was brought to me for examination. He had vomited a considerable quantity of coagulated blood. I happened to be particularly busy at the moment, and not observing anything peculiar in his countenance or manner, I ordered some astringent sedative medicine, and said that I would see him again in the afternoon.

In the course of the afternoon he was again brought. The vomiting had quite ceased. His mouth seemed to be swollen, and, on examining him, I found that some of his incisor teeth, both in the upper and lower jaw, had been torn out. This somewhat alarmed me; and, on inquiring of the servant, I was told that he suspected that they had had thieves about the house on the preceding night, for the dog had torn away the side of his kennel in attempting to get at them. I scolded him for not having told me of this in the morning; and then, talking of various things, in order to prolong the time and to be able closely to watch my patient, I saw, or thought I saw, but in a very slight degree, that the animal was tracing the fancied path of some imaginary object. I was then truly alarmed, and more especially since I had discovered that in the giving of the physic in the morning the man's hand had been scratched; a youth had suffered the dog to lick his sore finger, and the animal had also been observed to lick the sore ear of an infant. He was a remarkably affectionate dog, and was accustomed to this abominable and inexcusable nonsense.

I insisted on detaining the dog, and gave the man a letter to the surgeon, telling him all my fears. He promptly acted on the hint, and before evening, the proper means were taken with regard to all three.

I watched this dog day after day. He would not eat, but he drank a great deal more water than I liked. The surgeon was evidently beginning to doubt whether I was not wrong, but he could not dispute the occasional wandering of the eye, and the frequent spume upon the water. On the 26th of October, however, the sixth day after his arrival, we both of us heard the rabid howl burst from him: he did not, however, die until the 30th. I mention this as another instance of the great difficulty there is to determine the real nature of the case in an early stage of the disease.

M. Perquin relates an interesting case. A lady had a greyhound, nine years old, that was accustomed to lie upon her bed at night, and cover himself with the bed-clothes. She remarked, one morning, that he had torn the covering of his bed, and, although he ate but little, drank oftener, and in larger quantity, than he was accustomed to do. She led him to a veterinary surgeon, who assured her that there was nothing serious the matter. On the following day, he bit her fore-finger near the nail, as she was giving him something to eat. She led him again to the veterinary surgeon, who assured her that she needed not to be under the least alarm, and as for the little wound on her finger, it was of no consequence. On the following day, the 27th of December, the dog died. He had not ceased to drink most abundantly to the very last.

On the 4th of February, as the lady was dining with her husband, she found some difficulty in deglutition. She wished to take some wine, but was unable to swallow it.

On the 5th, she consulted a surgeon. He wished her to swallow a little soup in his presence. She attempted to do it, but could not accomplish her object after many an effort. She then fell into a state of violent agitation, with constriction of the pharynx, and the discharge of a viscid fluid from the mouth.

On the 7th, she died, four days after the first attack of the disease, and in a state of excessive loss of flesh.

There can be no doubt that both the dog and his mistress died rabid, the former having communicated the disease to the latter; but there is no satisfactory account of the manner in which the dog became diseased.[a]

Joseph Delmaire, of Looberghe, twenty-nine years old, was, on the 6th of October, 1836, bitten in the hand by a dog that he met with in the forest, and that was evidently rabid. On the following morning, he went to a medical man of some repute in the country, who washed the wound, and scarified it, and terminated the operation by tracing a bloody cross on the forehead of the patient.

He returned home, but he was far from being satisfied. The image of the dog that had attacked him was always before him, and his sleep was troubled with the most frightful dreams. So passed four-and-twenty days, when Delmaire, rising from his bed, felt the most dreadful trepidation; he panted violently; it seemed as if an enormous weight oppressed his chest, and from time to time there was profound sighing and sobbing. He complained every moment that he was smothered. He attempted to drink, but it was with great difficulty that a few drops of barley-water were swallowed. His mouth was dry, his throat burning, his thirst excessive, and all that he attempted to swallow was rejected with horror.

At nine o'clock at night he was largely bled. His respiration was more free, but the dread of every fluid remained. After an hour's repose, he started and felt the most fearful pain in every limb—his whole body was agitated with violent convulsions. The former place of bleeding was reopened, and a great quantity of blood escaped. The pulse became small and accelerated. The countenance was dreadful—the eyes were starting from their sockets—he continually sprung from his seat, and uttered the most fearful howling. A quantity of foam filled his mouth, and

[a] La Folie des Animaux, by M. Perquin.

compelled a continued expectoration. In his violent fits, the strength of six men was not sufficient to keep him on his bed. In the midst of a sudden recess of fury he would disengage himself from all that were attempting to hold him, and dash himself on the floor; there, freed from all control, he rolled about, beat himself, and tore everything that he could reach. In the short intervals that separated these crises, he regained possession of his reasoning powers: he begged his old father to pardon him, he talked to him and to those around with the most intense affection, and it was only when he felt that a new attack was at hand, that he prayed them to leave him. At length his mental excitation began to subside; his strength was worn out, and he suffered himself to be placed on his bed. The horrible convulsions from time to time returned, but the dread of liquors had ceased. He demanded something to drink. They gave him a little white wine, but he was unable to swallow it; it was returned through his nostrils. The poor fellow then endeavoured to sleep; but it was soon perceived that he had ceased to live.

The early symptoms of rabies in the dog are occasionally very obscure. In the greater number of cases, these are sullenness, fidgetiness, and continual shifting of posture. Where I have had opportunity, I have generally found these circumstances in regular succession. For several consecutive hours perhaps he retreats to his basket or his bed. He shows no disposition to bite, and he answers the call upon him laggardly. He is curled up and his face is buried between his paws and his breast. At length he begins to be fidgety. He searches out new resting-places; but he very soon changes them for others. He takes again to his own bed; but he is continually shifting his posture. He begins to gaze strangely about him as he lies on his bed. His countenance is clouded and suspicious. He comes to one and another of the family and he fixes on them a steadfast gaze as if he would read their very thoughts. "I feel strangely ill," he seems to say: "have you anything to do with it? or you? or you?" Has not a dog mind enough for this? If we have observed a rabid dog at the commencement of the disease, we have seen this to the very life.

There is a species of dog—the small French poodle—the essence of whose character and constitution is fidgetiness or perpetual motion.

If this dog has been bitten, and rabies is about to establish itself, he is the most irritative restless being that can be conceived of; starting convulsively at the slightest sound; disposing of his bed in every direction, seeking out one retreat after another in order to rest his wearied frame, but quiet only for a moment in any one, and the motion of his limbs frequently stimulating chorea and even epilepsy.

A peculiar delirium is an early symptom, and one that will never deceive. A young man had been bitten by one of his dogs; I was requested to meet a medical gentleman on the subject: I was a little behind my time; as I entered the room I found the dog eagerly devouring a pan of sopped bread. "There is no madness here," said the gentleman. He had scarcely spoken, when in a moment the dog quitted the sop, and, with a furious bark sprung against the wall as if he would seize some imaginary object that he fancied was there. "Did you see that?" was my reply. "What do you think of it?" "I see nothing in it," was his retort: "the dog heard some noise on the other side of the wall." At my serious urging, however, he consented to excise the part. I procured a poor worthless cur, and got him bitten by this dog, and carried the disease from this dog to the third victim: they all became rabid one after the other, and there my experiment ended. The serious matter under consideration, perhaps, justified me in going so far as I did.

This kind of delirium is of frequent occurrence in the human patient. The account given by Dr. Bardsley of one of his patients is very appropriate to our present purpose: "I observed that he frequently fixed his eyes with horror and affright on some ideal object, and then, with a sudden and violent emotion, buried his head beneath the bed-clothes. The next time I saw him repeat this action, I was induced to inquire into the cause of his terror. He asked whether I had not heard howlings and scratchings. On being answered in the negative, he suddenly threw himself on his knees, extending his arms in a defensive posture, and forcibly threw back his head and body. The muscles of the face were agitated by various spasmodic contractions; his eye-balls glazed, and seemed ready to start from their sockets; and, at the moment, when crying out in an agonizing tone, 'Do you not see that black dog?' his countenance and attitude exhibited the most dreadful picture of complicated horror, distress, and rage that words can describe or imagination paint."

I have again and again seen the rabid dog start up after a momentary quietude, with unmingled ferocity depicted on his countenance, and plunge with a savage howl to the end of his chain. At other times he would stop and watch the nails in the partition of the stable in which he was confined, and fancying them to move he would dart at them, and occasionally sadly bruise and injure himself from being no longer able to measure the distance of the object. In one of his sudden fits of violence a rabid dog strangled the Cardinal Crescence, the Legate of the Pope, at the Council of Trent in 1532.

M. Magendie has often injected into the veins of an hydrophobous dog as much as five grains of opium without producing any effect; while a single grain given to the healthy dog would suffice to send him almost to sleep.

One of Mr. Babington's patients thought that there was a cloud of flies about him. "Why do you not kill those flies?" he would cry; and then he would strike at them with his hand, and shrink under the bed-clothes, in the most dreadful fear.

There is also in the human being a peculiarity in this delirium which seems to distinguish it from every other kind of mental aberration. "The patient," in Mr. Lawrence's language, "is pursued by a thousand phantoms that intrude themselves upon his mind; he holds conversation with imaginary persons; he fancies himself surrounded with difficulties, and in the greatest distress. These thoughts seem to pass through his mind with wonderful rapidity, and to keep him in a state of the greatest distress, unless he is quickly spoken to or addressed by his name, and, then, in a moment the charm is broken; every phantom of imagination disappears, and at once he begins to talk as calmly and as connectedly as in perfect health."

So it is with the dog, whether he is watching the motes that are floating in the air, or the insects that are annoying him on the walls, or the foes that he fancies are threatening him on every side — one word recalls him in a moment. Dispersed by the magic influence of his master's voice, every object of terror disappears, and he crawls towards him with the same peculiar expression of attachment that used to characterize him.

Then comes a moment's pause—a moment of actual vacuity—the eye slowly closes, the head droops, and he seems as if his fore feet were giving way, and he would fall: but he springs up again, every object of terror once more surrounds him—he gazes wildly around — he snaps — he barks, and he rushes to the extent of his chain, prepared to meet his imaginary foe.

The expression of the countenance of the dog undergoes a considerable change, principally dependent on the previous disposition of the animal. If he was naturally of an affectionate disposition, there will be an anxious, inquiring countenance, eloquent, beyond the power of resisting its influence. It is made up of strange suppositions as to the nature of the depression of mind under which he labours, mingled with some passing doubts, and they are but passing, as to the concern which the master has in the affair; but, most of all, there is an affectionate and confiding appeal for relief. At the same time we observe some strange fancy, evidently passing through his mind, unalloyed, however, by the slightest portion of ferocity.

In the countenance of the naturally savage brute, or him that has been trained to be savage, there is indeed a fearful change; sometimes the conjunctiva is highly injected; at other times it is scarcely affected, but the eyes have an unusually bright and dazzling appearance. They are like two balls of fire, and there is a peculiar transparency of the hyaloid membrane, or injection of that of the retina.

A very early symptom of rabies in the dog, is an extreme degree of restlessness. Frequently, he is almost invariably wandering about, shifting from corner to corner, or continually rising up and lying down, changing his posture in every possible way, disposing of his bed with his paws, shaking it with his mouth, bringing it to a heap, on which he carefully lays his chest, or rather the pit of his stomach, and then rising up and bundling every portion of it out of the kennel. If he is put into a closed basket, he will not be still for an instant, but turn round and round without ceasing. If he is at liberty, he will seem to imagine that something is lost, and he will eagerly search round the room, and particularly every corner of it, with strange violence and indecision.

In a very great portion of cases of hydrophobia in the human being, there is, as a precursory symptom, uneasiness, pain, or itching of the bitten part. A red line may also be traced up the limb, in the direction of the lymphatics. In a few cases the wound opens afresh.

The poison is now beginning fatally to act on the tissue, on which it had previously lain harmless. When the conversation has turned on this subject, long after the bitten part has been excised, pain has darted along the limb. I have been bitten much oftener than I liked, by dogs decidedly rabid, but, proper means being taken, I have escaped; and yet often, when I have been over-fatigued, or a little out of temper, some of the old sores have itched and throbbed, and actually become red and swollen.

The dog appears to suffer a great deal of pain in the ear in common canker. He will be almost incessantly scratching it, crying piteously while thus employed. The ear is, oftener than any other part, bitten by the rabid dog, and, when a wound in the ear, inflicted by a rabid dog, begins to become painful, the agony appears to be of the intensest kind. The dog rubs his ear against every projecting body, he scratches it might and main, and tumbles over and over while he is thus employed.

The young practitioner should be on his guard there. Is this dreadful itching a thing of yesterday, or, has the dog been subject to canker, increasing for a considerable period. Canker both internal and external is a disease of slow growth, and must have been long neglected before it will torment the patient in the manner that I have described. The question as to the length of time that an animal has thus suffered will usually be a sufficient guide.

The mode in which he expresses his torture will serve as anotner direction. He will often scratch violently enough when he has canker, but he will not roll over and over like a football except he is rabid. If there is very considerable inflammation of the lining membrane of the ear, and engorgement and ulceration of it, this is the effect of canker; but if there is only a slight redness of the membrane, or no redness at all, and yet the dog is incessantly and violently scratching himself, it is too likely that rabies is at hand.

In the early stage of rabies, the attachment of the dog towards his owner seems to be rapidly increased, and the expression of that feeling. He is employed, almost without ceasing, licking the hands, or face, or any part he can get at. Females, and men too, are occasionally apt to permit the dog, when in health, to indulge this filthy and very dangerous habit with regard to them. The virus, generated under the influence of rabies, is occasionally deposited on a wounded or abraded surface, and in process of time produces a similar disease in the person that has been so inoculated by it. Therefore it is that the surgeon so anxiously inquires of the person that has been bitten, and of all those to whom the dog has had access, "Has he been accustomed to lick you? have you any sore places about you that can by possibility have been licked by him?" If there are, the person is in fully as much danger as if he had been bitten, and it is quite as necessary to destroy the part with which the virus may have come in contact. A lady once lost her life by suffering her dog to lick a pimple on her chin.

There is a beautiful species of dog, often the inhabitant of the gentleman's stable—the Dalmatian or coach dog. He has, perhaps, less affection for the human species than any other dog, except the greyhound and the bull-dog; he has less sagacity than most others, and certainly less courage. He is attached to the stable; he is the friend of the horse; they live under the same roof; they share the same bed; and, when the horse is summoned to his work, the dog accompanies every step. They are certainly beautiful dogs, and it is pleasing to see the thousand expressions of friendship between them and the horse; but, in their continual excursions through the streets, they are exposed to some danger, and particularly to that of being bitten by rabid dogs. It is a fearful business when this takes place. The coachman probably did not see the affray; no suspicion has been excited. The horse rubs his muzzle on the dog, and the dog licks the face of the horse, and in a great number of cases the disease is communicated from the one to the other. The dog in process of time dies, the horse does not long survive, and, frequently too, the coachman shares their fate. I have known at least twenty horses destroyed in this way.

A depraved appetite is a frequent attendant on rabies in the dog.

He refuses his usual food; he frequently turns from it with an evident expression of disgust; at other times, he seizes it with greater or less avidity, and then drops it, sometimes from disgust, at other times because he is unable to complete the mastication of it. This palsy of the organs of mastication, and dropping of the food, after it has been partly chewed, is a symptom on which implicit confidence may be placed.

Some dogs vomit once or twice in the early period of the disease: when this happens, they never return to the natural food of the dog, but are eager for everything that is filthy and horrible. The natural appetite generally fails entirely, and to it succeeds a strangely depraved one. The dog usually occupies himself with gathering every little bit of thread, and it is curious to observe with what eagerness and method he sets to work, and how completely he effects his object. He then attacks every kind of dirt and filth, horse-dung, his own dung, and human excrement. Some breeds of spaniels are very filthy feeders without its being connected with disease, but the rabid dog eagerly selects the excrement of the horse, and his own. Some considerable care, however, must be exercised here. At the period of dentition, and likewise at the commencement of the sexual affection, the stomach of the dog, and particularly that of the bitch, sympathises with, or shares in, the irritability of the gums, and of the constitution generally, and there is a considerably perverted appetite. The dog also feels the same propensity that influences the child, that of taking hard substances into the mouth, and seemingly trying to masticate them. Their pressure on the gums facilitates the passage of the new teeth. A young dog will, therefore, be observed gathering up hard substances, and, if he should chance to die, a not inconsiderable collection of them is sometimes found in the stomach. They are, however, of a peculiar character; they consist of small pieces of bone, stick, and coal.

The contents of the stomach of the rabid dog, are often, or generally, of a most filthy description. Some hair or straw is usually found, but the greater part is composed of horse-dung, or of his own dung, and it may be received as a certainty, that if he is found deliberately devouring it, he is rabid.

Some very important conclusions may be drawn from the appearance and character of the urine. The dog, and at particular times when he is more than usually salacious, may, and does diligently search the urining places; he may even, at those periods, be seen to lick the spot which another has just wetted; but, if a peculiar eagerness accompanies this strange employment, if, in the parlour, which is rarely disgraced by this evacuation, every corner is perseveringly examined, and licked with unwearied and unceasing industry, that dog cannot be too carefully watched, there is great

18*

danger about him; he may, without any other symptom, be pronounced to be decidedly rabid. I never knew a single mistake about this.

Much has been said of the profuse discharge of saliva from the mouth of the rabid dog. It is an undoubted fact that, in this disease, all the glands concerned in the secretion of saliva, become increased in bulk and vascularity. The sublingual glands wear an evident character of inflammation; but it never equals the increased discharge that accompanies epilepsy, or nausea. The frothy spume at the corners of the mouth, is not for a moment to be compared with that which is evident enough in both of these affections. It is a symptom of short duration, and seldom lasts longer than twelve hours. The stories that are told of the mad dog covered with froth, are altogether fabulous. The dog recovering from, or attacked by a fit, may be seen in this state; but not the rabid dog. Fits are often mistaken for rabies, and hence the delusion.

The increased secretion of saliva soon passes away. It lessens in quantity; it becomes thicker, viscid, adhesive, and glutinous. It clings to the corners of the mouth, and probably more annoyingly so to the membrane of the fauces. The human being is sadly distressed by it, he forces it out with the greatest violence, or utters the falsely supposed bark of a dog, in his attempts to force it from his mouth. This symptom occurs in the human being, when the disease is fully established, or at a late period of it. The dog furiously attempts te detach it with his paws.

It is an early symptom in the dog, and it can scarcely be mistaken in him. When he is fighting with his paws at the corners of his mouth, let no one suppose that a bone is sticking between the poor fellow's teeth; nor should any useless and dangerous effort be made to relieve him. If all this uneasiness arose from a bone in the mouth, the mouth would continue permanently open instead of closing when the animal for a moment discontinues his efforts. If after a while he loses his balance and tumbles over, there can be no longer any mistake. It is the saliva becoming more and more glutinous, irritating the fauces and threatening suffocation.

To this naturally and rapidly succeeds an insatiable thirst. The dog that still has full power over the muscles of his jaws continues to lap. He knows not when to cease, while the poor fellow labouring under the dumb madness, presently to be described, and whose jaw and tongue are paralysed, plunges his muzzle into the water-dish to his very eyes, in order that he may get one drop of water into the back part of his mouth to moisten and to cool his dry and parched fauces. Hence, instead of this disease being always characterised by the dread of water in the dog, it is marked by a thirst often perfectly unquenchable. Twenty years ago, this assertion would have been peremptorily denied. Even at the present day we occasionally meet with those who ought to know better, and who will not believe that the dog which fairly, or perhaps eagerly, drinks, can be rabid.

January 22*d*, 1815. — A Newfoundland dog belonging to a gentleman in Piccadilly was supposed to have swallowed a penny-piece on the 20th. On the evening of that day he was dull, refused his food, and would not follow his master. 21*st*. He became restless and panting, and continually shifting his position. He would not eat nor would he drink water, but followed his mistress into her bed-room, which he had never done before, and eagerly lapped the urine from her chamber-pot. He was afterwards seen lapping his own urine. His restlessness and panting increased. He would neither eat nor drink, and made two or three attempts to vomit. 22*d*. He was brought to me this evening. His eyes were wild, the conjunctiva considerably inflamed, and he panted quickly and violently. There was a considerable flow of saliva from the corners of his mouth. He was extremely restless and did not remain in one position half a minute. There was an occasional convulsive nodding motion of the head. The eyes were wandering, and evidently following some imaginary object; but he was quickly recalled from his delirium by my voice or that of his master. In a few moments, however, he was wandering again. He had previously been under my care, and immediately recognised me and offered me his paw. His bark was changed and had a slight mixture of the howl, and there was a husky choking noise in the throat.

I immediately declared that he was rabid, and with some reluctance on the part of his master, he was left with me. 23*d*, 8 A. M. The breathing was less quick and laborious. The spasm of the head was no longer visible. The flow of saliva had stopped and there was less delirium. The jaw began to be dependent; the rattling, choking noise in his throat louder. He carried straw about in his mouth. He picked up some pieces of old leather that lay within his reach and carefully concealed them under his bed. Two minutes afterwards he would take them out again, and look at them, and once more hide them. He frequently voided his urine in small quantities, but no longer lapped it. A little dog was lowered into the den, but he took no notice of it. 10 P. M. Every symptom of fever returned with increased violence. He panted very much, and did not remain in the same posture two seconds. He was continually running to the end of his chain and attempting to bite. He was eagerly and wildly watching some imaginary object. His voice was hoarser — more of the howl mixing with it. The lips were distorted, and the tongue very black. He was evidently getting weaker. After two or three attempts to escape, he would sit down for a second, and then rise and plunge to the end of his chain. He drank frequently, yet but little at a time, and that without difficulty or spasm. 12 P. M. The thirst strangely increased. He had drunk or spilled full three quarts of water. There was a peculiar eagerness in his manner. He plunged his nose to the very bottom of his pan, and then snapped at the bubbles which he raised. No spasm followed the drinking. He took two or three pieces from my hand, but immediately dropped them from want of power to hold them. Yet he was able for a moment suddenly to close his jaws. When not drinking he was barking with a harsh sound, and frequently started suddenly, watching, and catching at some imaginary object. *24th*, A. M. He was more furious, yet weaker. The thirst was insatiable. He was otherwise diligently employed in shattering and tearing everything within his reach. He died about three o'clock.

It is impossible to say what was the origin of this disease in him. It is not connected with any degree or variation of temperature, or any particular state of the atmosphere. It is certainly more frequent in the summer or the beginning of autumn than in the winter or spring, because it is a highly nervous and febrile disease, and the degree of fever, and irritability, and ferocity, and consequent mischief are augmented by increase of temperature. In the great majority of cases, the inoculation can be distinctly proved. In very few can the possibility be denied. The injury is inflicted in an instant. There is no contest, and before the injured party can prepare to retaliate, the rabid dog is far away.

It can easily be believed that when a favourite dog has, but for a moment, lagged behind, he may be bitten without the owner's knowledge or suspicion. A spaniel belonging to a lady became rabid. The dog was her companion in her grounds at her country residence, and it was rarely out of her sight except for a few minutes in the morning, when the servant took it out. She was not conscious of its having been bitten, and the servant stoutly denied it. The animal died. A few weeks afterwards the footman was taken ill. He was hydrophobous. In one of his intervals of comparative quietude he confessed that, one morning, his charge had been attacked and rolled over by another dog; that there was no appearance of its having been bitten, but that it had been made sadly dirty, and he had washed it before he suffered it again to go into the drawing-room. The dog that attacked it must have been rabid, and some of his saliva must have remained about the coat of the spaniel, by which the servant was fatally inoculated.

Another case of this fearful disease must not be passed over. A dog that had been docile and attached to his master and mistress, was missing one morning, and came home in the evening almost covered with dirt. He slunk to his basket, and would pay no attention to any one. His owners thought it rather strange, and I was sent for in the morning. He was lying on the lap of his mistress, but was frequently shifting his posture, and every now and then he started, as if he heard some strange sound. I immediately told them what was the matter, and besought them to place him in another and secure room. He had been licking both their hands. I was compelled to tell them at once what was the nature of the case, and besought them to send at once for their surgeon. They were perfectly angry at my nonsense, as they called it, and I took my leave, but went immediately to their medical man, and told him what was the real state of the case. He called, as it were accidentally, a little while afterwards, and I was not far behind him. The surgeon did his duty, and they escaped.

In May, 1820, I attended on a bitch at Pimlico. She had snapped at the owner, bitten the man-servant and several dogs, was eagerly watching imaginary objects, and had the peculiar rabid howl. I offered her water. She started back with a strange expression of horror, and fell into violent convulsions that lasted about a minute. This was repeated a little while afterwards, and with the same result. She was destroyed.

The horrible spasms of the human being at the sight of, or the attempt to swallow, fluids occur sufficiently often to prove the identity of the disease in the biped and the quadruped; but not in one in fifty cases is there, in the dog, the slightest reluctance to liquids, or difficulty in swallowing them.

In almost every case in which the dog utters any sound during the disease, there is a manifest change of voice. In the dog labouring under ferocious madness, it is perfectly characteristic. There is no other sound that it resembles. The animal is generally standing, or occasionally sitting, when the singular sound is heard. The muzzle is always elevated. The commencement is that of a perfect bark, ending abruptly and very singularly, in a howl, a fifth, sixth, or eighth higher than at the commencement. Dogs are often enough heard howling, but in this case it is the perfect bark, and the perfect howl rapidly succeeding to the bark.

Every sound uttered by the rabid dog is more or less changed. The huntsman, who knows the voice of every dog in his pack, occasionally hears a strange challenge. He immediately finds out that dog, and puts him, as quickly as possible, under confinement. Two or three days may pass over, and there is not another suspicious circumstance about the animal; still he keeps him under quarantine, for long experience has taught him to listen to that warning. At length the disease is manifest in its most fearful form.

There is another partial change of voice, to which the ear of the practitioner will, by degrees, become habituated, and which will indicate a change in the state of the animal quite as dangerous as the dismal howl; I mean when there is a hoarse inward bark, with a slight but characteristic elevation of the tone. In other cases, after two or three distinct barks, will come the peculiar one mingled with the howl. Both of them will terminate fatally, and in both of them the rabid howl cannot possibly be mistaken.

There is a singular brightness in the eye of the rabid dog, but it does not last more than two or three days. It then becomes dull and wasted; a cloudiness steals over the conjunctiva, which changes to a yellow tinge, and then to a dark green, indicative of ulceration deeply seated within the eye. In eight and forty hours from the first clouding of the eye, it becomes one disorganised mass.

There is in the rabid dog a strange embarrassment of general sensibility—a seemingly total loss of feeling.

Absence of pain in the bitten part is an almost invariable accompaniment of rabies. I have known a dog set to work, and gnaw and tear the flesh completely away from his legs and feet. At other times the penis is perfectly demolished from the very base. Ellis in his "Shepherd's Sure Guide," asserts, that, however severely a mad dog is beaten, a cry is never forced from him. I am certain of the truth of this, for I have again and again failed in extracting that cry. Ellis tells that at the kennel at Goddesden, some of the grooms heated a poker red hot, and holding it near the mad hound's mouth, he most greedily seized it, and kept it until the mouth was most dreadfully burned.

In the great majority of cases of furious madness, and in almost every case of dumb madness, there is evident affection of the lumbar portion of the spinal cord. There is a staggering gait, not indicative of general weakness, but referable to the hind quarters alone, and indicating an affection of the lumbar motor nerve. In a few cases it approaches more to a general paralytic affection.

In the very earliest period of rabies, the person accustomed to dogs will detect the existence of the disease.

The animal follows the flight, as has been already stated, of various imaginary objects. I have often watched the changing countenance of the rabid dog when he has been lost to every surrounding object. I have seen the brightening countenance and the wagging tail as some pleasing vision has passed before him; but, oftener has the countenance indicated the mingled dislike and fear with which the intruder was regarded. As soon as the phantom came within the proper distance he darted on it with true rabid violence.

A spaniel, seemingly at play, snapped, in the morning, at the feet of several persons. In the evening he bit his master, his master's friend, and another dog. The old habits of obedience and affection then returned. His master, most strangely, did not suspect the truth, and brought the animal to me to be examined. The animal was, as I had often seen him, perfectly docile and eager to be caressed. At my suggestion, or rather entreaty, he was left with me. On the following morning the disease was plain enough, and on the following day he died. A *post-mortem* examination took place, and proved that he was unequivocally rabid.

A lady would nurse her dog, after I had declared it to be rabid, and when he was dangerous to every one but herself, and even to her from the saliva which he plentifully scattered about. At length he darted at every one that entered the room, until a footman keeping the animal at bay with the poker, the husband of the lady dragged her from the room. The noise that the dog made was then terrific, and he almost gnawed his way through the door. At midnight his violence nearly ceased, and the door was partially opened. He was staggering and falling about, with every limb violently agitated. At the entreaty of the lady, a servant ventured in to make a kind of bed for him. The dog suddenly darted at him, and dropped and died.

A terrier, ten years old, had been ill, and refused all food for three days. On the fourth day he bit a cat of which he had been unusually fond, and he likewise bit three dogs. I was requested to see him. I found him loose in the kitchen, and at first refused to go in, but, after observing him for a minute or two, I thought that I might venture. He had a peculiarly wild and eager look, and turned sharply round at the least noise. He often watched the flight of some imaginary object, and pursued with the utmost fury every fly that he saw. He searchingly sniffed about the room, and examined my legs with an eagerness that made me absolutely tremble. His quarrel with the cat had been made up, and when he was not otherwise employed he was eagerly licking her and her kittens. In the excess or derangement of his fondness, he fairly rolled them from one end of the kitchen to another. With difficulty I induced his master to permit me to destroy him.

It is not every dog, that in the most aggravated state of the disease shows a disposition to bite. The finest Newfoundland dog that I ever saw became rabid. He had been bitten by a cur, and was supposed to have been thoroughly examined in the country. No wound, however, was found: the circumstance was almost forgotten, and he came up to the metropolis with his master. He became dull, disinclined to play, and refused all food. He was continually watching imaginary objects, but he did not snap at them. There was no howl, nor any disposition to bite. He offered himself to be caressed, and he was not satisfied except he was shaken by the paw. On the second day I saw him. He watched every passing object with peculiar anxiety, and followed with deep attention the motions of a horse, his old acquaintance; but he made no effort to escape, nor evinced any disposition to do mischief. I went to him, and patted and coaxed him, and he told me as plainly as looks and actions, and a somewhat deepened whine could express it, how much he was gratified. I saw him on the third day. He was evidently dying. He could not crawl even to the door of his temporary kennel; but he pushed forward his paw a little way, and, as I shook it, I felt the tetanic muscular action which accompanies the departure of life.

On the other hand there are rabid dogs whose ferocity knows no bounds. If they are threatened with a stick, they fly at, and seize it, and furiously shake it. They are incessantly employed in darting to the end of their chain, and attempting to crush it with their teeth, and tearing to pieces their kennel, or the wood work that is within their reach. They are regardless of pain. The canine teeth, the incisor teeth are torn away; yet, unwearied and insensible to suffering, they continue their efforts to escape. A dog was chained near a kitchen fire. He was incessant in his endeavours to escape, and, when he found that he could not effect it, he seized, in his impotent rage, the burning coals as they fell, and crushed them with his teeth.

If by chance a dog in this state effects his escape, he wanders over the country bent on destruction. He attacks both the quadruped and the biped. He seeks the village street, or the more crowded one of the town, and he suffers no dog to escape him. The horse is his frequent prey, and the human being is not always safe from his attack. A rabid dog running down Park-lane, in 1825, bit no fewer than five horses, and fully as many dogs. He was seen to steal treacherously upon some of his victims, and inflict the fatal wound. Sometimes he seeks the more distant pasturage. He gets among the sheep, and more than forty have been fatally inoculated in one night. A rabid dog attacked a herd of cows, and five-and-twenty of them fell victims. In July, 1813, a mad dog broke into the menagerie of the Duchess of York, at Oatlands, and although the palisades that divided the different compartments of the menagerie were full six feet in height, and difficult, or apparently almost impossible to climb, he was found asleep in one of them, and it was clearly ascertained that he had bitten at least ten of the dogs.

At length the rabid dog becomes completely exhausted, and slowly reels along the road with his tail depressed, seemingly half unconscious of surrounding objects. His open mouth, and protruded and blackened tongue, and rolling gait sufficiently characterise him. He creeps into some sheltered place and then he sleeps twelve hours or more. It is dangerous to disturb his slumbers, for his desire to do mischief immediately returns, and the slightest touch, or attempt to caress him, is repaid by a fatal wound. This should be a caution never to meddle with a sleeping dog in a way-side house, and, indeed, never to disturb him anywhere.

In an early period of the disease in some dogs, and in others when the strength of the animal is nearly worn away, a peculiar paralysis of the muscles of the tongue and jaws is seen. The mouth is partially open, and the tongue protruding. In some cases the dog is able to close his mouth by a sudden and violent effort, and is as ferocious and as dangerous as one the muscles of whose face are unaffected. At other times the palsy is complete, and the animal is unable to close his mouth or retract his tongue. These latter cases, however, are rare.

A dog must not be immediately condemned because he has this open mouth and fixed jaw. Bones constitute a frequent and a considerable portion of the food of dogs. In the eagerness with which these bones are crushed, spicula or large pieces of them become wedged between the molar teeth, and form an inseparable obstacle to the closing of the teeth. The tongue partially protrudes. There is a constant discharge of saliva from the mouth, far greater than when the true paralysis exists. The dog is continually fighting at the corners of his mouth, and the countenance is expressive of intense anxiety, although not of the same irritable character as in rabies.

I was once requested to meet a medical gentleman in consultation respecting a supposed case of rabies. There was protrusion and discoloration of the tongue, and fighting at the corners of the mouth, and intense anxiety of countenance. He had been in this state for four-and-twenty hours. This was a case in which I should possibly have been deceived had it been the first dog that I had seen with dumb madness. After having tested a little the ferocity or manageableness of the animal, I passed my hand along the outside of the jaws, and felt a bone wedged between two of the grinders. The forceps soon set all right with him.

It is time to inquire more strictly into the *post-mortem* appearances of rabies in the dog.

In dumb madness the unfailing accompaniment is, to a greater or less degree, paralysis of the muscles of the lower jaw, and the tongue is discoloured and swollen, and hanging from the mouth; more blood than usual also is deposited in the anterior and inferior portion of it. Its colour varies from a dark red to a dingy purple, or almost black. In ferocious madness it is usually torn and bruised, or it is discoloured by the dirt and filth with which it has been brought into contact, and, not unfrequently, its anterior portion is coated with some disgusting matter. The papillæ, or small projections on the back of the tongue, are elongated and widened, and their mucous covering evidently reddened. The orifices of the glands of the tongue are frequently enlarged, particularly as they run their course along the frœnum of the tongue.

The fauces, situated at the posterior part of the mouth, generally exhibit traces of inflammation. They appear in the majority of cases of ferocious madness, and they are never deficient after dumb madness. They are usually most intense either towards the palatine arch or the larynx. Sometimes an inflammatory character is diffused through its whole extent, but occasionally it is more or less intense towards one or both of the terminations of the fauces, while the intermediate portion retains nearly its healthy hue.

There is one circumstance of not unfrequent occurrence, which will at once decide the case—the presence of indigestible matter, probably small in quantity, in the back part of the mouth. This speaks volumes as to the depraved appetite of the patient, and the loss of power in the muscles of the pharynx.

Little will depend on the tonsils of the throat. They occasionally enlarge to more than double their usual size; but this is more in quiet than in ferocious madness. The insatiable thirst of the rabid dog is perhaps connected with this condition of them.

The epiglottis should be very carefully observed. It is more or less injected in every case of rabies. Numerous vessels increase in size and multiply round its edge, and there is considerable injection and thickening.

Inflammation of the edges of the glottis, and particularly of the membrane which covers its margin, is often seen, and accounts for the harsh guttural breathing which frequently accompanies dumb madness. The inflammatory blush of the larynx, though often existing in a very slight degree, deserves considerable attention.

The appearances in the trachea are very uncertain. There is occasionally the greatest intensity of inflammation through the whole of it; at other times there is not the slightest appearance of it. There is the same uncertainty with regard to the bronchial tubes and the lungs; but there is no characteristic symptom or lesion in the lungs.

Great stress has been laid on the appearance of the heart; but, generally speaking, in nine cases out of ten, the heart of the rabid dog will exhibit no other symptoms of disease than an increased yet variable deepness of colour in the lining membrane of the ventricles.

No dependence can be placed on any of the appearances of the œsophagus; and, when they are at the worst, the inflammation occupies only a portion of that tube.

With regard to the interior of the stomach, if the dog has been dead only a few hours the true inflammatory blush will remain. If four-and-twenty hours have elapsed, the bright red colour will have changed to a darker red, or a violet or a brownish hue. In a few hours after this, a process of corrosion will generally commence, and the mucous membrane will be softened and rendered thinner, and, to a certain extent, eaten through. The examiner, however, must not attribute that to disease which is the natural process of the cession of life.

Much attention should be paid to the appearance of the stomach and its contents. If it contains a strange mingled mass of hair, and hay, and straw, and horse-dung, and earth, or portions of the bed on which the dog had lain, we should seldom err if we affirmed that he died rabid; for it is only under the influence of the depraved appetite of rabies that such substances are devoured. It is not the presence of every kind of extraneous substance that will be satisfactory: pieces of coal, or wood, or even the filthiest matter, will not justify us in pronouncing the animal to be rabid; it is that peculiarly mingled mass of straw, and hair, and filth of various kinds, that must indicate the existence of rabies.

When there are no solid indigesta, but a fluid composed principally of vitiated bile or extravasated blood, there will be a strong indication of the presence of rabies. When, also, there are in the duodenum and jejunum small portions of indigesta, the detection of the least quantity will be decisive. The remainder has been ejected by vomit; and inquiry should be made of the nature of the matter that has been discharged.

The inflammation of rabies is of a peculiar character in the stomach. It is generally confined to the summits of the folds of the stomach, or it is most intense there. On the summits of the rugæ there are effusions of bloody matter, or spots of ecchymosis, presenting an appearance almost like crushed black currants. There may be only a few of them; but they are indications of the evil that has been effected.

From appearances that present themselves in the intestines, the bladder, the blood-vessels, or the brain, no conclusion can be drawn; they are simply indications of inflammation.

We now rapidly, and for a little while, retrace our steps. What is the cause of this fatal disease, that has so long occupied our attention? It is the saliva of a rabid animal received into a wound, or on an abraded surface. In horses, cattle, sheep, swine, and the human being, it is caused by inoculation alone; but, according to some persons, it is produced spontaneously in other animals.

I will suppose that a wound by a rabid dog is inflicted. The virus is deposited on or near its surface, and there it remains for a certain indefinite period of time. The wound generally heals up kindly; in fact, it differs in no respect from a similar wound inflicted by the teeth of an animal in perfect health. Weeks and months, in some cases, pass on, and there is nothing to indicate danger, until a degree of itching in the cicatrix of the wound is felt. From its long-continued presence as a foreign body, it may have rendered the tissue, or nervous fibre connected with it, irritable and susceptible of impression, or it may have attracted and assimilated to itself certain elements, and rabies is produced.

The virus does not appear to have the same effect on every animal. Of four dogs bitten by, or inoculated from, one that is rabid, three, perhaps, would display every symptom of the disease. Of four human beings, not more than one would become rabid. John Hunter used to say not more than one in twenty; but that is probably erroneous. Cattle appear to have a greater chance of escape, and sheep a still greater chance.

The time of incubation is different in different animals. With regard to the human being, there are various strange and contradictory stories. Some have asserted that it has appeared on the very day on which the bite was inflicted, or within two or three days of that time. Dr. Bardsley, on the other hand, relates a case in which twelve years elapsed between the bite and the disease. If the virus may lurk so long as this in the constitution, it is a most lamentable affair. According to one account, more than thirty years intervened. The usual time extends from three weeks to six or seven months.

In the dog I have never seen a case in which plain and palpable rabies occurred in less than fourteen days after the bite. The average time I should calculate at five or six weeks. In three months I should consider the animal as tolerably safe. I am, however, relating my own experience, and have known but two instances in which the period much exceeded three months. In one of these five months elapsed, and the other did not become affected until after the expiration of the seventh month.

The quality and the quantity of the virus may have something to do with this, and so may the predisposition in the bitten animal to be affected by the poison. If it is connected with œstrum, the bitch will probably become a disgusting, as well as dangerous animal; if with parturition ,there is a strange perversion of maternal affection—she is incessantly and violently licking her young, continually shifting them from place to place; and, in less than four-and-twenty hours, they will be destroyed by the reckless manner in which they are treated. In both cases the development of the disease seems to wait on the completion of her time of pregnancy. It appears in the space of two months after the bite, if her parturition is near at hand, or it is delayed for double that time, if the period of labour is so far distant.

The duration of the disease is different in different animals. In man it has run its course in twenty-four hours, and rarely exceeds seventy-two. In the horse from three to four days; in the sheep and ox from five to seven; and in the dog from four to six.

Of the real nature of the rabid virus, we know but little. It has never been analysed, and it would be a difficult process to analyse it. It is not diffused by the air, nor communicated by the breath, nor even by actual contact, if the skin is sound. It must be received into a wound. It must come in contact with some tissue or nervous fibre, and lie dormant there for a considerable, but uncertain period. The absorbents remove everything around; whatever else is useless, or would be injurious, is taken away, but this strange substance is unchanged. It does not enter into the circulation, for there it would undergo some modification and change, or would be rejected. It lies for a time absolutely dormant, and far longer than any other known poison; but, at length, the tissue on which it has lain begins to render it somewhat sensible, and assimilates to itself certain elements. The cicatrix begins to be painful, and inflammation spreads around. The absorbents are called into more powerful action; they begin to attack the virus itself, and a portion of it is taken up, and carried into the circulation, and acquires the property of assimilating other secretions to its own nature, or it is determined to one of the secretions only; it alters the character of that secretion, envenoms it, and gives it the power of propagating the disease.

Something like this is the history of many animal poisons. In variola and the vaccine disease the poison is determined to the skin, in glanders to the Schneiderian membrane, and in farcy to the superficial absorbents. Each in its turn becomes the depôt of the poison. So it is with the salivary glands of the rabid animal; in them it is formed, or to them it is determined, and from them, and them alone, it is communicated to other animals.

Professor Dick, in his valuable Manual of Veterinary Science, states some peculiar views, and those highly interesting, respecting the disease of rabies. He holds it to be essentially an inflammatory affection, attacking peculiarly the mucous membrane of the nose, and extending thence through the cribriform plate of the ethmoid bones to the interior part of the brain, and so giving rise to a derangement of the nervous system as a necessary consequence. This train of symptoms constitutes mainly, if not wholly, the essence of an occasional epidemic not unlike some forms of influenza or epizootic disease, and the bite of a rabid animal is not always, to an animal so bitten, the exciting cause of the disease, but merely an accidental concomitant in the prevailing disorder. Also the disease hydrophobia, produced in man, is not always the result of any poison introduced into his system, but merely the melancholy, and often fatal result of panic fear, and of the disordered state of the imagination. Those who are acquainted with the effects of sympathy, and imitation, and panic, in the production of nervous disorders, will readily apprehend the meaning of the Professor.

Some of these diseases speedily run their course and exhaust themselves. Cowpox and farcy, in many instances, have this character. Perhaps, to a certain degree, this may be affirmed of all of them. I have seen cases, which I could not mistake, in which the symptoms of rabies were one after another developed. The dog was plainly and undeniably rabid, and I had given him up as lost; but, after a certain period, the symptoms began to be less distinct; they gradually disappeared, and the animal returned to perfect health. This may have formed one ground of belief in the power of certain medicines, and most assuredly it gives encouragement to perseverance in the use of remedial measures.

It has then been proved, and I hope demonstratively, that rabies is propagated by inoculation. It has also been established that although every animal labouring under this disease is capable of communicating it, yet, with very few exceptions, it can be traced to the bite of the dog. It has still further been shown that the malady, generally appears at some period between the third and seventh month from the time of inoculation. At the expiration of the eighth month, the animal may be considered to be safe; for there is only one acknowledged case on record, in which the disease appeared in the dog after the seventh month from the bite had passed.

Then it would appear that if a species of quarantine could be established, and every dog confined separately for eight months, the disease would be annihilated in our country, or could only reappear in consequence of the importation of some infected animal. Such a course of proceeding, however, could never be enforced either in the sporting world or among the peasantry. Other measures, however, might be resorted to in order to lessen the devastations of this malady; and that which first presents itself to the mind as a powerful cause of rabies is the number of useless and dangerous dogs that are kept in the country for the most nefarious and, in the neighbourhood of considerable towns, the most brutal purposes; without the slightest hesitation, I will affirm that rabies is propagated, nineteen times out of twenty, by the cur and the lurcher in the country, and the fighting-dog in towns.

A tax should be laid on every useless dog, and doubly or trebly heavier than on the sporting-dog. No dog except the shepherd's should be exempt from this tax, unless, perhaps, it is the truck-dog, and his owner should be compelled to take out a license; to have his name in large letters on his cart; and he should be heavily fined if the animal is found loose in the streets, or if he is used for fighting.

The disease is rarely propagated by petted and house-dogs They are little exposed to the danger of inoculation; yet, we pity, or almost detest, the folly of those by whom their favourites are indulged, and spoiled even more than their children.

We will now suppose that a person has had the misfortune to be bitten by a rabid dog: what course is he to pursue? What preventive means are to be adopted? Some persons, and of no mean standing in the medical world, have recommended a ligature. The reply would be, that this ligature must be worn during a very inconvenient and dangerous period of time. The virus lies in the wound inert during many successive weeks and months.

Dr. Haygarth first suggested that a long-continued stream of warm water should be poured upon the wound from the mouth of a kettle. He says that the poison exists in a fluid form, and therefore we should suppose that water would be its natural solvent. Dr. Massey adds to this, that if the wound is small, it should be dilated, in order that the stream may descend on the part on which the poison is deposited. We are far, however, from being certain that this falling of water on the part, may not by possibility force a portion of the virus farther into the texture, or cause it to be entangled with other parts of the wound.[a]

There is a similar or stronger objection to the cupping-glass of Dr. Barry. The virus, forced from the texture with which it lies in contact by the rush of blood from the substance beneath, is too likely to inoculate, or become entangled with, other parts of the wound.

There is great objection to suction of the wound; for, in addition to this possible entanglement, the lips, or the mouth, may have been abraded, and thus the danger considerably aggravated. There also remains the undecided question as to the absorption of the virus through the medium of a mucous surface.

Excision of the part is the mode of prevention usually adopted by the human surgeon, and to a certain extent it is a judicious

[a] The physician Apollonius, having been bitten by a rabid dog, induced another dog to lick the wound, "ut idem medicus esset qui vulneris auctor fuit."

practice. If the virus is not received into the circulation, but lies dormant in the wound for a considerable time, the disease cannot supervene if the inoculated part is destroyed.

This operation, however, demands greater skill and tact than is generally supposed. It requires a determination fully to accomplish the desired object; for every portion of the wound with which the tooth could possibly have come into contact, must be removed. This is often exceedingly difficult to accomplish, on account of the situation and direction of the wound. The knife must not enter the wound, or it will be likely to be itself empoisoned, and then the mischief and the danger will be increased instead of removed. Dr. Massey was convinced of the impropriety of this when he advised that, "should the knife by chance enter the wound that had been made by the dog's tooth, the operation should be recommenced with a clean knife, otherwise the sound parts will become inoculated."

If the incision is made freely and properly round the wound, and does not penetrate into it, yet the blood will follow the knife, and a portion of it will enter into the wound caused by the dog, and will come in contact with the virus, and will probably be contaminated, and will then overflow the original wound, and will be received into the new incision, and will carry with it the seeds of disease and death: therefore it is, that scarcely a year passes without some lamentable instances of the failure of incisions. It has occurred in the practice of the most eminent surgeons, and seems scarcely or not all to impeach the skill of the operator.

Aware of this, there are very few human practitioners who do not use the caustic after the knife. Every portion of the new wound is submitted to its influence. They do not consider the patient to be safe without this second operation. But has the question never occurred to them, that if the caustic is necessary to give security to the operation by incision, the knife might have been spared, and the caustic alone used?

The veterinary surgeon, when operating on the horse, or cattle, or the dog, frequently has recourse to the actual cautery. I could, perhaps, excuse this practice, although I would not adopt it, in superficial wounds; but I do not know the instrument that could be safely used in deeper ones. If it were sufficiently small to adapt itself to the tortuous course of little wounds, it would be cooled and inert before it could have destroyed the lower portions of them. If it were of sufficient substance long to retain the heat, it would make a large and fearful chasm, and probably interfere with the future usefulness of the animal. The result of the cases in which the cautery has been used proves that in too many instances it is an inefficient protection. The rabid dog in Park Lane has already been mentioned. He bit several horses before he could be destroyed. Caustic was applied to one of them, and the hot iron to the others. The first was saved, almost all the others were lost. A similar case occurred last spring; the caustic was an efficacious preventive; the cautery was perfectly useless. What caustic then should be applied? Certainly not that to which the surgeon usually has recourse—a liquid one. Certainly not one that speedily deliquesces; for they are both unmanageable, and, what is a more important consideration, they may hold in solution, and not decompose the poison, and thus inoculate the whole of the wound. The application which promises to be successful, is that of the *lunar caustic*. It is perfectly manageable, and, being sharpened to a point, may be applied with certainty to every recess and sinuosity of the wound.

Potash and nitric acid form a caustic which will destroy the substances with which they come in contact, but the combination of this caustic and the animal fibre will be a soft or semi-fluid mass. In this the virus is suspended, and with this it lies or may be precipitated upon the living fibre beneath. Then there is danger of re-inoculation; and it would seem that this fatal process is often accomplished. The eschar formed by the lunar caustic is dry, hard, and insoluble. If the whole of the wound has been fairly exposed to its action, an insoluble compound of animal fibre and the metallic salt is produced, in which the virus is wrapped up, and from which it cannot be separated. In a short time the dead matter sloughs away, and the virus is thrown off with it.

Previous to applying the caustic it will sometimes be necessary to enlarge the wound, in order that every part may be fairly got at; and the eschar having sloughed off, it will always be prudent to apply the caustic a second time, but more slightly, in order to destroy any part that may not have received the full influence of the first operation, or that, by possibility, might have been inoculated during the operation.

Mr. Smerdon, in the Medical and Physical Journal, March 1820, thus reasons:—"All the morbid poisons that require to lie dormant a certain time before their effects are manifested, pass into the system through the medium of the absorbents," (we somewhat differ from Mr. Smerdon here, but his reasoning is equally applicable to the nervous system,) "and if the absorbents are excited, their action is increased. I am satisfied that even in a venereal sore the application of a caustic, instead of destroying the disease, causes its rapid extension. Then," asks he, "if the virus on a small venereal sore is rendered more active by the caustic, is it not highly probable that the same law holds good with respect to the poison of rabies?"

The sooner the caustic is applied the better; but I should not hesitate to have recourse to it even after the constitution has become affected. It is related in the Medico-Chirurgical Annals of Altenburg (Sept. 1821), that two men were bitten by a rabid dog. One became hydrophobous and died; the other had evident symptoms of hydrophobia a few days afterwards. A surgeon excised the bitten part, and the disease disappeared. After a period of six days the symptoms returned. The wound was examined; considerable fungus was found sprouting from its bottom. This was extirpated. The hydrophobic symptoms were again removed, and the man did well. This is a most instructive case.

In the Journal Pratique de Médecine Vétérinaire, M. Damalix gives an interesting account of the effect of a bite of a rabid dog on a horse. On the 8th of July, 1828, a fowl-merchant, proceeding to the market of Colmar, was attacked by a dog, who, after some fruitless efforts to get into the cart, bit the horse on the left side of the face, and fled precipitately. A veterinary surgeon was sent for, who applied the cautery to the horse, gave him some populeum ointment, and bled him. Everything appeared to go on well, and on the 16th the wounds were healed.

On the 25th a great alteration took place. The horse was careless and slow; he sometimes refused to go at all, and would not attend in the least to the whip, which had never occurred before. In the evening the wounds opened spontaneously, an ichorous and infectious pus run from them; there was salivation and utter loss of appetite: strange fancies seemed to possess him; he showed a desire to bite his master. The veterinary surgeon might approach him with safety; but the moment his owner or the children appeared, he darted at them, and would have torn them in pieces. The disease now took on the appearance of acute glanders; livid and fungous wounds broke out; the stable was saturated with an infectious smell, the horse refused his food, or was unable to eat The mayor at last interfered, and the animal was destroyed. In the Treatises on The Horse, Cattle, and Sheep, in former volumes, accounts are fully given of this dreadful malady in these animals. It may not be uninteresting to give a hasty sketch of it in some of the inferior classes.

Rabies in the Rabbit.—I very much regret that I never instituted a course of experiments on the production and treatment of rabies in this animal. It would have been attended with little expense or danger, and some important discoveries might have been made. Mr. Earle, in a case in which he was much interested, inoculated two rabbits with the saliva of a dog that had died rabid. They were punctured at the root of the ears. One of the rabbits speedily became inflamed about the ears, and the ears were paralysed in both rabbits. The head swelled very much, and extensive inflammation took place around the part where the virus was inserted. One of them died without exhibiting any of the usual symptoms of the disease; the other, after a long convalescence, survived, and eventually recovered the use of his ears. Mr. Earle very properly doubted whether this was a case of rabies.

Dr. Capello describes, but in not so satisfactory a manner as could be wished, a case of supposed rabies in one of these animals. A rabbit and a dog lived together in a family. They were strange associates; but such friendships are not unfrequent among animals. The dog became rabid, and died. A man bitten by that dog became hydrophobous, and died. No one dreamed of the rabbit being in danger, and he ran about the house as usual; but, one day, he found his way to the chamber of the mistress of the house, with a great deal of viscid saliva running from his mouth, furiously attacked her, and left the marks of his violence on her leg. He then ran into a neighbouring stable, and bit the hind-legs of a horse several times. Finally, he retreated to a corner of the stable, and was there found dead. Neither the lady nor the horse eventually suffered.

Rabies in the Guinea-pig.—A man suspected of being hydrophobous was taken to the Middlesex Hospital. He was examined before several of the medical students; one of whom, in order to make more sure of the affair, inoculated a guinea-pig with the saliva taken from the man's mouth. The guinea-pig had been usually very playful, and fond of being noticed; but, on the eleventh day after this inoculation, he began to be dull and sullen, retiring into his house, and hiding himself as much as he could in a corner. On the following day he became out of temper, and even ferocious in his way; he bit at everything that was presented to him, gnawed his cage, and made the most determined efforts to escape. Once or twice his violence induced convulsions of his whole frame; and they might be produced at pleasure by dashing a little water at him. In the course of the night following he died.

Rabies in the Cat.—Fortunately for us, this does not often occur; for a mad cat is a truly ferocious animal. I have seen two cases, one of them to my cost; yet, I am unable to give any satisfactory account of the progress of the disease. The first stage seems to be one of sullenness, and which would probably last to death; but from that sullenness it is dangerous to rouse the animal. It probably would not, except in the paroxysm of rage, attack any one; but during that paroxysm it knows no fear, nor has its ferocity any bounds.

A cat, that had been the inhabitant of a nursery, and the playmate of the children, had all at once become sullen and ill-tempered. It had taken refuge in an upper room, and could not be coaxed from the corner in which it had crouched.

It was nearly dark when I went. I saw the horrible glare of her eyes, but I could not see so much of her as I wished, and I said that I would call again in the morning.

I found the patient, on the following day, precisely in the same situation and the same attitude, crouched up in a corner, and ready to spring. I was very much interested in the case; and as I wanted to study the countenance of this demon, for she looked like one, I was foolishly, inexcusably imprudent. I went on my hands and knees, and brought my face nearly on a level with hers, and gazed on those glaring eyes, and that horrible countenance, until I seemed to feel the deathly influence of a spell stealing over me. I was not afraid, but every mental and bodily power was in a manner suspended. My countenance, perhaps, alarmed her, for she sprang on me, fastened herself on my face, and bit through both my lips. She then darted down stairs, and, I believe, was never seen again. I always have nitrate of silver in my pocket, even now I am never without it; I washed myself, and applied the caustic with some severity to the wound; and my medical adviser and valued friend, Mr. Millington, punished me still more after I got home. My object was attained, although at somewhat too much cost, for the expression of that brute's countenance will never be forgotten.

The later symptoms of rabies in this animal, no one, perhaps, has had the opportunity of observing: we witness only the sullenness and the ferocity.

Rabies in the Fowl.—Dr. Ashburner and Mr. King inoculated a hen with the saliva from a rabid cow. They made two incisions through the integument, under the wings, and then well rubbed into these cuts the foam taken from the cow's mouth. She was after this let loose among other fowls in the poultry-yard. The incisions soon healed, and their places could with difficulty be discovered. Ten weeks passed over, when she was observed to refuse her food, and to run at the other fowls. She had a strange, wild appearance, and her eyes were blood-shot. Early on the following morning her legs became contracted, so that she very soon lost the power of standing upright. She remained sitting a long time, with the legs rigid, refusing food and water, and appearing very irritable when touched. She died in the evening, immediately after drinking a large quantity of water which had been offered to her.

Rabies in the Badger. — Hufeland, in his valuable Journal of Practical Medicine, relates a case of a rabid female badger attacking two boys. She bit them both, but she fastened on the thigh of one of them, and was destroyed in the act of sucking his blood. The poor fellow died hydrophobous, but the other escaped. This fact, certainly, gives us no idea of the general character of the disease in this animal; but it speaks volumes as to its ferocity.

Rabies in the Wolf.—Rabies is ushered in by nearly the same symptoms, and pursues the same course in the wolf as in the dog, with this difference, which would be readily expected, that his ferocity and the mischief which he accomplishes are much greater. The dog hunts out his own species, and his fury is principally directed against them; although, if he meets with a flock of sheep, or a herd of cattle, he readily attacks them, and, perhaps, bites the greater part of them. The dog, however, frequently turns out of his way to avoid the human being, and seldom attacks him without provocation. The wolf, on the contrary, although he commits fearful ravages among the sheep and cattle, searches out the human being as his favourite prey. He conceals himself near the entrance to the village, and steals upon and wounds every passenger that he can get at. There are several accounts of more than twenty persons having been bitten by one wolf; and there is a fearful history of sixteen persons perishing from the bite of one of these animals. This is in perfect agreement with the account which I have given of the connexion between the previous temper and habits of the rabid dog, and the mischief that he effects under the influence of this malady. The wolf, as he wanders in the forest, regards the human being as his persecutor and foe; and, in the paroxysm of rabid fury, he is most eager to avenge himself on his natural enemy. Strange stories are told of the arts to which he has recourse in order to accomplish his purpose. In the great majority of cases he steals unawares upon his victim, and the mischief is effected before the wood-cutter or the villager is conscious of his danger.

The following observations and experiments respecting rabies, by Dr. Hertwich, Professor at the Veterinary School at Berlin, are well worthy of attention.

1. Out of fifty dogs that had been inoculated with virůs taken from a rabid animal of the same species, fourteen only were infected.

2. In the cases where inoculation had been practised without effect, no reason could be assigned why the disease should not have taken place. This consequently proves that the malady is similar to others of a contagious nature, and that there must exist a predisposition in the individual to receive the disease before it can occur. In one experiment, a mastiff dog, aged four years, was inoculated without exhibiting any symptoms of the malady, while seven others, who had been inoculated at the same time and place, soon became rabid. Several of these animals had been inoculated several times before any symptoms showed themselves, while in others, on the contrary, once was sufficient.

3. It appears that in a state of doubtful rabies, one or two accidental or artificial inoculations are not sufficient to create a negative proof of its existence.

4. This disease has never been communicated to an individual from one infected by means of the perspirable matter; this, therefore, is a proof that the contagious part of the disease is not of a volatile nature.

5. It does not only exist in the saliva and the mucus of the mouth, but likewise in the blood and the parenchyma of the salivary glands; but not in the pulpy substance of the nerves.

6. The power of communicating infection is found to exist in all stages of the confirmed disease, even twenty-four hours after the decease of the rabid animal.

7. The morbid virus, when administered internally, appears to be incapable of communicating this disease; inasmuch as of twenty dogs to whom was given a certain quantity, not one exhibited the least symptom of rabies.

8. The application of the saliva upon recent wounds appears to have been as often succeeded by confirmed rabies as when the dog had been bitten by a rabid animal.

9. It cannot now be doubted that the disease is produced by the wound itself, as was supposed by M. Girard of Lyons, not by the fright of the individual, according to the opinion of others, but only from the absorption of the morbid virus from its surface.

10. Several experiments have proved to me the little reliance there is to be placed on the opinions of Baden and Capello, who believe that, in those dogs who become rabid after the bite of an animal previously attacked with this disease, the contagious properties of the saliva is not continued, but only exists in those primarily bitten.

11. During the period of incubation of the virus there are no morbid, local, or general alterations of structure or function to be seen in the infected animal; neither are there any vesicles to be perceived on the inferior surface of the tongue, nor any previous symptoms which are found in other contagious diseases.

12. This disease is generally at its height at the end of fifty days after either artificial or accidental inoculation; and the author has never known it to manifest itself at a later period.

13. It is quite an erroneous idea to suppose that dogs in a state of health are enabled to distinguish, at first sight, a rabid animal, inasmuch as they never refuse their food when mixed with the secretions of those infected.[a]

The following singular trial respecting the death of a child by hydrophobia is worth quoting:—

---

[a] Journal Pratique de Méd. Vét.

Jones v. *Parry.*—The plaintiff is a labourer, who gets only fourteen shillings a week to support himself and his family. The defendant is his neighbour, and keeps a public-house. This was an action brought by the plaintiff to recover damages against the defendant for the loss of his son, seven years of age, who was bitten by the defendant's dog, and afterwards became affected with rabies, of which disease he died.

It appeared in the evidence that the defendant's dog had, some time ago, been bitten by another dog; in consequence of which this dog was tied in the cellar, but the length of the rope which was allowed him enabled him to go to a considerable distance. The plaintiff's child knew the dog, having often played with him when he was at large. Some time ago the child crossed the street, near to the place where the dog was fastened, who rushed out of the place in which he was confined to where the child stood, sprung upon him, and bit him sadly in the face, and afterwards violently shook him. The child being thus wounded, a surgeon was sent for, who, after having dressed him, and attended him for a certain time, gave directions that he should be taken to the sea-side, and bathed in the salt water.

This having been continued for some time, the child was brought home, and, at the expiration of a month from the day on which he was bitten, became evidently and strangely ill. The surgeon proved beyond all shadow of doubt that the child laboured under rabies; that he had the never-failing symptoms of that dreadful affliction; and that, a little while before he expired, he even barked like a dog. The surgeon's charge to the father for his attendance was 1*l.* 6*s.* 6*d.*, which, together with the charge of the undertaker for the funeral of the child, amounted to between six and seven pounds. Application was made to the defendant to defray this expense, which at first he expressed a willingness to comply with, but afterwards refused; upon which this action was brought.

After some time the defendant offered to pay the plaintiff the sum of 6*l.* 3*s.* 6*d.*, and the expense of the funeral and the surgeon, provided the plaintiff would bear the expenses of the lawsuit, which he was not in a condition to do, as probably it would amount to more than that money. On this account, therefore, the action was now brought into court. There was no proof that the defendant knew or suspected his dog to be mad, previously to his attacking the boy; but an animal known to have been bitten by a mad dog, ought either to have been at once destroyed, or so secured that it was impossible for him to do mischief.

Lord Kenyon observed to the jury, that this was one of those causes which came home to the feelings of all, yet must not be carried farther than justice demanded. A cause like this never, perhaps, before occurred in a court of justice; but there had been many resembling it in point of principle. If a dog, known to be ill-tempered and vicious, did any person an injury without provocation, there could be no question that the owner of the dog was answerable, in a court of justice, for the injury inflicted. Here was a worse case. The dog by whom the child was bitten had been attacked by another that was undeniably rabid. His master was aware of this, and placed him in a state of partial confinement—a confinement so lax, and so inefficient, that this poor child had broken through it, and was bitten and died. What other people would have done in such a situation he could not tell; but, if he were asked what he would do, he answered, he certainly would kill the dog, however much of a favourite he had been, because no atonement was within the reach of his fortune to make to the injured party for such a dreadful visitation of Providence as this. It was not enough for the owner of such a dog to say, he took precaution to prevent mischief: he ought to have made it impossible that mischief could happen; and, therefore, as soon as there was any reasonable suspicion that the dog was rabid, he ought to have destroyed him.

But, if the owner wished to save the animal, until he was satisfied of the actual state of the case, he ought to have secured him, so that every individual might be safe. Whether the defendant thought he had done all that was necessary, his lordship did not know; but this he knew, that the dog was not perfectly secured, otherwise this misfortune could not have happened.

The care which the defendant took in this case was not enough, and, therefore, he had no doubt that this action was maintainable. The jury would judge what damages they ought to give. He would refer this to their feelings. They could not avoid commiserating the distress of the family of this poor man. He should, however, observe to the jury, that they must not give vindictive damages; but still he did not think that damages merely to the amount of 6*l.* or 7*l.*, which was stated to be the expense of the funeral, &c., would at all meet the justice of the case. He was inclined to advise them to go beyond that, although he did not plead vindictive damages. There would be costs to be defrayed by the plaintiff, well known in the profession under the head of "extra costs," even although he had a verdict. If the verdict had been at his disposal, he would have taken care that these costs should have been borne by the party that had been the cause of the injury. That appeared to him to be the justice of the case.

He trusted that none who heard him would doubt his sincerity, when he said, he lamented the misfortune which had given birth to this action; and, with that qualification of the case, he must say that he was not sorry that this action had been brought. He thanked the plaintiff for bringing it; for it might be of public benefit. It would teach a lesson that would not soon be forgotten, "That a person, who knowingly keeps a vicious, dangerous animal, should be considered to be answerable for all the acts of that animal." There were instances in which very large damages had been given to repair such injuries. He did not say that the present case called for large damages; but, if other cases of the same kind should be brought into court after this had been made public, he hoped the jury would go beyond the ordinary limits, and give verdicts which might operate *in terrorem* on the offending parties.

Verdict for the plaintiff—damages 36*l*.[a]

A child was bitten by a rabid dog at York, and became hydrophobous. All possibility of relief having vanished, the parents, desirous of putting an end to the agony of their child, or fearful of its doing mischief, smothered it between two pillows. They were tried for murder, and found guilty. They were afterwards pardoned; but the intention of the prosecutor was that of deterring others from a similar practice, in a like unfortunate situation.[b]

In 1821, a physician, at Poissy, was sentenced to pay 8000 francs (320*l*.) to a poor widow whose husband died of hydrophobia, in consequence of a bite from the physician's dog, he knowing that the dog had been bitten, yet not confining him.

[Our author having written so extensively upon the subject of rabies, it would seem superfluous in us to attempt to add anything more upon a subject so ably and practically handled by one having so great opportunities to make personal observations. However, to allay the feelings of many of our dogkilling citizens, we will not hesitate to assert that we do not place as much credence in the frequency of rabies as is generally done; but, on the other hand, are strongly led to believe that the accounts of this much-dreaded malady are greatly exaggerated both in this country and in England.

That there may be a few cases of rabies in our country in the course of a year, we do not doubt: but, at the same time, we are satisfied that the affection in its genuine form is quite rare, and that the great hue and cry made every season about mad dogs, is more the result of ignorance and fright than of reality.

Our limits in this publication would not allow us sufficient space to enlarge upon the many pathological questions naturally arising from a minute examination of this subject, more particularly as our views are somewhat at variance with the generally received opinion, and which, of course, we would be forced to express with considerable diffidence, owing to the impossibility of collecting such evidence as might seem necessary to substantiate any peculiar doctrine.

---

[a] Sporting Magazine, vol. xviii. p. 186. [b] Daniel's Rural Sports, vol. i. p. 220.

That tetanus, hysteria, and other spasmodic affections have often been mistaken for rabies, there is no doubt, and we can easily imagine the mental effect produced upon an individual of a highly nervous temperament, by the knowledge of his being bitten by an animal known to be hydrophobic; and we can, without difficulty, reconcile with our best judgment the belief *that the workings of such an individual's imagination, occasioned by the never-ceasing dread of the horrid malady to which he is now exposed, might be sufficient to produce a train of symptoms somewhat resembling the actual state of rabies.*

For the benefit of these nervous unfortunates, we might say to them, that the statistics of this affection show a very considerable ratio in favour of escape from inoculation when bitten, or of entire recovery even after the developement of the disease, and that there are many other ills in the catalogue of medicine that they should take equal pains to provide against as lyssa canina. We doubt not that the minds of many will be relieved, when informed that John Hunter mentions an instance, in which, out of twenty persons bitten by a rabid dog, only one suffered from the malady; and that of fifty-nine dogs inoculated by Professor Hertwick at the veterinary school of Berlin, only fourteen were affected; and of eleven patients entrusted to the care of M. Blaise of Cluny, seven recovered after exhibiting greater or less degrees of spasmodic symptoms.

It may prove interesting to our readers, to insert in these pages an account of the first two cases of rabies known in Philadelphia, and as related to us by a venerable and much-esteemed citizen, who is well known in the scientific world as a gentleman of deep research, and we agree with him in opinion, that this much-dreaded disease is most frequently the result of like causes, or rather that like symptoms often induce the belief of the presence of this malady, when, in fact, no such disease does exist.

Towards the close of the last century, there lived a tailor in Front street, near Market, in the midst of the most respectable people of that period; among the number was our esteemed friend Mr. Hembel, as also Judge Tilghman. This tailor possessed an ill-tempered little spaniel, who, lounging about the street-door, attacked every one that passed by, snapping and snarling in the most worrisome manner, more particularly at every little urchin that invaded his "right of pavement," and not unfrequently biting them or tearing their clothes from their back. The owner of the dog was appealed to on many occasions by the neighbours, begging that the quarrelsome brute should either be disposed of or kept within doors. To all these solicitations and warnings the little tailor paid no heed, but continued stitching his breeches and cribing his customers' goods, while the ugly little spaniel, without interruption, amused himself by snapping at and biting the heels of the passers-by.

The nuisance at last became insufferable, and Judge Tilghman applied to Mr. Hembel to assist him in getting rid of this troublesome brute; the latter gentleman advised the administration of a small quantity of strychnia, concealed in a portion of meat, which proposition was agreed upon and immediately carried into execution. A short time after the administering of this dose the spaniel sickened, and retired from his post to the kitchen, which was in the basement, and where an Irish domestic was engaged in washing; the dog appeared uneasy for a time, and suddenly, being taken with the involuntary muscular convulsions that so frequently follow the administration of this powerful drug, ran around the kitchen yelping and howling at a most terrible rate, and ultimately, to the no small discomfiture and amazement of the maid, sprang up into the wash-tub, at which unceremonious caper, on the part of the dog, the woman became greatly alarmed and ran out into the street, followed by the whole household, crying mad dog, which soon produced an uproar in the neighbourhood, no one daring to satisfy himself as to the correctness of the report, and all, perhaps, too ignorant of the subject to discern the real cause of the animal's singular behaviour. The tailor, still bearing a strong attachment to his unfortunate favourite, and being somewhat more daring than his neighbours, ventured, at length, to peep into the kitchen to see the state of affairs, and seeing the dog still convulsed and foaming at the mouth, was more than ever confirmed in the belief of hydrophobia, and knowing full well the biting propensities of the animal, independent of rabies, concluded, much to the relief of every one, to shoot him. The next step in the programme was the dragging out and consigning of the patient to a watery grave, which was accomplished by placing, with a pair of tongs, a noose over the head of the animal, and thus hawling him out of the basement window amid the cheers of the assembled populace who soon cast him into the Delaware.

The second case of rabies as related to us by Mr. Hembel was as follows:—In 1793 the barbers of the city were in the habit of going around to the various boarding-houses for the purpose of shaving the visitors in their apartments, instead of accommodating them, as at the present time, in their own establishments.

One of these knights of the razor, living also in Front street, when going to and from a fashionable boarding-house in the vicinity, was not unfrequently assailed by a small cur who often took him by the heels when hurrying along.

To get rid of this annoying little animal as speedily and secretly as possible, he had recourse to the powers of strychnia, which produced in a very short time similar effects upon the poor victim, and tne result was another great hue and cry about mad dogs.

These authentic and remarkable cases of hydrophobia were heralded in all the papers of the day, which, from that time forward, were filled with notes of caution to all dog-owners.

Of the *treatment* of rabies we will make but a few remarks, as of the immense number of specifics proposed for this disease, amounting in all to several hundred, few or none can be relied on to the exclusion of the others; but those medicines, perhaps, known as opiates or anti-spasmodics, claim a larger share of attention than any others in combating the disease after its development. In looking over the very original works of Jacques Du Fouilloux, a worthy cynegetical writer of the sixteenth century, we find a prescription that was supposed by many to be an infallible specific for this disease, and as it appears to us quite as certain in its effects on the animal economy as many others of the inert substances that have been lauded to the skies both in our country and in other parts of the world as antidotes, we take the liberty of transcribing it, as also of adding a translation of his quaint French.

Autre recepte par mots preservants la rage.

'Ay appris vne recepte d'vn Gentil-homme, en Bretaigne, lequel faisoit de petits escriteaux, où n'y auoit seulement que deux lignes, lesquels il mettoit en vne omellette d'œufs, puis les faisoit aualer aux chiens qui auorient esté mords de chiens enragez, et auoit dedans l'escriteau, *Y Ran Qviran Cafram Cafratrem, Cafratrosqve.* Lesquels mots disoit estre singuliers pour empescher les chiens de la rage, mais quant à moi ie n'y adiouste pas foy.

I have learned a recipe from a nobleman of Brittany, which is composed of a written charm, in which there are only two lines; these he put in an omelet of eggs, he then made the dogs that had been bitten by a rabid animal swallow them. There was on the paper "*Y Ran Quiran Cafram, Cafratrem Cafratrosque.*" These words were said to be singularly efficacious in preventing madness in dogs, but for my part I do not credit it.

Although our quaint author considered the above charm even too marvellous for his belief, we give below his own prescription in which he placed implicit confidence, but, no doubt, on trial it would prove "*as singularly efficacious" as the other.*

Baing pour lauer, les chiens, quand ils ont esté mords des chiens enragez, de peur qu'ils enragent.

Qvand les chiens sont mords ou desbrayez de chiens enragez, il faut incontinent emplir vne pippe d'eau, puis prendre quatre boisseaux de sel et les ietter dedans, en meslaut fort le sel auec vn baston pour le faire fondre soudainement: et quand il sera fondu, faut mettre le chien dedans, et le plonger tout, sans qu'il paroisse rien, par neuf fois: puis quand il sera bien laué, faut le laisser aller, celà l'empeschera d'enrager.

When a dog has been bitten or scratched by another affected with madness, we must immediately take a tub of water and throw into it four bushels of salt, stirring it briskly with a stick to make it dissolve quickly. When the salt shall be dissolved, put the dog into the bath, and plunge him well nine times, so that the bath shall cover him each time; now that he is well washed you may let him go, as this will prevent his becoming rabid.

Having given publicity to the two preceding valuable receipts, we must be pardoned for adding our own views upon this point, as a caution to those who may not feel sufficient faith in the remedies above mentioned.

The wound should be thoroughly washed and cleansed as soon as possible after the bite is inflicted: no sucking of the parts, as is advised by many, for the purpose of extracting the poison, as the presence of a small abrasion of the lips or interior of the mouth would most assuredly subject the parts to inoculation. If the wound be ragged, the edges may be taken off with a pair of sharp scissors; the wound must then be thoroughly cauterized with nitrate of silver (lunar caustic), being sure to introduce the caustic into the very depths of the wound, so that it will reach every particle of poison that may have insinuated itself into the flesh. If the wound is too small to admit of the stick of caustic, it may be enlarged by the knife, taking care, however, not to carry the poison into the fresh cut, which can be avoided by wiping the knife at each incision. Should the wound be made on any of the limbs, a bandage may be placed around it during the application of these remedies, the more effectually to prevent the absorption of the virus. Nitrate of silver is a most powerful neutralizer of specific poisons, and the affected parts will soon come away with the slough, no dressings being necessary, except perhaps olive oil, if there should be much inflammation of the parts. If the above plan be pursued, the patient need be under no apprehension as to the result, but make his mind perfectly easy on the point. This is the course generally pursued by all the veterinary surgeons of Europe, and there are but few of them who have not, some time in their practice, been bitten and often severely lacerated by rabid animals; nevertheless, we never hear of their having suffered any bad effects from such accidents. If caustic be not at hand, the wound may be seared over with red-hot iron, which will answer as good a purpose, although much more painful in its operation. Mr. Blaine, in closing his able and scientific article on this subject, very justly remarks, "Would I could instil into such minds the *uncertainty* of the disease appearing at all; that is, even when no means have been used; and the *perfect security* they may feel who have submitted to the preventive treatment detailed. I have been bitten several times, Mr. Youatt several also; yet in neither of us was any dread occasioned: our experience taught us the *absolute certainty* of the *preventive* means; and such I take on me to pronounce they always prove, when performed with dexterity and judgment." We acknowledge ourselves a convert to this gentleman's doctrine; and feel satisfied that if the above course be adopted, there need be no fear whatever of the developement of this frightful affection.—L.]

CHAPTER VIII.

THE EYE AND ITS DISEASES.

The diseases that attack the same organ are essentially different, in different animals, in their symptoms, intensity, progress, and mode of treatment. In periodic ophthalmia — that pest of the equine race and opprobrium of the veterinary profession—the cornea becomes suddenly opaque, the iris pale, the aqueous humour turbid, the capsule of the lens cloudy, and blindness is the result. After a time, however, the cornea clears up, and becomes as bright as ever; but the lens continues impervious to light, and vision is lost.

Ophthalmia in the dog presents us with symptoms altogether different. The conjunctiva is red; that portion of it which spreads over the sclerotica is highly injected, and the cornea is opaque. As the disease proceeds, and even at a very early period of its progress, an ulcer appears on the centre; at first superficial, but enlarging and deepening until it has penetrated the cornea, and the aqueous humour has escaped. Granulations then spring from the edges of the ulcer, rapidly enlarge, and protrude through the lids. Under proper treatment, however, or by a process of nature, these granulations cease to sprout; they begin to disappear; the ulcer diminishes; it heals; scarcely a trace of it can be seen; the cornea recovers its perfect transparency, and vision is not in the slightest degree impaired.

There is a state of the orbit which requires some consideration. It is connected with the muscles employed in mastication. Generally speaking, the food of the dog requires no extraordinary degree of mastication, nor is there usually any great time employed in this operation. That muscle which is most employed in the comminution of the food, namely, the temporal muscle, has its action very much limited by the position of the bony socket of the eye; yet sufficient room is left for all the force that can be required. In some dogs, either for purposes of offence or defence, or the more effectual grasping of the prey, a sudden violent exertion of muscular power, and a consequent contraction of the temporal muscle, are requisite, but for which the imperfect socket of the orbit does not seem to afford sufficient scope and room. There is an admirable provision for this in the removal of a certain portion of the orbital process of the frontal bone on the outer and upper part of the external ridge, and the substitution of an elastic cartilage. This cartilage momentarily yields to the swelling of the muscles; and then, by its inherent elasticity, the external ridge of the orbit resumes its pristine form. The orbit of the dog, the pig, and the cat, exhibits this singular mechanism.

The horse is, to a certain extent, also an illustration of this. He requires an extended field of vision to warn him of the approach of his enemies in his wild state, and a direction of the orbits somewhat forward to enable him to pursue with safety the headlong course to which we sometimes urge him; and for this purpose his eyes are placed more forward than those of cattle, sheep, or swine. That which Mr. Percivall states of the horse is true of our other domesticated animals:—"The eyeball is placed within the anterior or more capacious part of the orbit, nearer to the frontal than to the temporal side, with a degree of prominence peculiar to the individual, and, within certain limits, variable at his will."

In many of the carnivorous animals the orbit encroaches on the bones of the face. A singular effect is also produced on the countenance, both when the animal is growling over his prey and when he is devouring it. The temporal muscle is violently acted upon; it presses upon the cartilage that forms part of the external ridge; that again forces itself upon and protrudes the eye, and hence the peculiar ferocity of expression which is observed at that time. The victims of these carnivorous animals are also somewhat provided against danger by the acuteness of sight with which they are gifted. Adipose matter also exists in a considerable quantity in the orbit of the eye, which enables it to revolve by the slightest contraction of the muscles.

We should scarcely expect to meet with cases of fracture of the orbital arch in the dog, because, in that animal, cartilage, or a cartilago-ligamentous substance, occupies a very considerable part of that arch; but I have again and again, among the cruelties that are practised on the inferior creation, seen the cartilage partly, or even entirely, torn asunder. I have never been able satisfactorily to ascertain the existence of this during life; but I have found it on those whom I have recommended to be destroyed on account of the brutal usage which they had experienced. Blows somewhat higher, or on the thick temporal muscle of this animal, will very rarely produce a fracture.

A few cases of disease in the eye may be interesting and useful.

Case I.—The eyes of a favourite spaniel were found inflamed and impatient of light. Nothing wrong had been perceived on the preceding day. No ulceration could be observed on the cornea, and there was but a slight mucous discharge. An infusion of digitalis, with twenty times the quantity of tepid water, was employed as a collyrium, and an aloetic ball administered. On the following day the eyes were more inflamed. The collyrium and the aloes were employed as before, and a seton inserted in the poll.

Three or four days afterwards the redness was much diminished, the discharge from the eye considerably lessened, and the dog was sent home. The seton, however, was continued, with an aloetic ball on every third or fourth day.

Two or three days after this the eyes were perfectly cured and the seton removed.

Case II.—The eye is much inflamed and the brow considerably protruded.

This was supposed to be caused by a bite. I vainly endeavoured to bring the lid over the swelling. I scarified the lid freely, and ordered the bleeding to be encouraged by the constant application of warm water, and a physic-ball to be given.

On the following day the brow was found to be scarcely or at all reduced, and the eye could not be closed. I drew out the haw with a crooked needle, and cut it off closely with sharp scissors. The excised portion was as large as a small-kidney-bean. The fomentation was continued five days afterwards, and the patient then dismissed cured.

Case III. — A pointer was brought in a sad state of mange. Redness, scurf, and eruptions were on almost every part. Apply the mange ointment and the alterative and physic balls. On the following day there was an ulcer on the centre of the cornea, with much appearance of pain and impatience of light. Apply an infusion of digitalis, with the liquor plumbi diacetatis. He was taken away on the twelfth day, the mange apparently cured, and the inflammation of the eye considerably lessened. A fortnight afterwards this also appeared to be cured.

Case IV.—A spaniel had been bitten by a large dog. There was no wound of the lids, but the eye was protruded from the socket. I first tried whether it could be reduced by gentle pressure, but I could not accomplish it. I then introduced the blunt end of a curved needle between the eye and the lid; and thus drawing up the lid with the right hand, while I pressed gently on the eye with the left hand, I accomplished my object. I then subtracted three ounces of blood and gave a physic-ball. On the following day the eye was hot and red, with some tumefaction. The pupil was moderately contracted, but was scarcely affected by any change of light. The dog was sent home, with some extract of goulard, and a fortnight afterwards was quite well.

Case V.—A dog received a violent blow on the right eye. Immediate blindness occurred, or the dog could apparently just discern the difference between light and darkness, but could not distinguish particular objects. The pupil was expanded and immovable. A pink-coloured hue could be perceived on looking earnestly into the eye. A seton was introduced into the poll, kept there nearly a month, and often stimulated rather sharply. General remedies of almost every kind were tried: depletion was carried to its full extent, the electric fluid was had recourse to; but at the expiration of nine weeks the case was abandoned and the dog destroyed. Permission to examine him was refused.

I have, in two or three instances, witnessed decided cases of dropsy of the eye, accumulation of fluid taking place in both the anterior and posterior chambers of the eye; there was also effusion of blood in the chambers, but in one case only was there the slightest benefit produced by the treatment adopted, and in that there was gradual absorption of the effused fluid.

About the same time there was another similar case. A pointer had suddenly considerable opacity of one eye, without any known cause: the other eye was not in the least degree affected. The dog had not been out of the garden for more than a week. The eye was ordered to be fomented with warm water.

On the following day the inflammation had increased, and the adipose matter was protruded at both the inner and outer canthus. The eye was bathed frequently with a goulard lotion. On the fourth day the eyeball was still more inflamed, and the projections at both canthi were increased. A curved needle was passed through both eyes, and there was considerable bleeding. On the following day the inflammation began to subside. At the expiration of a week scarcely any disease remained, and the eye became as transparent as ever.

A curious case of congenital blindness was brought to my infirmary. A female pointer puppy, eight weeks old, had both her eyes of their natural size and formation, but the inner edge of the iris was strangely diseased. The pupil was curiously four-cornered, and very small. There hung out of the pupil a grayish-white fibrous matter, which appeared to be the remainder of the pupillary membrane.

Six months afterwards we examined her again, and found that the pupil was considerably enlarged, and properly shaped, and the white skin had vanished. In the back-ground of the eye there was a faint yellow-green light, and the dog not only showed sensibility to light, but some perception of external objects. At this period we lost sight of her.

A very considerable improvement has taken place with regard to the treatment of the enlarged or protruded ball of the eye. A dog may get into a skirmish, and have his eye forced from the socket. If there is little or no bleeding, the case will probably be easily and successfully treated.

The eye must, first, be thoroughly washed, and not a particle of grit must be left. A little oil, a crooked needle, and a small piece of soft rag should be procured. The blunt end of the needle should be dipped into the oil, and run round the inside of the lid, first above and then below. The operator will next — his fingers being oiled — press upon the protruded eye gently, yet somewhat firmly, changing the pressure from one part of the eye to the other, in order to force it back into the socket.

If, after a couple of minutes' trial, he does not succeed, let him again oil the eye on the inside and the out, and once more introduce the blunt end of the needle, attempting to carry it upwards under the lid with two or three fingers pressing on the eye, and the points of pressure being frequently changed. In by far the greater number of cases, the eye will be saved.

If it is impracticable to cause the eye to retract, a needle with a thread attached must be passed through it, the eye being then drawn as forward as possible and cut off close to the lids. The bleeding will soon cease and the lids perfectly close.

Ophthalmia is a disease to which the dog is often liable. It is the result of exposure either to heat or to cold, or violent exertion: it is remedied by bleeding, purging, and the application of sedative medicines, as the acetate of lead or the tincture of opium. When the eye is considerably inflamed, in addition to the application of tepid or cold water, either the inside of the lids or the white of the eye may be lightly touched with the lancet. From exposure to cold, or accident or violence, inflammation often spreads on the eye to a considerable degree, the pupil is clouded, and small streaks of blood spread over the opaque cornea. The mode of treatment just described must be pursued.

The crystalline lens occasionally becomes opaque. There is cataract. It may be the result of external injury or of internal predisposition. Old dogs are particularly subject to cataract. That which arises from accident, or occasionally disease, may, although seldom, be reinstated, especially in the young dog, and both eyes may become sound; but, in the old, the slow-growing opacity will, almost to a certainty, terminate in cataract.

There is occasionally an enlargement of the eye, or rather an accumulation of fluid within the eye, to a very considerable extent. No external application seems to have the slightest effect in reducing the bulk of the eye. If it is punctured, much inflammation ensues, and the eye gradually wastes away.

In *amaurosis*, the eye is beautifully clear, and, for a little while, this clearness imposes upon the casual observer; but there is a peculiar pellucid appearance about the eye — a preternatural and unchanging brightness. In the horse, the sight occasionally returns, but I have never seen this in the dog.

The occasional glittering of the eyes of the dog has been often observed. The cat, the wolf, some carnivora, and also sheep, cows, and horses, occasionally exhibit the same glittering. Pallas imagined that the light of these animals emanated from the nervous membrane of the eye, and considered it to be an electrical phenomenon. It is found, however, in every animal that possesses a *tapetum lucidum*. The shining, however, never takes place in complete darkness. It is neither produced voluntarily, nor in consequence of any moral emotion, but solely from the reflection that falls on the eye.

[The eye and its diseases being so concisely treated by Mr. Youatt, we are emboldened to add a more full and particular treatise on this interesting subject, couched in language the most simple, and we trust sufficiently plain to be understood by the most unscientific patron of the canine race.

THE EYE AND ITS DISEASES.

THE NICTITATING MEMBRANE.

It is somewhat astonishing that an organ, so delicate and so much exposed as the eye of the hunting dog necessarily is, should not more frequently be attacked with disease, or suffer from the thorns, poisonous briars, and bushes that so constantly oppose their progress while in search of game. Nature, ever wise in her undertakings, while endowing this organ with extreme sensibility, also furnished it with the means of protecting itself in some measure against the many evils that so constantly threaten its destruction.

The plica semilunaris, haw or nictitating membrane, though not as largely developed in the dog as in some other animals, is, nevertheless, of sufficient size to afford considerable protection to the ball of the eye, and assists materially in preventing the accumulation of seeds and other minute particles within the conjunctiva. This delicate membrane is found at the inner canthus of the eye, and can be drawn at pleasure over a portion of the globe, so as to free its surface from any foreign substances that might be upon it. Although the eye of the dog is attacked by many diseases, almost as numerous as those of the human being, still they are much less frequent and far more tractable.

OPHTHALMIA—SIMPLE INFLAMMATION OF THE EYE.

In its mild form this disease is frequently met with, and easily yields to the administration of the proper remedies, but when it appears as an epidemic, in a kennel, it proves more stubborn. The discharge in epidemic ophthalmia, when carried from one dog to the eyes of another, no doubt is contagious, and, therefore, it is necessary to separate dogs as much from each other as possible during any prevalent epidemic of this nature.

The disease announces itself by slight redness of the conjunctiva, tenderness to light, and increased flow of the secretions.

The eyeball appears retracted in its socket, and more moist and transparent than usual. The infected vessels of the conjunctiva form a species of net-work, and can be moved about with this membrane, showing that the inflammation is entirely superficial, and not penetrating the other coverings of the eye. Extravasation of blood within the conjunctiva, (bloodshot,) is also not an uncommon appearance, but is frequently the first symptom that draws our attention to the malady.

As the disease progresses, the conjunctiva becomes more vascular, the photophobia intolerable, the cornea itself becomes opaque, and sometimes exhibits a vascular appearance. There is considerable itching of the ball, as evinced by the disposition of the dog to close the eye. If the disease progresses in its course, unchecked by any remediate means, the cornea may lose its vitality, ulceration commence, and the sight be for ever destroyed by the bursting and discharge of the contents of the eye.

Causes.—Simple canine ophthalmia proceeds from many causes, distinct in their character, but all requiring pretty much the same treatment. Bad feeding, bad lodging, want of exercise, extremes of heat and cold, are the most active agents in producing this affection.

Treatment.—The disease in its mild form is very tractable, and requires but little attention; soothing applications, in connexion with confinement to an obscure apartment and low diet, will generally correct the affection in its forming stage.

In all inflammations of the eye, tepid applications we consider preferable to cold, the latter producing a temporary reaction, but no permanent good, while the former exerts a soothing and relaxing influence over the tissues and parts to which they are applied.

Weak vinegar and water, with a small proportion of laudanum, we have frequently seen used with advantage as a wash in this complaint.

When there is fever, it will be necessary to bleed and purge. Scarifying the conjunctiva with the point of a lancet, has been resorted to by some veterinary surgeons with success.

CHRONIC OPHTHALMIA.

When the disease assumes this form, the discharge from the eyes is lessened, and becomes more thick, the conjunctiva is not of such a bright arterial red, but more of a brick-dust colour, and the inner side of the lids when exposed will present small prominences and ulcerations.

Treatment.—More stimulating collyria will now be necessary, as solutions of sulphate of zinc, copper, acetate of lead, &c. See No. 1, 2, 3, of the Collyria. The direct application of sulphate of copper, or nitrate of silver, will often be of great benefit in changing the action of the parts.

The lids should be turned down and brushed over two or three times with the above articles in substance, and the dog restrained for a few moments to prevent him from scratching during the temporary pain inflicted upon him by the application.

Laudanum dropped in the eye will also prove very beneficial, allaying the itching and pain, at the same time stimulating the organs to renewed action. If the disease does not succumb under this treatment, a seton placed in the pole will generally conquer it.

TRAUMATIC OPHTHALMIA

is produced by wounds of poisoned briars, stings of insects, bites of other dogs, the scratching of cats, or the actual presence of foreign bodies in the eye itself, which latter cause frequently occurs, and is often overlooked by the sportsman.

Treatment.—This species of ophthalmia is best subdued by the application of emollient poultices, depletion, purgation and cooling washes. If a seed, small briar, or other substance has got in under the lids, or inserted itself in the globe of the eye, the dog keeps the eye closed, it waters freely, and in a short time becomes red and inflamed. The removal of the article alone, will generally produce a cure; sometimes it is necessary to use a cooling wash and administer a purge or two. Great care should be had for the extraction of extraneous substances from the eyes of dogs, as their presence often causes great suffering to the animal even while diligently employed in the field. The writer has seen dogs more than once rendered useless while hunting, by grass, clover-seeds, or other small particles burying themselves under the lids.

Ophthalmia of Distemper.—This species of inflammation will be spoken of when treating of this latter affection.

SYMPATHETIC OPHTHALMIA

arises from the presence of some other disease located in another portion of the body, as derangement of the stomach, mange, surfeit, &c. The presence of one of these affections will indicate the cause of the other.

Treatment.—Soothing applications to the organ itself, and remedies for the removal of the primary affection.

HYDROPHTHALMIA,

though not a common affection in the canine race, is occasionally met with; several cases have come under the observation of the writer, and no doubt there are but few dog-fanciers who have not seen the eyeballs of some dog suffering with this malady, ready to start from their sockets.

This affection depends upon a superabundance of the humours of the eye, occasioned by over-secretion, or a want of power in the absorbent vessels to carry off the natural secretions of the parts.

Old dogs are more apt to suffer from this disease than young dogs: nevertheless, the latter are not by any means exempt; we once saw a pup, a few days old, with the globe of the eye greatly extended by this affection.

As the disease progresses, the eye becomes more hard and ten der, the sight is greatly impaired, and ultimately, if not arrested, the eye bursts, discharges its contents, and total blindness ensues, greatly to the relief of the poor animal.

Treatment.—This disease is very intractable, and is to be combated by saline purges, bleeding, and stimulating application to the organ itself. Mercurial ointment, rubbed over the eyebrow, will assist in stimulating the absorbents.

When the disease has progressed for a long time, and the pain, as is often the case, seems intense, it will save the animal great suffering, by opening the ball and allowing the humours to escape. This may be done by puncturing the cornea or the sclerotic coat with a needle. Setons introduced along the spine would have a good effect.

CONGENITAL BLINDNESS

occasionally occurs throughout a whole litter, no doubt being entailed upon the progeny of those dogs who have defective vision, or who are old and infirm at the time of copulation. The best and only remedy is speedy drowning.

CATARACT

consists in the partial or complete opacity of the crystalline lens;

it results from numerous causes, and is more frequent in the old than the young subject. In old dogs both eyes are usually attacked, producing absolute blindness, while in young animals one eye alone is generally attacked.

Causes.—Old age, hard work, and bad feeding, are the agents most active in the production of this affection; it generally comes on slowly, but sometimes very quickly.

When the disease occurs in young dogs, it is generally the result of wounds or blows over the head, convulsions and falls.

Treatment.—Little can be accomplished towards curing this disease either in the old or young dog, as the disease, in spite of all our efforts, will run its course, and terminate in total opacity of the lens. Mild purging, blistering on the neck, introduction of the seton, and blowing slightly stimulating powders into the eye, will sometimes arrest the progress of the disease in the young dog.

ULCERATIONS ON THE CORNEA

are sometimes very troublesome, and if not put a stop to, will often cause opacity and blindness, if not total destruction of the eye.

Slightly stimulating washes and purges are useful; the careful application of nitrate of silver will often induce the ulcer to heal; it must be put on very nicely and gently.

SPOTS ON THE CORNEA

are the result of ulcers and inflammation. If they do not materially interfere with vision, they had better be left alone.

Powdered sugar and a small quantity of alum blown into the eye daily through a quill, we have seen used with much success.

AMAUROSIS—GUTTA SERENA OR GLASS EYE.

A partial or complete paralysis of the optic nerves of either side is not a frequent disease. It usually comes on gradually, but sometimes may appear in the course of a few hours from the effects of wounds or convulsions. When the paralysis is complete, total blindness of course ensues. The intimate connection, or sympathy, existing between the nerves of either eye, is so peculiar that disease of one is quickly followed by a corresponding disease in the other.

Amaurosis, therefore, ordinarily ends in total blindness. The disease is characterized by a dilated state of the pupil, which seldom contracts under the effect of any degree of light thrown upon it. The coats and humours of the eye are perfectly transparent, in fact appear to be more pellucid than natural.

Causes.—This affection is produced in many different ways; among the most common causes may be mentioned wounds on the head, or of the parts surrounding the nerve, strains, falls, disease of the bone, convulsions, and epileptic fits.

We have seen a case produced by a tumour, which occupied the posterior portion of the orbit, and caused the organ to be somewhat protruded from its proper position, giving the eye the appearance of hydrophthalmia, for which it was taken, the existence of the tumour never for a moment being suspected. In this case there was partial amaurosis in both sides, although nothing of disease could be discovered in the left eye.

Amaurosis is a very deceptive disease, the nerves alone being affected; the humours and coverings of the eye remaining perfectly transparent and natural, imposes upon the inexperienced observer, but is easily detected by those who have witnessed the disease in others. There is a singular watery appearance and vacant stare about the eye of the dog that cannot be mistaken. This peculiarity is owing, no doubt, to the enlargement of the pupil, as before observed.

Treatment.—When proceeding from blows, convulsions, or inflammation of the nerve itself, bleeding will be serviceable, as also purging and blistering. If the disease should appear without any symptom, or other cause, to lead us to believe that there is any local affection, the antiphlogistic course should be laid aside, and resort be had to local and constitutional tonic applications, and revulsive frictions to the nape of the neck and spine. A seton may also be applied; and electricity has been recommended in such cases, no doubt arising from want of tone in the general system.

This affection, in spite of every effort, is very unmanageable, and but seldom yields to any course of treatment. Strychnia has been used lately, both internally and externally, in the cure of this complaint; it may be sprinkled over a blistered surface immediately above the eye, in the proportion of a grain morning and evening; it may also be administered inwardly at the same time, in doses from the half a grain to a grain twice a day.

EXTIRPATION OF THE EYE.

It sometimes becomes necessary, from the diseased state of this organ, that it should be taken completely from its socket. This operation, though frightful, perhaps, to consider, is very simple in its application, and may be performed without difficulty by any one accustomed to the use of the knife. The animal is to be held firmly, as before directed, and an assistant to keep the lids widely extended.

If the lids cannot be drawn well over the eye, owing to enlargement of the ball caused by disease, they may be separated by an incision at the external angle. A curved needle armed with a thread is now to be passed entirely through the eye, being careful to include sufficient of the sound parts within its grasp to prevent its tearing out. This finished, the needle may be detached, and the ends of the thread being united, the movements of the eye can be governed by means of this ligature: then proceed as follows:

1st. The assistant keeping the lids well separated, the operator draws the eye upward and outward, and then inserting the scalpel at the inner and lower angle of the eye, with a gentle sweep separates the ball from the lids, extending the incisions through to the external canthus.

2d. The ball is now to be drawn inwardly and downward, while the scalpel, continuing the circular movement as far as the internal canthus, separates the upper lid.

3d. The muscles and optic nerves still bind this organ to the orbit, which attachments can easily be destroyed by the scalpel, by pulling the eye forward sufficiently to reach them. If the eye has been extirpated on account of any malignant disease, it is necessary to remove every particle of muscle from the orbit; and when the disease has extended itself to the lids, it will also be proper to remove that portion of them included in the affection.

The hemorrhage from the operation is trifling, and may generally be arrested by the pressure of the fingers, or the insertion of a conical ball of lint within the socket, which may be allowed to remain two or three days if necessary. If there is nothing to apprehend from hemorrhage, it is only necessary to draw the lids together, and unite that portion which has been separated by a suture, and place a hood over the whole.

We do not recommend the stuffing of the orbit with lint, except in case of hemorrhage, as its presence will sometimes produce violent inflammation, which may extend to the brain. The cavity of the eye will, in a measure, be filled up by newly formed matter. The dog must be restricted to a low cooling diet, and have administered two or three saline purges.

ULCERATIONS OF THE EYELIDS

are often met with in old mangy, ill-fed animals, and are difficult to overcome, except by curing the primary affection, which is often no easy task. The lids become enlarged, puffy, and tender, the lashes fall out, and the edges present an angry reddish appearance.

Treatment—Must be directed, in the first place, to the curing of the old affection, by which, in connection with blisters, purging, stimulating washes, &c., a cure may be effected. When the swelling of the lids is considerable, scarifying them with the point of a lancet will often be of much service. Ointment of nitrate of silver may also be smeared on the edges.

WARTS ON THE EYELIDS

sometimes make their appearance; they may be lifted up with the forceps, and excised with a knife or scissors, and the wound touched with nitrate of silver. The same treatment will answer for those warts, or little excrescences, that sometimes come on the inside of the lids.

ENTROPIUM—INVERSION OF THE EYELIDS.

This disease we do not find mentioned by any of the writers on canine pathology: nevertheless, we are led to believe that it is not an uncommon form of ophthalmia, and we must express our surprise that it should have escaped the attention of such close observers as Blain and Youatt.

The acute form of the disease resulting from, or attending, simple ophthalmia, we have often witnessed, but the chronic form, of which we more particularly speak, is more rare. We have seen three cases of the latter, and, no doubt, might have found many more if our opportunities of studying canine pathology were equal to those of the English writers. The inversion of the eyelids upon the globe is accompanied with pain and irritation, swelling and inflammation, both of the lids and eye, which ultimately renders the dog almost useless, if not entirely blind.

Causes.—Neglected chronic ophthalmia was, no doubt, the cause of the disease in two cases, a setter and a pointer, while the other, in a hound, was the result of an acute attack of ophthalmia brought on by scalding with hot pitch thrown upon the animal. Some of this substance entered the eye, while a large portion adhered to the muzzle and lids. The eye, as well as the lids, became inflamed; the latter, being puffed up and contracted on their edges, were necessarily drawn inwards from the tension of the parts, and double eutropium was thus produced. The inflammation and tumefaction of the parts continued for a considerable time, and when ultimately reduced by the application of tepid fomentations, the skin appeared greatly relaxed; and the muscular fibres having lost their power of support or contractility, owing to their long quiescence, seemed no longer able to keep their lids in their proper situation; the edges therefore remained in the abnormous position previously assumed.

By this strange condition of the parts, the eyeball continued greatly irritated by the constant friction of the lashes; water was continually flowing over the lids, and from its irritating character produced considerable excoriation of the face and muzzle. The conjunctiva remained inflamed, the cornea in due course became ulcerous, and the eye was ultimately destroyed by the discharge of its contents. This was the course and final termination of the disease in the case of the hound above referred to, all of which disastrous results might have been prevented by proper management.

Treatment.—When in England, we sent to the United States a fine bred pointer dog, designed as a present for one of our sporting friends. This animal travelled from Leeds to Liverpool, chained on top of the railroad cars; the journey occupied several hours, during which the weather was cold and boisterous, and we noticed on his arrival at the latter place that his eyes were watering and somewhat inflamed. On examining them more particularly, we were enabled to extract several pieces of cinder from under the lids, which seemed to relieve him somewhat. He went to sea, in the care of the steward, on the following day; and remained on deck exposed to the inclemency of the weather during a long voyage. When he arrived in Philadelphia, the inflammation, we were informed, was very considerable, occasioned by the presence of some other small particles of cinder that may have escaped our attention before shipping him. The presence of these foreign substances in the eye, in connection with the salt spray and irritating atmosphere, greatly aggravated the ophthalmia, and resolved it into a chronic affection, which ultimately resulted in entropium.

"Fop" was hunted during the same autumn, which no doubt increased the malady to a considerable extent; and before the hunting season was over, the dog was rendered almost useless: the lids becoming so much swollen and the irritation so considerable, that it was deemed cruel to allow him to go into the field.

When we saw him some time in the course of the same winter, the lower lids of both eyes were completely inverted on their globes, and the conjunctival inflammation and flow of tears considerable.

The eyes seemed contracted within their sockets, and at times were nearly hidden from view, the corneas were somewhat opaque, the photophobia intolerable, and the animal showed evident signs of extreme pain, by his restless anxiety and constant efforts at scratching and rubbing the eyes.

Under the judicious application of cooling astringent collyria, and other remediate means, the irritation and pain of the parts were relieved, and the lids somewhat retracted.

"Fop" remained in this condition till the following autumn, suffering at times considerably from the increased inflammation and tumefaction of the lids, which continued obstinately to persist, insomuch that when turned out by the pressure of the fingers on them, they immediately contracted, and were forced inwards on the ball when freed from the fingers.

Finding that no external application was of any permanent

benefit, we resolved to have resort to the same operation we saw practised in the Parisian hospitals for the cure of a similar malformation in the human subject.

To insure quiet we enclosed the body of the dog in a case, made stationary and sufficiently small to prevent struggling, with the head firmly fixed by a sliding door, as represented in the accompanying drawing.

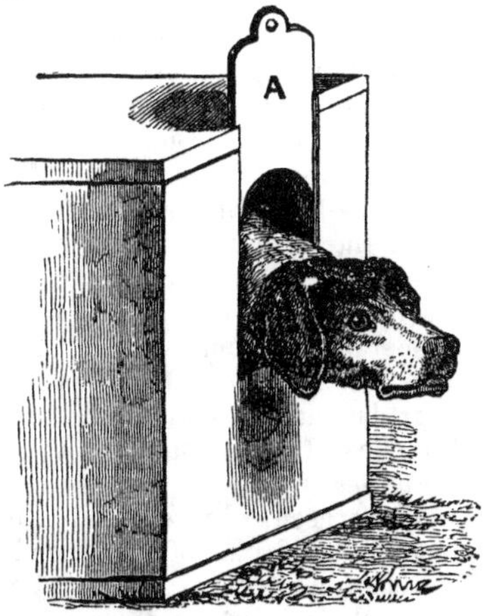

The mouth was kept closed by a small strap passed around the muzzle. This method of fixing a strong dog, we consider the best ever adopted for all nice operations on the face. The first step in the operation was to pinch up a portion of the lax skin of the diseased lid and pass three needles, armed with silk ligatures, successively through the base of the upraised integuments.

One needle approximating the external canthus, another the internal, and a third midway between these two points, as represented in the annexed drawing.

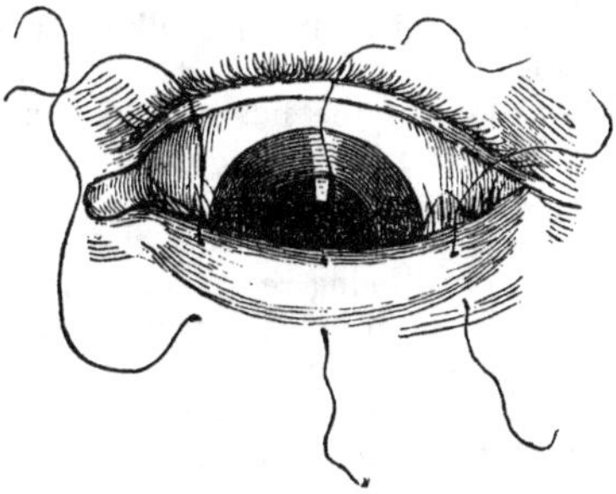

The next step was to raise up the integuments included in the ligature, and, by means of a pair of sharp scissors, cut off the superabundant skin as near to the ligatures as possible; having care however to leave sufficient substance included in the ligatures, to prevent their sloughing out before adhesion has taken place. The next and last step of the operation was, to draw the edges of the wound together by tying each ligature, which procedure immediately secured the lid and held it firmly in its natural position. The ligatures were now cut short, and a large wire muzzle, covered over with some dark substance on the operated eye, being put on him, and his legs hobbled with a piece of strong twine, more effectually to prevent his scratching the head, "Fop" was then set at liberty, and soon became reconciled to this eye-shade.

The hemorrhage was trifling, the wound healed up by the first intention and the ligatures were drawn away in a few days, when a perfect cure was effected—the conjunctiva having lost its inflammatory appearance, and the cornea having again become quite transparent.

The other eye was operated on in the same way and with like success. In the first operation we cut away the loose flaccid teguments only; whereas, in the second, we snipped small longitudinal fibres from the cartilage itself, and the operation consequently was more perfect, if possible, than in the first instance.

The eyes were now perfectly restored, and remained well during the whole of the shooting season, after which we lost sight of our patient, he having accompanied one of our friends as a "compagnon de voyage" on a commercial expedition to Santa Fé, and, when on his return, had the misfortune to lose "Fop," who was carried off into captivity by some prowling Camanches, who no doubt have long since sacrificed him to the Great Spirit in celebrating the buffalo or wolf dance.

PROTRUSION OF THE EYE.

The eye may be forced from its orbit by wounds or the bites of other animals.

If not materially injured, the ball should be cleaned with a little tepid water, or by wiping off with a fine silk or cambric handkerchief, and immediately replaced within its socket; otherwise the inflammation and swelling of the lids will soon prevent its easy admission. When handling the protruded eye, the fingers should be dipped in olive oil or warm water.

When sufficient time has elapsed from the occurrence of the accident to prevent the ball being replaced, owing to the swelling and contraction of the lids, an incision may be made at the external angle of the eye, so as to divide the lids, which will then admit the eye into its natural position. If not, the lid itself can be raised up and slit far enough to allow its being drawn over the globe.

As considerable inflammation generally follows this accident, it will be prudent to bleed the animal and confine him.

We have seen eyes replaced, that have been out of their sockets for several hours, perfectly recover their strength and brilliancy.

WEAK EYES.

Some dogs, particularly several breeds of spaniels, have naturally weak eyes, attended by an over-secretion and constant flow of tears, more particularly when exposed to the sun. When there is no disease of the lachrymal duct, the secretion may be diminished and the eyes strengthened by the daily application of some slightly tonic wash, as No. 1, 2, 3, &c.

FISTULA LACHRYMALIS.

The lachrymal duct is a small canal, leading from the internal angle of the eye to the nostrils, and is the passage through which the tears escape from the eye. This duct may become closed by inflammation of the lining membrane of the nose, caries of the bone, ulcers, fungous growths, or by the presence of some extraneous substance impacted in it. The tears, no longer having a natural outlet, are necessarily forced over the lids, accompanied, not unfrequently, by a good deal of purulent matter.

This canal, when thus obstructed from some one of the above causes, often forms an ulcerous opening at its upper extremity, just below the internal canthus, for the escape of the pus that usually collects in a sac at that point. This perforation is called "Fistula Lachrymalis." The tears, entering the canal at its punctum, are carried along till they pass out at the fistulous opening.

Treatment.—This is a very troublesome affection, and has been pronounced incurable by some writers. However, we would not hesitate making an attempt at relieving a favourite or valuable dog of this disagreeable deformity. We should first endeavour to clear out the nasal canal, either by means of a minute flexible probe, or by directing a stream of water from a suitable syringe through its course. A small silver or copper style may then be placed in the canal to keep it open, as also to direct the tears through the natural route. This being done, and the dog confined in such a way as not to be able to scratch or rub the eye, the fistulous opening might close up in a short time. However, it might be necessary to wear the style for many months. In such a case, we see no reason why a wire muzzle, such as used by us after the operation for Entropium, might not be worn for an indefinite period, without any inconvenience to the animal.

CARUNCULA LACHRYMALIS AND PLICA SEMILUNARIS, OR HAW.

The caruncula lachrymalis is a small glandular body situated at the internal commissure of each eye. This little gland often becomes greatly enlarged from inflammation or fungous growths—old dogs are much more subject to the disease than young ones.

Treatment.—The application of cooling collyria and a weak solution of nitrate of silver, will generally suppress the further growth of this gland. If, however, it continues much swollen and runs on to suppuration, it may be punctured with a lancet and poultices applied. If the affection be of a malignant character, the gland may be drawn out by passing a ligature through its base, and then excised.

The haw is most frequently concerned in the disease, and may also be removed.

Collyria.

No. 1.

℞ Vinegar .... ℥ i.
Laudanum .... ℈ i.
Water .... ℥ vii.

Mix.—The eyes to be frequently bathed with the mixture.

No. 2.

℞ Sulphate of zinc (white vitriol) .... ℈ i.
Water .... ℥ vi.

M.—To be used as above.

No. 3.

℞ Sulphate of copper (blue vitriol) .... ℈ i.
Water .... ℥ vi.

M.—To be used as above.

No. 4.

℞ Acetate of lead (sugar of lead) .... ℈ ii.
Water .... ℥ vi.

M.—To be used as above.

No. 5.

℞ Argenti nitrat. (nitrate of silver).............. ℈ i.
Water .... ℥ vi.

M.—To be dropped in the eye 2 or 3 times daily.

No. 6.

℞ Sub-muriate of mercury (corrosive sublimate) ... grs. x.
Water .... ℥ vi.

M.—To be used as the preceding.

No. 7.

℞ Argenti nitrat (nitrate of silver).............. grs. v.
Fresh butter or lard .... ℥ i.

No. 8.

℞ Powdered alum............................ grs. xv.
Calomel.................................. grs. vii.

M.—Blown in the eye, will often have a most excellent effect, more particularly in old chronic ophthalmia.

No. 9.

Infusions of slippery elm bark, sassafras or elder pith, infusions of green tea, flaxseed, &c., are all excellent emollient applications.—L.]

CHAPTER IX.

THE EAR AND ITS DISEASES.

Canker in the Ear.—All water-dogs, and some others, are subject to a disease designated by this name, and which, in fact, is inflammation of the integumental lining of the inside of the ear. When the whole of the body, except the head and ears, is surrounded by cold water, there will be an unusual determination of blood to those parts, and consequent distension of the vessels and a predisposition to inflammation. A Newfoundland dog, or setter, or poodle, that has been subject to canker, is often freed from a return of the disease by being kept from the water.

The earliest symptom of the approach of canker is frequent shaking of the head, or holding of the head on one side, or violent scratching of one or both ears. Redness of the integument may then be observed, and particularly of that portion of it which lines the annular cartilage. This is usually accompanied by some enlargement of the folds of the skin. As soon as any of these symptoms are observed, the ear should be gently but well washed, two or three times in the day, with lukewarm water, and after that a weak solution of the extract of lead should be applied, and a dose or two of physic administered.

If the case is neglected, the pain will rapidly increase; the ear will become of an intenser red; the folds of the integument will enlarge, and there will be a deposition of red or black matter in the hollow of the ear. The case is now more serious, and should be immediately attended to. This black or bloody deposit should be gently but carefully washed away with warm water and soap; and the extract of lead, in the proportion of a scruple to an ounce of water, should be frequently applied, until the redness and heat are abated. A solution of alum, in about the same quantity of alum and water as the foregoing lotion, should then be used.

Some attention should be paid to the method of applying these lotions. Two persons will be required in order to accomplish the operation. The surgeon must hold the muzzle of the dog with one hand, and have the root of the ear in the hollow of the other, and between the first finger and the thumb. The assistant must then pour the liquid into the ear; half a tea-spoonful will usually be sufficient. The surgeon, without quitting the dog, will then close the ear, and mould it gently until the liquid has insinuated itself as deeply as possible into the passages of the ear. Should not the inflammation abate in the course of a few days, a seton should be inserted in the poll, between the integument and the muscles of the occiput, reaching from ear to ear. The excitement of a new inflammation, so near to the part previously diseased, will materially abate the original affection. Physic is now indispensable. From half a drachm to a drachm of aloes, with from one to two grains of calomel, should be given every third day.

Should the complaint have been much neglected, or the inflammation so great as to bid defiance to these means, ulceration will too often speedily follow. It will be found lodged deep in the passage, and can only be detected by moulding the ear; the effused pus will occasionally occupy the inside of the ear to its very tip. However extensive and annoying the inflammation may be, and occasionally causing so much thickening of the integument as perfectly to close the ear, it is always superficial. It will generally yield to proper treatment, and the cartilage of the ear may not be in the slightest degree affected. Still, however, the animal may suffer extreme pain; the discharge from the ulcer may produce extensive excoriation of the cheek; and, in a few cases, the system may sympathise with the excessive local application, and the animal may be lost.

The treatment must vary with circumstances. If the ulceration is deep in the ear, and there is not a very great degree of apparent inflammation, recourse may be had at once to a stimulating and astringent application, such as alum or the sulphate of zinc, and in the proportion of six grains of either to an ounce of water. If, however, the ulceration occupies the greater part of the hollow of the ear, and is accompanied by much thickening of the integument, and apparent filling up of the entrance to the ear, some portion of the inflammation must be first subdued.

The only chance of getting rid of the disease is to confine the ear A piece of strong calico must be procured, six or eight inches in width, and sufficiently long to reach round the head and meet under the jaw. Along each side of it must be a running piece of tape, and a shorter piece sewed at the centre of each of the ends. By means of these the cap may be drawn tightly over the head, above the eyes, and likewise round the neck behind the ears, so as perfectly to confine them.

After all, no mild ointment will dispose such an ulcer to heal, and recourse must be had at once to a caustic application. A scruple of the nitrate of silver must be rubbed down with an ounce of lard, and a little of it applied twice every day, and rubbed tolerably hard into the sore until it assumes a healthy appearance; it may then be dressed with the common calamine ointment.

If the discharge should return, the practitioner must again have recourse to the caustic ointment.

The cartilage will never close, but the integument will gradually cover the exposed edges, and the wound will be healed. The ear will, however, long continue tender, and, if it should be much beaten, by the shaking of the head, the ulcer will reappear. This must be obviated by occasionally confining the ears, and not overfeeding the dog.

Some sportsmen are accustomed to *round* the ears, that is to cut off the diseased part. In very few instances, however, will a permanent cure be effected, while the dog is often sadly disfigured. A fresh ulcer frequently appears on the new edge, and is more difficult to heal than the original one. Nine times out of ten the disease reappears.

The Newfoundland dog is very subject to this disease, to remedy which recourse must be had to the nitrate of silver.

Spaniels have often a mangy inflammation of the edges of the ear. It seldom runs on to canker; but the hair comes off round the edges of the ear, accompanied by much heat and scurfiness of the skin. The common sulphur ointment, with an eighth part of mercurial ointment, will usually remove the disease.

From the irritation produced by canker in or on the ear, and the constant flapping and beating of the ear, there is sometimes a considerable effusion of fluid between the integument and the cartilage occupying the whole of the inside of the flap of the ear. The only remedy is to open the enlarged part from end to end, carefully to take out the gossamer lining of the cyst, and then to insert some bits of lint on each side of the incision, in order to prevent its closing too soon. In a few days, the parietes of the cyst will begin to adhere, and a perfect cure will be accomplished

If the tumour is simply punctured, the incision will speedily close, and the cyst will fill again in the space of four-and-twenty hours. A seton may be used, but it is more painful to the dog, and slower in its operation.

The ear should be frequently fomented with a decoction of white poppies, and to this should follow the Goulard lotion; and, after that, if necessary, a solution of alum should be applied. To the soreness or scabby eruption, which extends higher up the ear, olive oil or spermaceti ointment may be applied. In some cases, portions of the thickened skin, projecting and excoriated, and pressing on each other, unite, and the opening into the ear is then mechanically filled. I know not of any remedy for this. It is useless to perforate the adventitious substance, for the orifice will soon close; and, more than once, when I have made a crucial incision, and cut out the unnatural mass that closed the passage, I have found it impossible to keep down the fungous granulations or to prevent total deafness.

The following is a singular case of this disease:—1st July, 1820 a dog was sent with a tumour, evidently containing a fluid, in the flap of the ear. A seton had been introduced, but had been sadly neglected. The hair had become matted round the seton, and the discharge had thus been stopped. Inflammation and considerable pain had evidently followed, and the dog had nearly torn the seton out. I removed it, washed the ear well, and applied the tincture of myrrh and aloes. The wound soon healed. On the 14th the ear began again to fill. On the 17th the tumour was ripe for the seton, which was again introduced, and worn until the 9th of August, when the sides of the abscess appeared again to have adhered, and it was withdrawn. Canker had continued in the ear during the whole time; and, in defiance of a cold lotion daily applied, the ear was perceived again to be disposed to fill. The seton was once more inserted, and the cyst apparently closed. The seton was continued a fortnight after the sinus was obliterated, and then removed. Six weeks afterwards the swelling had disappeared, and the canker was quite removed. This anecdote is an encouragement to persevere under the most disheartening circumstances.

All dogs that are foolishly suffered to become gross and fat are subject to canker. It seems to be a natural outlet for excess of nutriment or gross humour; and, when a dog has once laboured under the disease, he is very subject to a return of it. The fatal power of habit is in few cases more evident than in this disease. When a dog has symptoms of mange, the redness or eruption of the skin, generally, will not unfrequently disappear, and bad canker speedily follow. The habit, however, may be subdued, or at least may be kept at bay, by physic and the use of Goulard lotion or alum.

Sportsmen are often annoyed by another species of canker Pointers and hounds are particularly subject to it.

This species of canker commences with a scurfy eruption and

thickening of the edges of the ear, apparently attended by considerable itching or pain. The dog is continually flapping his ear, and beating it violently against his head. The inflammation is thus increased, and the tip of the ear becomes exceedingly sore. This causes him to shake his head still more violently, and the ulcer spreads and is indisposed to heal, and at length a fissure or crack appears on the tip of the cartilage, and extends to a greater or less distance down the ear.

The narration of one or two cases may be useful, as showing the inveteracy of the disease.

8th Feb. 1832.—A Newfoundland dog, very fat, had dreadful canker in both ears, and considerable discharge of purulent matter. He was continually shaking his ears, lying and moaning. Apply the canker lotion, and give the alterative balls.

13th. The discharge considerably lessened from one ear, but that from the other has increased. Continue the lotion and apply a seton.

22d. The dog, probably neglected at home, was sent to me. Both ears were as bad as ever.

25th. The dog is perfectly unmanageable when the lotion is poured into the ear, but submits when an ointment is applied. Use ung. sambuci, ℥j. cerus. acet. ʒj., mix well together. Continue the alteratives.

30th. Slowly amending; the whining has ceased, and the animal seldom scratches. Continue the lotion, alteratives, and purgatives.

10th Oct.—Slowly improving. Continue the treatment.

17th. One ear well, the other nearly so.

24th. Both ears were apparently well. Omit the lotion.

28th. One ear was again ulcerated. Applied the ærugo æris.

31st. This has been too stimulating, and the ulceration is almost as great as at first. Return to the ung. sambuci and cerusa acetata.

From this time to the 24th February, 1833, we continued occasionally taking out the seton, but returning to it every two or three days; applying the canker lotion until we were driven from it, mixing with it variable quantities of tinctura opii, having recourse to mercurial ointment, and trying a solution of the sulphate of copper. With two or three applications we could keep the disease at bay; but with none could we fairly remove the evil. The sulphate of zinc, the acetate of lead, decoctions of oak bark, a very mild injection of the nitrate of silver,—all would do good at times; but at other times we were set at complete defiance.

Another gentleman brought his dog about the same time. This was also a Newfoundland dog. He had always been subject to mangy eruptions, and had now mange in the feet, the inside of the ear covered with scaly eruptions, the skin red underneath, considerable thickening of the ear, and a slight discharge from its base. A seton was inserted and a physic-ball given every second day. The canker lotion had little good effect. Some calamine ointment, with a small portion of calomel, was then had recourse to.

In ten days the dog had ceased to scratch himself or shake his head, and the ear was clean and cool. The seton was removed; but the animal being confined, a little redness again appeared in the ear, which the lotion soon removed.

At the expiration of a month he was dismissed apparently cured; but he afterwards had a return of his old mangy complaints, which bade defiance to every mode of treatment.

Herr Maassen, V. S., Würtemburg, has lately introduced, and with much success, the use of creosote for the cure of canker in the ear.

The first experiment was on a setter with canker in his ear. The owner of the dog had ordered it to be hanged, as all remedies had failed in producing a cure. Herr Maassen prescribed creosoti ʒss. et spirit. vini rectificat. ℥ij. This mixture was applied once in every day to the diseased part. In a few weeks the dog was completely cured, and has since had no return of the complaint. In a terrier, and also in three spaniels, the effect of this application was equally satisfactory. In some cases, where the disease showed itself in a less degree, the creosote was dissolved in water, instead of spirit of wine. It is always necessary to take away the collar while the dog is under treatment, in order that the flap of the ear may not be injured by striking against it.

Vegetating Excrescences in the Ear. (By F. J. J. Rigot.)—Productions of this kind, which he had the opportunity of observing only once, are sometimes united in masses, and completely close the auditive canal. The surface is granulated and black, and there escapes from it an unctuous fetid discharge. On both sides the animal is exceedingly susceptible of pain, and the excrescences bleed if the slightest pressure is brought to bear upon them.

He thought it right to cut away these excrescences bodily, which he found to be composed of a strong dense tissue, permitting much blood to escape through an innumerable quantity of vascular openings. They were reproduced with extreme promptitude after they had been cut off or cauterized. Some of them appeared no more after being destroyed by the nitrate of mercury.

Sometimes, however, twenty-four hours after a simple incision, not followed by cauterization, these productions acquire an almost incredible size. It seemed, in M. Rigot's case, to be impossible to conquer the evil, and the patient was destroyed.

Eruptions in the Ear.—A Newfoundland dog had long been subject to mangy eruptions on the back and in the feet. They had suddenly disappeared, and the whole of the inside of the ear became covered with scaly eruptions. The skin was red; there was considerable thickening of the ear, and a discharge from the base of it. The canker-lotion was used, a physic-ball given every second day, and a seton inserted in the poll reaching from ear to ear. No apparent benefit resulted. A little calamine ointment, to which was added one-eighth part of mercurial ointment, was then tried, and considerable benefit immediately experienced. The dog no longer continued to scratch himself or to shake his head, and the ear became clean and cool. The seton was removed, and nothing remained but a little occasional redness, which the lotion very soon dispersed.

The owner, however, became ultimately tired of all this doctoring, and the animal was destroyed.

A poodle had had exceedingly bad ears during several months. There was considerable discharge, apparently giving much pain. The dog was continually shaking his head and crying. A seton was introduced, the canker-lotion was resorted to, and alterative and purgative medicines exhibited. On the 29th of December the discharge from the ear ceased; but, owing to the neglect of the servant, it soon broke out again, and there was not only much excoriation under the ear, but, from the matting of the hair, deep ulcers formed on either side, the edges of the wound were ragged, and the skin was detached from the muscular parts beneath. Probes were introduced on each side, which passed down the neck and nearly met. The smell was intolerably offensive, and the dog was reduced almost to a skeleton. I was, for the second time, sent for to see the case. I immediately recommended that the animal should be destroyed; but this was not permitted. I then ordered that it should daily be carefully washed, and diluted tincture of myrrh be applied to the wounds. They showed no disposition to heal, and the dog gradually sunk under the continued discharge and died.

Violent Affection of the Ear. *20th May*, 1828.—A spaniel screamed violently, even when it was not touched, and held its head permanently on one side, as if the muscles were contracted. The glands beneath the ear were enlarged, but the bowels were regular; the nose was not hot; there was no cough. A warm bath was ordered, with aperient medicine.

On the 22d she was no better. I examined the case more carefully. The left ear was exceedingly hot and tender: she would scarcely bear me to touch it. I continued the aperient medicine, and ordered a warm lotion to be applied, consisting of the liquor plumbi acetatis and infusion of digitalis. She improved from the first application of it, and in a few days was quite well. A fortnight afterwards the pain returned. The lotion was employed, but not with the same success. A seton was then applied. She wore it only four days, when the pain completely disappeared.

I have an account in my records of the conduct of a coward, who, coming from such a breed, was not worthy of the trouble we took with him. He was a Newfoundland dog, two years old, with considerable enlargement, redness, and some discharge from both ears. He was sent to our hospital for treatment. When no one was near him, he shook his head and scratched his ears, and howled dreadfully. Many times in the course of the day he cried as if we were murdering him. We sent him home thoroughly well, and glad we were to get rid of him.

Cropping of the Ears.—I had some doubt, whether I ought not to omit the mention of this cruel practice. Mr. Blaine very properly says, that "it is one that does not honour the inventor, for nature gives nothing in vain. Beauty and utility appear in all when properly examined, but in unequal degrees. In some, beauty is pre-eminent; while, in others, utility appears to have been the principal consideration. That must, therefore, be a false taste, that has taught us to prefer a *curtailed* organ to a perfect one, without gaining any convenience by the operation." He adds, and it is my only excuse for saying one word about the matter, that "custom being now fixed, directions are proper for its performance."

The owner of the dog commences with maiming him while a puppy. He finds fault with the ears that nature has given him, and they are rounded or cut into various shapes, according to his whim or caprice. It is a cruel operation. A great deal of pain is inflicted by it, and it is often a long time before the edge of the wound will heal: a fortnight or three weeks at least will elapse ere the animal is free from pain.

It has been pleaded, and I would be one of the last to oppose the plea, that the ears of many dogs are rounded on account of the ulcers which attack and rend the conch; because animals with short ears defend themselves most readily from the attacks of others; because, in their combats with each other, they generally endeavour to lay hold of the neck or the ears; and, therefore, when their ears are shortened, they have considerable advantage over their adversary. There is some truth in this plea; but, otherwise, the operation of cropping is dependent on caprice or fashion.

If the ears of dogs must be cropped, it should not be done too early. Four, five, or six weeks should first pass; otherwise, they will grow again, and the second cropping will not produce a good appearance.

The scissors are the proper instruments for accomplishing the removal of the ear; the tearing of the cartilages out by main force is an act of cruelty that none but a brute in human shape would practise; and, if he attempts it, it is ten to one that he does not obtain a good crop. If the conch is torn out, there is nothing remaining to retain the skin round the auricular opening: it may be torn within the auditory canal, and as that is otherwise very extensible in the dog, it is prolonged above the opening, which may then probably be closed by a cicatrix. The animal will in this case always remain deaf, at least in one ear. In the mean time, the mucous membrane that lines the *meatus auditorius* subsists, the secretion of the wax continues; it accumulates and acquires an irritating quality; the irritation which it causes produces an augmentation of the secretion, and soon the whole of the subcutaneous passage becomes filled, and seems to assume the form of a cord; and it finishes by the dog continuing to worry himself, shaking his head, and becoming subject to fits.

Mr. Blaine very naturally observes, that, "it is not a little surprising that this cruel custom is so frequently, or almost invariably, practised on pug-dogs, whose ears, if left alone to nature, are particularly handsome and hang very gracefully. It is hardly to be conceived how the pug's head — which is not naturally beautiful except in the eye of perverted taste—is improved by suffering his ears to remain.

If the cropping is to be practised, the mother should have been previously removed. It is quite erroneous, that her licking the wounded edges will be serviceable. On the contrary, it only increases their pain, and deprives the young ones of the best balsam that can be applied—the blood that flows from their wounds.

Polypi in the Ears.—Dr. Mercer, in The Veterinarian, of July, 1844, gives an interesting account of the production of polypi in the meatus of the ear. He considers that there are two kinds of polypi—first, the soft, vascular and bleeding polypus, usually produced from the fibro-cartilaginous structure of the outer half of the tube; and, secondly, the hard and cartilaginous polypus or excrescence produced from the lining membrane of its inner half. The first is termed the hæmatoid polypus, and the other the chondromatous. The dog suffering under either generally has a dull, heavy, and rather watery eye. He moans or whines at intervals. If his master is present he feels a relief in pressing and rubbing his aching ear against him. At other times he presses and rubs his ear against the ground, in order to obtain a slight relief, flapping his ears and shaking his head; the mouth being opened and the tongue protruded, and the affected ear pointing to the ground. Then comes a sudden, and often a profuse, discharge of fetid pus. The local discharge of pus and blood becomes daily more and more fetid, and the poor animal becomes an object of disgust.

In the first variety of polypus, where it is practicable, the soft and vascular excrescence should be excised with a pair of scissors or a small knife, or it may be noosed by a ligature of silk or of silver wire, or twisted off with a pair of forceps. Immediately after its removal, the base of the tumour should be carefully destroyed by the nitrate of silver, and this should be repeated as long as there is any appearance of renewed growth. Any ulcer or carious condition of the meatus should be immediately removed.

In order to protect the diseased parts, a soft cap should be used, and within the ear a little cotton wadding may defend the ear from injury.

Dr. Mercer very properly remarks that, in the second or chondromatous variety of polypus of the meatus, the treatment must depend upon the concomitant circumstances. If the tumour is seated close to the membrana tympani, and has a broad and sessile base, then it cannot be excised or noosed with any degree of success. It must therefore be treated by the daily application of the solid nitrate of silver, applied exactly to its surface; and, in the intervals of application, the use of any collyria may be had recourse to. If the substance of the growth be firm and solid, and possess little sensibility, then a very speedy mode of getting rid of it is to divide its substance with a small knife; and afterwards, by applying the solid nitrate of silver, the tumour will soon be sloughed away.

The dog is liable to polypi in the nasal cavity, in the anus, and in the vagina, which it will not be out of place to mention here.

The polypi of the nasal and of the anal cavities often show themselves under the form of rounded bodies, projecting from the nose or anus. Their size and consistence are variable—sometimes soft, tearing with the greatest facility, and bleeding at the slightest touch; at other times, solid and covered with pituitary membrane. They are generally the result of ulcerations, wounds, fractures, perforations of the turbinated bones, sinuses, &c. These polypous productions obstruct the passage of the air, and more or less impede the breathing. They are best extirpated by means of a ligature, or circular compression, on the pedicle of the polypus, and tightened every second day.

We may discover the presence of a tumour of this nature in one of the nasal passages, when, on putting our hand to the orifice of the nostril, there issues little or no air; or when we sound the nostril with the finger or a probe, or examine it on a bright day.

The methods of destroying polypi in the nasal cavity vary with the texture, size, form, and position of these excrescences. Excision with the bistoury, or with scissors, may be tried when the polypus is near the orifice of the nostril, and particularly when it is not large at the base. Excision should be followed by cauterization with the red-hot iron, by which a portion of the base of the tumour is destroyed, and which could not be reached by a sharp instrument. To succeed in these operations, it is frequently necessary to cut through the false nostril. The edges of the wound may afterwards be united by a suture.

The ligature, or circular compression, excised immediately on the pedicle of the polypus, by means of a wire or waxed string, and directed into the nasal cavity by means of a proper instrument, may be tried when the polypus is deeply situated, and particularly when its base is narrow. But, for this operation, which is difficult to perform, and which may be followed by a new polypous production, when the base is not perfectly destroyed, we may substitute the forcible detachment, especially when we have to act on vascular and soft excrescences.

The Italian greyhound is strangely subject to these polypi in the matrix or vagina. The reason it is difficult to explain.

A bitch, ten years old, was brought to the author on the 20th December, 1843, with an oval substance, as large as a thrush's egg, occasionally protruding from the vagina. I advised that it should be removed by means of a ligature; but the owner was afraid, and a fortnight was suffered to pass before she was brought again. The tumour had rapidly increased; it was as large as a pigeon's egg, considerably excoriated, and the pedicle being almost as large as the tumour itself. The operation was now consented to. I passed a ligature as firmly round the pedicle and as high up as I could. The bitch scarcely seemed to suffer any pain. 3*d Jan.*—The circulation is evidently cut off, and the tumour is assuming a thoroughly black hue, but it appears to cause no inconvenience to the dog. I tightened the ligature. 4th. The tumour is now completely black, considerably protruded, and apparently destitute of feeling. I again tightened the ligature. 5th. The tumour not appearing disposed to separate, and the uterus seeming to be drawn back by its weight, I cut off the tumour close to the ligature. Not the slightest pain seemed to be given, and the tumour was hard and black. There was, however, a very little oozing of bloody fluid, which continuing to the 8th, I injected a slight solution of alum into the vagina, and three days afterwards the discharge was perfectly stopped.

[Although our author has given us several interesting and practical pages upon the diseases of the ear and its appendages, it seems to us that the arrangement of the matter is rather objectionable, and not sufficiently explicit to be easily comprehended by sportsmen, not before familiar with the subject; we therefore add a concise resumé or epitome of these troublesome affections, which we trust will be found of practical utility to the reader.

SIMPLE OTORRHÆA,

or running from the ear, produced by inflammation of the mucous membrane of the external auditory canal, is of frequent occurrence. The dog should be purged with salts, and the ear washed with castile soap and tepid water. The following solution may be in-introduced several times a day:

℞ Sulphate of zinc ....℈ i.
Water.................................℥ i.
Mix. or,

℞ Sugar of lead...........................℈ i.
Water.................................℥ i.

If the discharge be fetid, the following may be applied often:

℞ Chloride of lime ....℥ i.
Water ....1 pint.

This affection in old dogs is very troublesome, and in most cases impossible to cure. Alum, zinc, copper, lead, and other astringent applications may be used in powder, as a local application in these cases. A seton and blisters will also be serviceable.

TUMOURS OF THE FLAP.

A tumour, particularly in old dogs, is often seen extending from the tip of the flap even to the base of the ear. It progresses slowly but surely, if not interfered with in its career, and will become eventually enormously large and very painful. These tumours are most common in old setters, Newfoundlands, and hounds.

Treatment.—The tumour, at its commencement, may be discussed by the application of astringent washes, as warm vinegar, water, and laudanum, or sugar of lead. When, however, it has become more extensive, the only remedy is opening it through its whole extent, and pressing out its purulent contents. A poultice may then be applied, and tepid fomentations used for several days. It is often extremely difficult to heal up the abscess, or arrest the fetid discharge that is constantly collecting: a seton placed in the poll, in connexion with washes of a stimulating character, will, however, effect a cure, if patiently persevered in. Either of the following will answer this purpose:

℞ Chloride of lime ... .℥ i.
Water........ ....℥ vi.
Mix. or,

℞ Sulphate of zinc .... ℈ i.
Water .... ℥ jii.
Mix.

We used on one occasion tincture of iodine with perfect success in an old and obstinate case.

CANKER OF THE EAR.

This is a rather indefinite term, as applied to the diseased ear of a dog; in fact, any malignant corroding sore may be called a canker, no matter where situated. Some writers describe, under the head of canker, a violent chronic otitis, attended by a purulent sanguinoid discharge. Others understand by canker a species of erysipelatous inflammation, that makes its appearance on the inside of the flap, and extends itself to the interior of the ear. What we understand by canker, is an acute inflammation of the lining membrane of the ear, destroying the tympanum or drum, and producing total deafness. The secretion is often considerable, and if not removed, will soon fill up the cavity of the ear with a dark reddish deposit, which greatly increases the irritation and inflammation of the parts. Mr. Blaine states that he has seen this disease take a very malignant character, and extend its ravages over the face, destroying the soft parts, and even penetrating through the bone into the interior of the head.

Causes.—This disease may be excited by any of those causes that produce a general or local inflammatory action; exposure to cold, the presence of malignant diseases on other portions of the body, high living, heat, confinement, or extraneous substances lodged in the organ itself.

Water-dogs are most subject to this affection, owing, no doubt, to the frequent afflux of blood to these parts, while the remainder of the body is immersed in the water. A tendency to this peculiar inflammation may also be produced in these animals by the action of the water upon the delicate membranes of the ear, which occasions a violent shaking of the head and beating of the flaps, which not unfrequently bruises them considerably. Dogs that seldom or never go into the water are not, however, by any means exempt from the disease; as we have often seen it developed in terriers, mastiffs, and every species of mongrel.

Treatment.—When the disease appears in its acute form, and without any apparent cause beyond luxurious living and confinement, bleeding, purging, low diet, and regular exercise, together with tepid and soothing washes, will generally relieve the inflammatory action of the parts. The ear should be carefully and tenderly washed out with castile soap, and a small quantity of the following solution poured into it two or three times daily, and the ear worked about gently in the hand to secure the percolation of the fluid through its structure.

℞	Goulard's extract....................	℥ sj.
	Water..............................	1 pint.
	Mix.	or,

℞	Sugar of lead..........................	℈ i.
	Water..............................	℥ i.
	Mix.	or,

℞	Powdered alum.........................	℈ i.
	Water..............................	℥ i.
	Mix.	

The above mixtures should be warmed before using, otherwise the dog may resist their introduction.

When the disease from bad treatment or neglect has subsided into the chronic form, and ulceration and suppuration have commenced, it will be necessary to pursue a somewhat different treatment, and remain more patient, awaiting the result.

At this time the auditory passage is filled with a dark purulent secretion, which forms a thick and irritating crust.

This deposit should first be removed by washing with castile soap and tepid water, and the daily application of a hop poultice. If there be much inflammatory action of the parts, the dog may be bled, and alterative or purgative balls administered. The following wash must be used two or three times daily.

℞	Sugar of lead.................	℈ i.
	Laudanum	gtt.—20 (drops.)
	Water......................	℥ i.
	Mix.	

As the discharge is usually very offensive, the following solution will correct its fetor, and should be injected or poured in the ear every morning and evening.

℞	Chloride of lime	ʒ i.
	Water.............................	℥ vi.
	Mix.	

If granulations have sprung up, touch them with a camel's hair brush, dipped in the following mixture:

℞	Sulphate of copper	℈ i.
	Water.......................... ..	℥ i.
	Mix.	

If, however, the excrescences continue to sprout from the cartilage, and the discharge continues unabated and offensive, they may be excised and the parts brushed over with nitrate of silver in substance. After this operation the flap often becomes extremely tender and much swollen; poultices of poppy-heads or hops will often afford much relief.

Setons are of much value in the treatment of obstinate cases, and should be placed in the poll, and kept open till a cure is effected, or the case abandoned.

All greasy applications to the parts should be discarded; the only one we consider allowable would be a very nice preparation of fresh butter, alum, and laudanum, smeared over the surface of the ulcers when very indolent and painful.

The following wash will be found very soothing in the same case:

℞	Opium	gtt. 20.
	Gum arabic	iss.—
	Lime water	℥ iv.

If the disease has progressed far enough to destroy a considerable portion of the cartilages, and perforate the tympanum, more care is necessary in using the above washes, as the fluid will enter the internal ear through this opening, and cause much uneasiness to the animal, if not fatal consequences.

WOUNDS OF THE EAR.

Wounds of the flap are often occasioned by the tearing of poisonous briars, while hunting in close cover, or in conflicts with other dogs.

The former will generally heal up without much trouble, but the latter, when extensive, sometimes two or three inches in length, require uniting by one or more sutures, to prevent deformity.

WARTS.

When these little excrescences appear on the external or internal portions of the flap, they may be taken off with the knife, and caustic applied to the wound, to induce them to heal, and keep down further granulations.

CANKER OF THE EDGE OF THE FLAP.

When a corroding sore of this nature attacks the edges of the ear, and refuses to yield to the application of a few stimulating washes, such as sulphate of copper, alum, borax, nitrate of silver, &c., the diseased edges may be paired off, and the actual cautery applied to the parts. This will frequently arrest its further progress.

POLYPUS OF THE EAR.

Polypi often spring up from the interior of the ear; they may be cut off with the scissors, or by the application of a fine wire, or horse-hair ligature. The wound should be touched with caustic, tincture of iodine, or the actual cautery.

DISEASES OF THE EAR—MANGY EDGES.

This affection generally accompanies the same disease in other portions of the body, but may occasionally make its appearance independent of this cause. The edges of the flap become rough, thickened, and furrowed, the itching intolerable; and the dog perpetually shaking and scratching the head, occasions a constant oozing of blood from the wound. Smooth-haired dogs are most subject to this disease, such as pointers, hounds, and terriers.

Treatment.—Slightly stimulating washes, such as castile soap, alum-water, or infusion of oak-bark, will, in the majority of cases, induce these sores to heal up. If these do not answer, it will be necessary to use the mange ointment, keeping the animal hobbled to prevent him from scratching. Old inveterate cases are best cured by trimming off the affected parts.—L.]

CHAPTER X.

ANATOMY OF THE NOSE AND MOUTH; AND DISEASES OF THE NOSE AND OTHER PARTS OF THE FACE.—THE SENSE OF SMELL; THE TONGUE; THE LIPS; THE TEETH; THE LARYNX; BRONCHOCELE; PHLEGMONOUS TUMOUR.

The Ethmoid Bones.—There is some difficulty in describing the ethmoid bones; but we shall not, however, deviate far from the truth if we give the following account:

A great number of small hollow pedicles proceed from and form around the cribriform plate; as they move downwards, they project into distinct vesicles or cavities, smaller and more numerous behind, fewer in number and larger in front; and each of them not a simple cavity, but more or less convoluted, while the long walls of those cells are of gossamer thinness, and as porous as gauze. They even communicate, and are lined, and externally wrapped together, by the same membrane; the whole assuming a pear-like form, attached by its base or greater extremity, and decreasing in size as it proceeds downwards; the cells becoming fewer, and terminating at length in a kind of apex, which passes under the superior turbinated bone, and forms a valve between the nasal cavity and the maxillary sinuses. If to this is added, that the olfactory or first pair of nerves abut on these cribriform plates, and pass through their minute openings, and spread themselves over every one of these cells, we have a tolerably correct picture of this portion of the ethmoid bones. This nerve has different degrees of development in different animals, in proportion to their acuteness of smell. There is comparatively but little necessity for acuteness in the horse. The ox has occasion for somewhat more, especially in the early part of the spring, when the plants are young, and have not acquired their peculiar scent. In the sheep it is larger, and fills the superior portion of the nasal cavity; but in the dog it seems to occupy that cavity almost to the exclusion of the turbinated bones. It is also much more fragile in the dog than in the ox, and the plates have a considerably thinner structure.

The ethmoid bone of the horse or the ox may be removed from its situation with little injury; but that of the dog can scarcely be meddled with without fracture. Below it are the two turbinated bones; but they are reduced to insignificance by the bulk of the ethmoid bone. The inferior turbinated bone in the dog is very small, but it is curiously complicated.

The *meatus* contains three distinct channels; and the air, loitering, as it were, in it, and being longer in contact with the sensitive membrane by which it is lined, contributes to the acuter sense of smell. The larger cavity is along the floor of the nasal duct. It is the proper air-passage; and because it has this important function to discharge, it is out of the way of violence or injury.

The *lachrymal duct* is the channel through which the superfluous tears are conveyed to the lower parts of the nostril. A long canal here commences, and runs down and along the maxillary bone. It is very small, and terminates in the cuticle, in order that the highly sensitive membrane of the nose may not be excoriated by the tears occasionally rendered acrimonious in inflammation of the eye. The oval termination of this duct is easily brought into view by lifting the nostril.

From some occasional acrimony of the tears, the lining of this duct may be inflamed and thickened, or some foreign body, or some unctuous matter from the ciliary glands, may insinuate itself into the duct, and the fluid accumulates in the sac and distends it, and it bursts; or the ulcer eats through the integument, and there is a small fistulous opening beneath the inner canthus of the eye, or there is a constant discharge from it. It is this constant discharge that prevents the wound from healing. In some cases the lachrymal bone is involved in the ulcerative process and becomes carious. In the dog, and particularly in the smaller spaniel, the watery eye, *fistula lacrymalis*, is of no unusual occurrence. The fistula will be recognised by a constant, although perhaps slight, discharge of pus.

The structure and office of the *velum palati*, or veil of the palate, is in the horse a perfect interposed section between the cavity of the mouth and the nose, and cutting off all communication between them. In the dog, who breathes almost entirely through the mouth, the velum palati is smaller; the tensor muscle, so beautifully described by Mr. Percivall, is weak, but the circumflex one is stronger and more developed. When *coryza* in the dog runs on to catarrh, and the membrane of the pharynx partakes of the inflammation, the velum palati becomes inflamed and thickened, but will not act as a perfect communication between the mouth and the nose. When there is a defluxion from the nose, tinged by the colour of the food, and particles of food mingle with it, we have one of the worst symptoms that can present itself, because it proves the extent and violence of the inflammation.

In inflammatory affections of the membrane of the nose in the dog, we often observe him snorting in a very peculiar way, with his head protruding, and the inspiration as forcible as the expiration. An emetic will usually afford relief, or grain doses of the sulphate of copper.

The Nasal Bones.—The nasal bones of the dog (see fig. 2, in the head of the dog, page 181) are very small, as they are in all carnivorous animals. Instead of constituting the roof, and part of the outer wall of the cavity, as in other animals, the nasal bones form only a portion, and a small one, of the roof.

The *superior maxillaries* here swell into importance, and constitute the whole of the outer wall, and, sometimes, a part of the roof. The jaws are the weapons of offence and defence; and as much space as possible is devoted to the insertion of those muscles that will enable the animal to seize and to hold his prey. One of the most powerful of them, the *masseter*, rises from the superior maxillary bone, and spreads over its whole extent: therefore, that bone is developed, while the nasal bone is compressed into a very small space. The substitution of a portion of cartilage, instead of bone, at the posterior part of the orbital ring, in order to give more play for the coracoid process of the posterior maxillary, round which the temporal bone is wrapped, is a contrivance of the same nature.

The scent of the dog is not sacrificed or impaired by the apparent diminution of the nasals; for the cavity enlarges considerably upward, and is occupied chiefly by the *ethmoid bone*, which, having the greater portion of nervous pulp spread on it, seems to have most to do with the sense of smell.

The nasal bones of the dog are essentially different from those of the horse, cattle, and sheep. They commence, indeed, as high up in the face as those of the horse, their superior extremities being opposite to the lachrymal gland; but that commencement is an apex or point varying materially in different breeds. They form, altogether, one sharp projection, and are received within lengthened processes of the frontal bone on either side. In some breeds these processes extend nearly one-third of the length of the nasals.

The superior maxillary (3.3.) takes the situation of the nasal (2.), pushes the lachrymal bone (4.) out of its place, and almost annihilates it, reaches the frontal bone (7.) and expands upon it, and forms with it the same denticulated suture which is to be seen in the nasal. The action of the muscle between these bones, and for the development of which all this sacrifice is made, is exceedingly powerful. The strength of this muscle in a large dog is almost incredible: the sutures between these bones must possess corresponding strength; and so strong is the union between them, that, in many old dogs, the suture between the superior maxillary and frontal bones is nearly obliterated, and that between the nasal and frontal maxillary quite effaced.

As the nasal bones proceed downward they become somewhat wider. They unite with a long process of the anterior maxillary for the purpose of strength, and then terminate in a singular way. They have their apexes or points on the outer edge of the bone; and these apexes or points are so contrived, that, lying upon, and seemingly losing themselves, on the processes of the anterior maxillary, they complete, superiorly and posteriorly, that elliptical bony opening into the nose which was commenced by the maxillary anteriorly and inferiorly. The nasal cavity of the dog, therefore, and of all carnivorous animals, terminates by a somewhat circular opening, more or less in the form of an ellipse. This bony aperture varies in size in different dogs, and, as we should expect from what we have seen of the adaptation of structure to the situation and wants of the animal, it is largest in those on whom we are most dependent for speed and stoutness.

The *olfactory*, or first pair of nerves, have a double origin, namely, from the *corpus striatum* and the base of the *corpus callosum*. They are prolongations of the medullary substance of the central portion of the brain. They are the largest of the cerebral nerves. Their course is exceedingly short; and they have not a single anastomosis, in order that the impression made on them may be conveyed undisturbed and perfect to the brain.

The olfactory nerve is a prolongation of the substance of the brain, and it abuts upon the cribriform bone, of which mention has been made. I will not speak of the singular cavities which it contains, nor of their function; this belongs to the sensorial system: but its pulpy matter has already been traced to the base of the ethmoid bone, and the under part of the septum, and the superior turbinated bone. Although we soon lose it in the mucous membrane of the nose, there is little doubt that in a more filmy form it is spread over the whole of the cavity, and probably over all the sinuses of the face and head. It is, however, so mingled with the mucous membrane, that no power of the lens has enabled us to follow it so far. It is like the *portio mollis* of the seventh pair, eluding the eye, but existing in sufficient substance for the performance of its important functions.

We have frequent cases of *ozæna* in old dogs, and sometimes in those that are younger. The discharge from the nostril is abundant and constant, and sometimes fetid. The Schneiderian membrane, of more than usual sensibility in this animal, is exposed to many causes of irritation, and debilitated and worn out before its time. Pugs are particularly subject to ozæna. I scarcely ever knew a very old pug that had it not to a greater or less degree. The peculiar depression between the nasal and frontal bones in this breed of dogs, while it almost totally obliterates the frontal sinuses, may narrow the air-passage at that spot, and cause greater irritation there from the unusual rush of the air, and especially if the membrane becomes inflamed or any foreign body insinuates itself.

Little can be done in these cases, except to encourage cleanliness about the face and nostrils. It is, in the majority of these cases, a disease of old age, and must take its course.

A terrier uttered a continual loud stertorous sound in breathing, which could be plainly heard in our parlour when the dog was in the hospital. The animal was evidently much oppressed and in considerable pain. He made continual, and generally ineffectual, efforts to sneeze. When he did succeed, a very small quantity of pus-like fluid was discharged; the dog was then considerably relieved, but a quarter of an hour afterwards he was as bad as ever. I ordered a slight emetic every third day. There was some relief for seven or eight hours, and then he was as bad as ever. I could neither feel nor see any cause of obstruction. The owner became tired, and the dog was taken away; but we could not learn what became of it.

Another terrier was occasionally brought for consultation. The dog breathed with considerable difficulty, and occasionally snorted with the greatest violence, and bloody purulent matter was discharged; after which he was somewhat relieved; but, in the course of a few days, the obstruction was as great as ever. I am not aware of a single instance of this affection of the pug being completely removed. The discharge from the nostrils of the bull-dog is often considerable, and, once being thoroughly established, is almost as obstinate as in the pug.

[OZÆNA.

Ozæna, or fetid discharge from the nose, is, perhaps, the most troublesome and frequent affection that this organ is subject to; it is attended, at first, with slight fever, swelling of the parts, and a fetid discharge from the nostrils, which, if not corrected in the early stage of the disease, subsides into a chronic purulent secretion, that not only weakens the dog, but renders him peculiarly offensive. Caries and destruction of the bones of the nose will ultimately take place.

Causes.—Inflammation of the lining membrane of the nose, either idiopathic, or arising from distemper, or other morbid disturbance of the system. It may also be a symptom, or the produce, of polypi in this organ.

Treatment.—In commencing the treatment of this disease, it will be necessary first to prescribe some alterative medicines, as balls of aloes and rhubarb, and protect the animal from all severe atmospherical vicissitudes. This precaution, in connexion with mild astringent injections into the seat of the disorder, will generally effect a cure.

Injections for Ozæna.

No. 1.

℞ Sulphate of Zinc....................grs. v to x.
Water ....℥ i.
Mix.

No. 2.

℞ Alum................................℈ ii.
Water ....℥ i.
Mix.

No. 3.

℞ Chloride of Soda...................grs. v. to x.
Water ....℥ i.
Mix.

No. 4.

℞ Teneriffe, Madeira or Sherry wine ....℥ i.
Extract of Tannin ....grs. iv.
Mix.

Any of the above injections will answer a good purpose. No. 3 is particularly useful to correct the fetidness of the discharge. When the disease is an old chronic affection, it should not be arrested too suddenly by astringent injections; in such cases it will be better to insert a seton in the poll, and thus keep up a drain from the system after the suppression of the other.—L.]

THE SENSE OF SMELL.

In the dog we trace the triumph of *olfactory power*. How indistinct must be that scent which is communicated to, and lingers on, the ground by the momentary contact of the foot of the hare, the fox, or the deer; yet the hound, of various breeds, recognises it for hours, and some sportsmen have said for more than a day. He also can not only distinguish the scent of one species of animal from another, but that of different animals of the same species. The fox-hound, well broken-in, will rarely challenge at the scent of the hare, nor will he be imposed upon when the crafty animal that he pursues has taken refuge in the earth, and thrusts out a new victim before the pack.

The sense of smelling is, to a certain degree, acute in all dogs. It is a provision wisely and kindly made, in order to guide them to their proper food, or to fit them for our service. It may possibly be the medium through which much evil is communicated. Certain particles of a deleterious nature may be, and doubtless are, arrested by the mucous membrane of the nose, and there absorbed, and the constitution, to a considerable degree, becomes affected. Hence appears the necessity for attention to ventilation, and especially to prevent the membrane of the nose from being habitually stimulated and debilitated by the effluvia generated in a close and hot kennel.

M. Majendie instituted some curious experiments on the sense of smelling, and he was led to believe that it depended more on the fifth pair of nerves than on the olfactory nerve. He divided the fifth pair, and from that moment no odour, no puncture, produced the slightest apparent impression on the membrane of the nose. In another dog he destroyed the two olfactory nerves, and placed some strong odours beneath the nostrils of the animal. The dog conducted himself as he would have done in his ordinary state. Hence he concluded it probable that the olfactory nerve was not that of smelling.

The simple fact, however, is, that there are two species of nerves here concerned—those of common and of peculiar sensation. The olfactory nerve is the nerve of smelling, the fifth pair is that of common sensation. They are to a certain degree necessary to each other.

Scent.—This leads us to the consideration of the term "scent." It expresses the odour or effluvium which is constantly issuing from every animal, and especially when that animal is in more than usual exercise. In a state of heat or excitement, the pores of the skin appear relaxed, and a fluid or aqueous vapour is secreted, which escapes in small or large quantities, adheres to the persons or substances on which it falls, and is, particularly, received on the olfactory organs. The hound, at almost the earliest period, begins to comprehend the work which he has to perform. The peculiar scent which his nostrils imbibe urges him eagerly to pursue; but the moment he ceases to be conscious of the presence of the effluvium, he is at a perfect loss.

Mr. Daniel, in his work on the Chase, very properly observes, that "the scent most favourable to the hound is when the effluvium, constantly perspired from the game as it runs, is kept by the gravity of the air at the height of his breast. It is then neither above his reach nor does he need to stoop for it. This is what is meant when the scent is said to be breast-high."

When the leaves begin to fall, the scent does not lie well in the cover. It frequently alters materially in the same day. This depends principally on the condition of the ground and the temperature of the air, which should be moist but not wet. When the ground is hard and the air dry, there will seldom be much scent. The scent rarely lies with a north or east wind. A southerly wind without rain is the best. Sudden storms are sure to destroy the scent. A fine sunshiny day is not good; but a warm day without sun is always a good one. If, as the morning advances, the drops begin to hang on the bushes, the scent will not lie. During a white frost the scent lies high, and also when the frost is quite gone; but at the time of its going off the scent never lies. In a hard rain, if the air is mild, the scent will sometimes be very good. A wet night often produces the best chases. In heathy countries, where the game brushes the grass or the boughs as it goes along, the scent seldom fails. It lies best on the richest soils; but the countries that are favourable to horses are not always so to hounds. The morning usually affords the best scent, and the game is then least able to escape. The want of rest, added perhaps to a full belly, gives the hounds a decided superiority over an early-found fox; and the condition of the ground and the temperature of the air are circumstances of much importance.

Such are the results of the best observations on scent; but, after all, we have much to learn concerning it. Many a day that predicated to be a good one for scent has turned out a very bad one, and *vice versâ*. An old or experienced sportsman, knowing this, will never presume to make sure of his scent.

We shall be forgiven if we pursue this subject a little at length.

There is not only a constant appropriation of new matter to repair the losses that animals are continually sustaining, but there is a constant elaboration of gaseous or fluid matter maintaining the balance of the different systems, and essential to the continuance of life. This effluvium, as the animal moves from place to place, is attracted and detained for a while by the substances with which it comes into contact, or it remains floating in the atmosphere

There is a peculiar smell or scent belonging to each individual, either generally or under peculiar circumstances.

The sportsman takes advantage of this; and, as most species of dogs possess great acuteness of olfactory power, they can distinguish, or are readily taught to distinguish, not only the scent of the hare from that of the fox, but that of the hare or fox which they are pursuing from that of half a dozen others that may be started during the chase.

The dogs that are selected for this purpose are those the conformation of whose face and head gives ample room for the development of the olfactory apparatus, and these are the different species of hounds; but a systematic education, and too often a great deal of unnecessary cruelty, is resorted to, in order to make them perfect in their work. The distinction between the scent of the fox and that of the hare is soon learned by the respective packs; and, when it is considered that the hunted hare is perspiring at every pore, and her strength being almost exhausted, she is straining every limb to escape from her pursuers, the increasing quantity of vapour which exudes from her will prevent every other newly started animal from being mistaken for her.

It has been well observed that when the atmosphere is loaded with moisture, and rain is at hand, the gas is speedily dissolved and mingles with the surrounding air. A storm dissipates it at once, while the cessation of the rain is preceded by the return and increased power of scent. A cold, dry easterly wind condenses and absorbs it, and this is even more speedily and irretrievably done by superabundant moisture. On fallows and beaten roads the scent rarely lies well, for there is nothing to detain it, and it is swept away in a moment; while over a luxuriant pasture, or by the hedge-row, or on the coppice, it lingers, clinging to the grass or the bushes. In a sunshiny day the scent is seldom strong; for too much of it is evaporated by the heat. The most favourable period is a soft southerly wind without rain, the scent being of the same temperature and gravity with the atmosphere. Although it spreads over the level, it rises not far above the ground, and, being *breast high*, enables the hound, keeping his muzzle in the midst of it, to run at his greatest speed. The different manners or attitudes in which the dog runs afford pleasing and satisfactory illustrations of the nature of the scent. Sometimes they will be seen galloping with their noses in the air, as if their game had flown away, and, an hour or two afterwards, every one of them will have his muzzle on the ground. The specific gravity of the atmosphere has changed, and the scent has risen or fallen in proportion.

A westerly wind stands next to a southerly one, for a hunting morning. This is all simple enough, and needs not the mystification with which it has been surrounded. A valuable account of this may be found in Johnson's Shooting Companion, a work that is justly and highly approved.

Mr. Delmé Radcliffe has also, in his splendid work on "the noble science," some interesting remarks on the scent of hounds. He says that there is an idiosyncracy, a peculiarity, in their several dispositions. Some young hounds seem to enter on their work instinctively. From their first to their last appearance in the field they do no wrong. Others, equally good, will take no notice of anything; they will not stoop to any scent during the first season, and are still slack at entering even at the second; but are ultimately distinguished at the head of the pack; and such usually last some seasons longer than the more precocious of the same litter.

THE TONGUE.

The manner of drinking is different in the different animals. The horse, the ox, and the sheep do not plunge their muzzles into the water, but bring their lips into contact with it and sip it gradually. The dog, whose tongue is longer, plunges it a little way into the fluid, and, curving its tip and its edges, laps, in the language of Johnson, with a "quick reciprocation of the tongue." The horse sucks the water that is placed before him, the dog laps it; and both of them are subject to inflammation of the tongue, to enlargement of that organ, and to a considerable or constant flow of saliva over it.

Extending from the base to the tip of the tongue there is on either side a succession of tendons, which help to retain the tongue in the mouth, and to curve the edge of it, so as to convey the food or the water to the posterior part of the mouth. These all spring from one central cord, and ramify over the membrane of the tongue. On opening the mouth, and keeping it open by means of two pieces of tape, one behind the upper canine teeth, and the other behind the lower ones, and drawing the tongue from the mouth and exposing its under surface, a cuticular fold or ridge will present itself, occupying a middle line from the base of the tongue to its very point. If this is opened with a lancet, a minute fibrous cord will be exposed through its whole extent. It is the cord which governs the motions of the tongue.

This cord is, sometimes, foolishly and uselessly detached from its adhesions, so far as we can effect it, and drawn forward with a tenaculum and divided. There is one abominable course pursued in effecting this. The violence used in stripping down the tendon is so great, and the lacerated fibrous substance is put so much on the stress, and its natural elasticity is so considerable, that it recoils and assumes the appearance of a dying worm, and the dog is said to have been wormed. For the sake of humanity, as well as to avoid the charge of ignorance, it is to be hoped that this practice will speedily cease.

The Blain.—The blain is a vesicular enlargement on the lateral and under part of the tongue in horses, oxen, and dogs, which, although not of unfrequent occurrence, or peculiarly fatal result, has not been sufficiently noticed by veterinary authors. In the horse and the dog it is often unaccompanied by any previous indisposition, or by other disease; but suddenly there is a copious discharge of saliva, at first limpid and without smell, but soon becoming purulent, bloody, and exceedingly fetid. On examination, the tongue is found apparently enlarged. It is elevated from its base between the maxillary bones, and on the side and towards the base of it are seen large vesicles, pellucid, red, livid, or purple; and, if the discharge is fetid, having near their bases ulcers, irregular, unhealthy, and gangrenous.

In the horse and the dog the progress of the disease is slow, and seldom extends beyond the sides of the tongue. The vesicles are not of such magnitude as to interfere with respiration, and the ulcers are neither many nor foul.

In cattle it is sadly different. The vesicles attain an enormous size. They quickly break and form deep ulcerations, which are immediately succeeded by other vesicles still larger. The whole membrane of the mouth becomes affected; the inflammation and swelling extend to the cellular substance of the neighbouring parts, and the head and neck are considerably, and sometimes enormously, enlarged; the respiratory passages are obstructed; the animal breathes with the greatest difficulty, and is, in some cases, literally suffocated.

The primary seat of blain, is the cellular substance beneath the integument of the part. As the sublingual glands stretch along the under part of the tongue, and their ducts open on the side of the frænum, it is possible that this disease may proceed from, or be connected with, obstruction or inflammation of these ducts. Dissection, however, has not proved this; and the seat of the disease, when the swellings are first discovered, is chiefly the cellular tissue between the integument and the lateral parts of the tongue, and also that between the membrane of the mouth and the sublingual glands.

Post-mortem examination shows intense disease: the small intestines are highly inflamed with red and black patches, which are also found in the cœcum, colon, and rectum.

The blain is more frequent in spring and summer than at other seasons of the year. These are the times when the animal is debilitated by the process of moulting, and is then more than usually disposed to inflammatory complaints. It is usually an epidemic disease. Many cases of it occur about the same time in certain districts, and over a great extent of country. When it appears in towns, the country is rarely exempt from it. I am not prepared to say that it is contagious either in the horse or the dog. I have not seen any instance of it. At all events, it is not so virulent in these animals as it is in cattle.

The vesicles should be freely lanced from end to end. There will not, perhaps, be much immediate discharge; for the vesicle will be distended by a substance imperfectly organised, or of such a glassy or inspissated nature as not readily to escape. It will, however, soon disappear; and in four-and-twenty hours, in the majority of cases, the only vestige of the disease will be an incision, not, perhaps, looking very healthy, but that will soon become so and heal. If there have been any previous ulcerations, or the slightest fetor, the mouth should be frequently washed with a diluted solution of the chloride of lime; one part of the saturated solution, and eleven of water. This will act as a powerful and useful stimulus to the foul and indolent ulcer. When all unpleasant smell is removed, the mouth should be bathed with a lotion composed of equal parts of tincture of myrrh and water, or half an ounce of alum dissolved in a quart of water, and two ounces of the tincture of catechu added to the solution. I do not recollect a case in the horse or dog, in which these medicines were not employed with advantage. In cattle, before there has been fetor attending the discharge, or the constitution has been materially affected, these simple means will perfectly succeed.

If the practitioner is consulted somewhat too late, when the constitution has become affected, and typhoid fever has ensued, he should still lance the tumours, and apply the chloride of lime and the tincture of myrrh, and give a gentle aperient. He should endeavour to rouse and support the system by tonic medicines, as gentian and colomba with ginger, adding to two drachms of the first two, and one drachm of the last, half an ounce of nitre; but he should place most dependence on nourishing food. Until the mouth is tolerably sound, it is probable that the animal will not be induced to eat; but it will occasionally sip a little fluid, and, therefore, gruel should be always within its reach. More should occasionally be given, as thick as it will flow, with a spoon or small horn.

[*Inflammation of the Tongue.*—Glossitis or inflammation of the tongue is not an unfrequent disease, but is occasionally met with in its simple form or in connexion with inflammatory affections of the throat. Under all and any circumstances this affection must be considered a dangerous malady, as it not unfrequently proves fatal in the course of a few hours from suffocation, occasioned by the swelling of the organ itself and other portions of the throat. The disease comes on suddenly with fever, heat, swelling and redness of the tongue. The tongue protrudes from the mouth and exhibits a dry, hot, inflammatory appearance, the respiration is hurried, and the animal expresses great uneasiness, and constant desire to lap water, which he can with difficulty accomplish. If not arrested, the inflammation may terminate in suppuration, by which process the swelling is relieved, and a cure often effected.

Causes.—Independent of the natural agents before referred to in the production of inflammatory affections, there are some few causes to which we can especially attribute this disease. Direct injuries done to the member itself, either by wounds or stings of insects, the taking of poisonous or irritating substances into the mouth, want of water while hunting in hot weather, &c.

Several years ago we witnessed the death of a very valuable pointer, suffering from this disease produced by poison maliciously administered. He was affected so suddenly and violently with inflammation of the throat and tongue that his owner, Mr. F——, was lead to believe that a bone had lodged in the throat, which was the occasion of all the trouble. After proper examination and considerable delay, he was forced to abandon this erroneous idea, but not in time to save the poor animal, who soon died from strangulation or congestion of the lungs. This valuable dog might have been saved if promptly and energetically treated.

The stings of wasps or bees may also produce this affection.

Treatment.—Nothing can be done with this malady without the use of the lancet, by which six or eight ounces of blood should be drawn at the commencement of the disease. If the tongue is much swollen and very tender, longitudinal incisions should be made in it, extending as far back as possible, and their bleeding assisted by sponging the mouth out with tepid water. Astringent applications may then be used as washes, such as alum water, strong vinegar, infusions of oak bark or solutions of nitrate of silver, four or six grains to the ounce, to be applied once or twice a day. A large blister may also be placed under the throat, and when the inflammation is sufficiently reduced to allow the introduction of articles into the stomach, a powerful purge of aloes should be given. Nothing, however, can be done without copious bleeding.—L.]

THE LIPS

of the dog discharge, with somewhat less efficiency, the same office as in the horse, cattle, and sheep; and are usefully employed in gathering together the food, and conveying it to the mouth. The lips also secrete the saliva, a fluid that is indispensably necessary for the proper comminution of the food.

Swellings on the inside of the cheek or upper lip, and extending nearly to the angle of the lip, are of frequent occurrence. A superficial sore spreads over it, slightly covered by a yellowish, mattery pellicle; and on the teeth, and extending down the gums, there is a deposition of hardened tartarous matter, which is scaled off with a greater or less degree of difficulty. It must be removed, or the sore will rapidly spread over the cheek. A lotion of equal parts of tincture of myrrh and water, with a few drops of the tincture of cantharides, will be usually sufficient to cause the swelling to subside, and the pellicle to be detached. The lip, however, will generally remain slightly thickened. A little soreness will sometimes return, but be easily reduced.

THE TEETH

next claim attention.

According to the dentition of the dog by M. Girard and Linnæus, the following is the acknowledged formula:—

$$\text{Incisors, } \frac{6}{6}; \text{ Canines, } \frac{1-1}{1-1}; \text{ Molars, } \frac{6-6}{7-7}, =42.$$

The following cuts exhibit the front teeth of the dog in various stages of growth and decay:

Fig. 1.

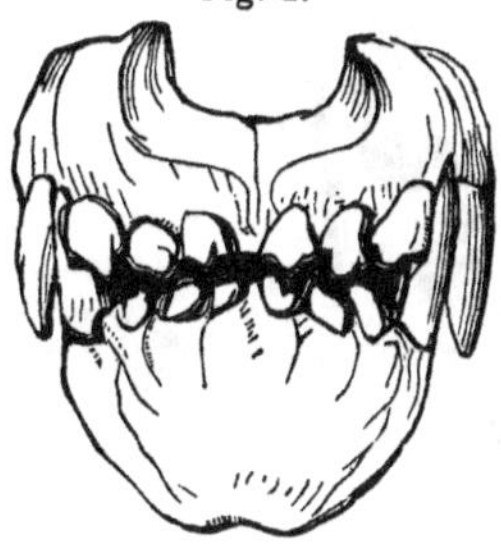

Fig. 2.

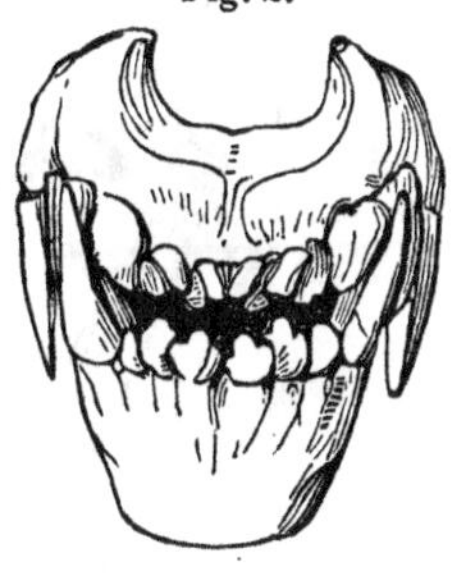

Fig. 3.

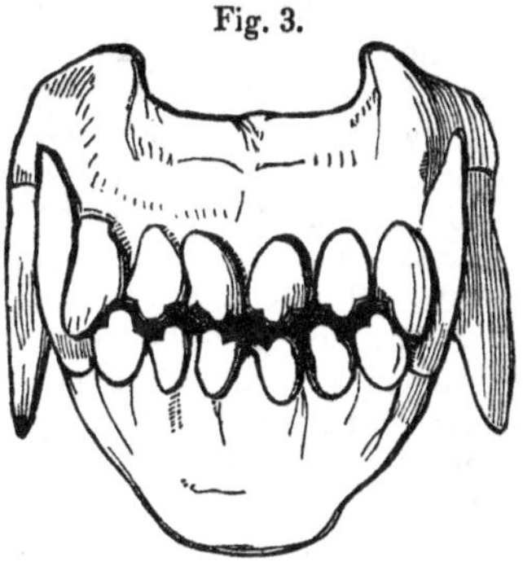

Fig. 4.

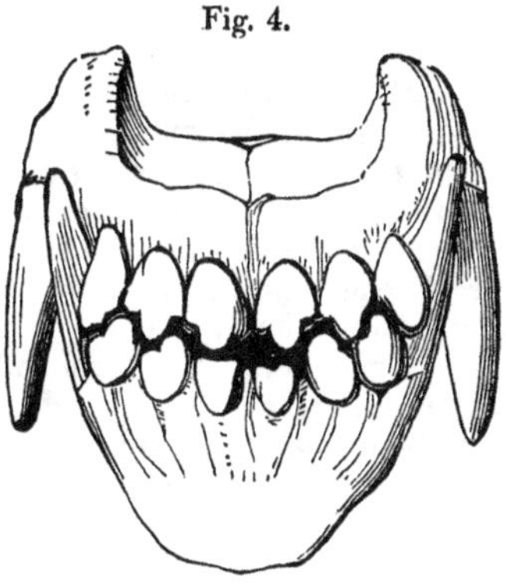

Fig. 5.

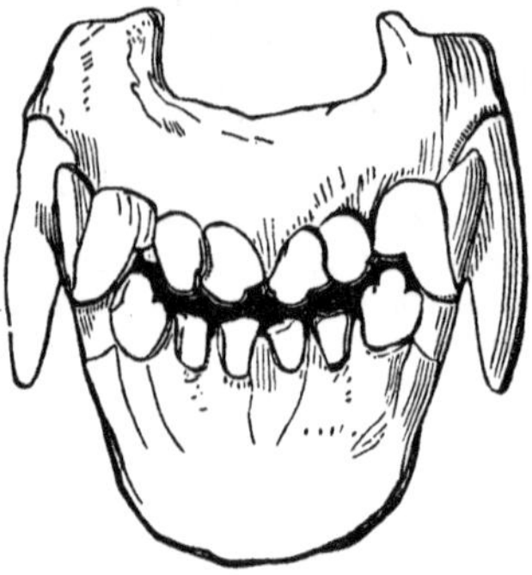

Fig. 6.

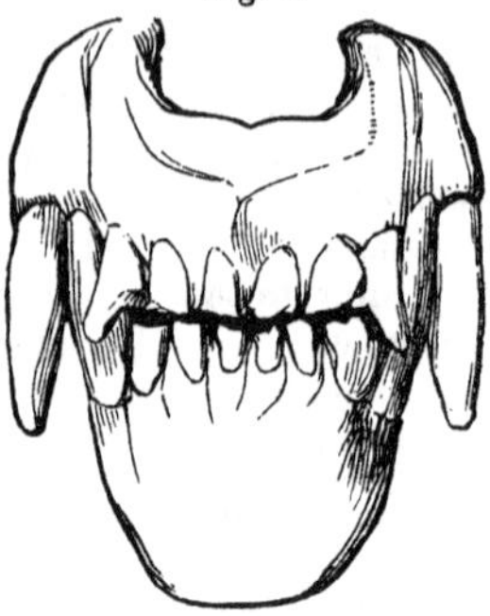

Fig. 7.

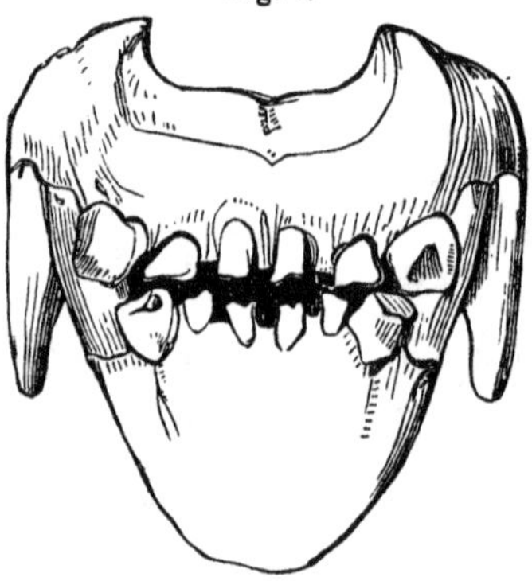

The full-grown dog has usually 20 teeth in the upper, and 22 in the lower jaw, with two small supernumerary molars. All of them, with the exception of the tushes, are provided with a bony neck covered by the gums, and separating the body of the tooth from the root. The projecting portion of the teeth is more or less pointed, and disposed so as to tear and crush the food on which the dog lives. They are of a moderate size when compared with those of other animals, and are subject to little loss of substance compared with the teeth of the horse. In most of them, however, there is some alteration of form and substance, both in the incisors and the tushes; but this depends so much on the kind of food on which the animal lives, and the consequent use of the teeth, that the indication of the age, by the altered appearance of the mouth, is not to be depended upon after the animal is four or five years old. The incisor teeth are six in number in each jaw, and are placed opposite to each other. In the lower jaw, the pincers, or central teeth, are the largest and the strongest; the middle teeth are somewhat less; and the corner teeth the smallest and the weakest. In the upper jaw, however, the corner teeth are much larger than the middle ones; they are farther apart from their neighbours, and they terminate in a conical point curved somewhat inwards and backwards.

As long as the teeth of the full-grown dog are whole, and not injured by use, they have a healthy appearance, and their colour is beautifully white. The surface of the incisors presents, as in the ruminants, an interior and cutting edge, and a hollow or depression within. This edge or border is divided into three lobes, the largest and most projecting forming the summit or point of the tooth. The two lateral lobes have the appearance of notches cut on either side of the principal lobe; and the union of the three resembles the *fleur de lis*, which, however, is in the process of time effaced by the wearing out of the teeth. (Figs. 3 and 4.)

While the incisor teeth are young, they are flattened on their sides, and bent somewhat backwards, and there is a decided cavity, in which a pulpy substance is enclosed. This, however, is gradually contracted as the age of the dog increases.

M. F. Cuvier speaks of certain supernumerary teeth occasionally developed in each of the jaws. There is much irregularity accompanying them; and they have even been supposed to have extended to seven or eight in number.

The Indications of Age.—The dog displays natural indications of age. The hair turns gray to a certain extent as in the human being. This commences about the eyes, and extends over the face, and weakens the sight; and, at ten years old, or earlier, in the majority of dogs, this can scarcely be mistaken. At fifteen or sixteen years the animal is becoming a nuisance, yet he has been known to linger on until he has reached his two-and-twentieth year.

Among the diseases from which the dog suffers, there are few of more frequent occurrence than decayed teeth, especially in towns, or in the habitations of the higher classes of society: the carious teeth, in almost every case, becoming insufferably fetid, or so loose as to prevent mastication; or an immense accumulation of tartar growing round them.

The course which the veterinary surgeon pursues is an exceedingly simple one. If any of the teeth are considerably loose, they must be removed. If there is any deposit of tartaric acid, it must be got rid of by means of the proper instruments, not very different from those which the human surgeon employs. The teeth must be perfectly cleaned, and every loose one taken away. Without this the dog will be an almost insufferable nuisance.

The decayed and loose teeth being removed, chlorinated lime diluted with 15 or 20 times its bulk of water should be applied to the gums. By the use of this the ulcers will quickly heal; the fetor will be removed, and the deposition of the tartar prevented. Mr. Blaine first introduced the chlorinated lime for the accomplishment of these purposes.

Two little histories out of a great number will sufficiently illustrate these cases. A terrier had scarcely eaten during more than a week. He dropped his meat after attempting to chew it, and the breath was very offensive. Several of the teeth were loose, and the rest were thickly encrusted with tartar. The gums had receded from the teeth, and were red, sore, and ulcerated.

I removed all the loose teeth; for experience had taught me that they rarely or never became again fixed. I next, with the forceps and knife, cleaned the others, and ordered the diluted chlorinated lime to be alternated with tincture of myrrh and water. The extraction of the loose teeth, and the removal of the tartar from those that were sound, occupied a full hour; for the dog resisted with all his might. He, however, soon began to eat; the lotions were continued; and five months afterwards, the mouth of the dog was not in the slightest degree offensive.

An old dog should not be quite abandoned. A pug had only four teeth remaining beside the canines. They were all thickly covered with tartar, and two of them were very loose. The gums and lips were in a dreadfully cankerous state, and the dog was unable to eat. All that he could do was to lap a little milk or broth.

I extracted the two loose teeth, cleaned the others, and ordered a lotion of equal parts of tincture of myrrh and water to be applied.

13*th August*, 1842.—A very considerable discharge of pus was observed, with blood from the mouth, apparently proceeding from the cavity whence one of the teeth had been extracted. The dog is exceedingly thirsty, and walks round and round the water-dish, but is afraid to lap. He has not eaten for two days. Use the lotion as before, and force him with strong soup.

15*th*. The dog has not voluntarily eaten, but is still forced with soup. He is very costive. Give two grains of calomel and an equal quantity of antimonial powder.

18*th*. He has eaten a very little, but gets thinner and weaker. Continue the lotion.

27*th*. The ulcers are nearly healed, and the discharge of pus has ceased.

31*st*. The mouth is clean, the gums are healed, and there is no longer anything offensive about the dog.

THE LARYNX

is placed at the top of the windpipe, the exit from the lungs, and is also connected with the Schneiderian membrane. At its upper part is the epiglottis, the main guard against the passage of the food into the respiratory tubes, and, at the same time, of the instrument of the voice. It consists of five cartilages united together by a ligamentous substance, and, by distinct and perfect articulations, adapting itself to every change of the respiratory process and the production of the voice.

At the base is the *cricoid cartilage,* the support and bond of union of the rest. Above are the *arytenoid cartilages,* resting on the *chordæ vocales* and influencing their action. The *epiglottis* is placed at the extremity of the opening into the windpipe, with its back opposed to the pharynx, so that when a pellet of food passes from the pharynx in its way to the œsophagus, the epiglottis is applied over the glottis, and by this means closes the aperture of the larynx, and prevents any portion of the food from passing into it. The food having passed over the epiglottis, that cartilage, from its elastic power, again rises and resumes its former situation.

The *thyroid cartilage* envelopes and protects all the rest, and particularly the lining membrane of the larynx, which vibrates from the impulse of the air that passes. The vibrations spread in every direction until they reach the delicate membrane of the tympanum of the ear. That membrane responds to the motion without, and the vibration is carried on to the pulp of the auditory nerve, deep in the recesses of the ear. The loudness of the tone —its acuteness or graveness—depends on the force of the expired air and the shortening or lengthening of the chord. Hence it is, that the tone of the bark of the dog, or the neighing of the horse, depends so much on the age or size of the animal. Thus we compare the shrill bark of the puppy with the hoarse one of the adult dog; the high-toned but sweet music of the beagle with the fuller and lower cry of the fox-hound, and the deep but melodious baying of the mastiff. I may, perhaps, be permitted to add to these, the whinnying of the colt and the neighing of the horse.

Each animal has his peculiar and intelligible language. He who has long lived among them will recognise the tone of delight at meeting, rising into and terminating in a sharper sound; the strong and elevated tone when they are calling to or challenging each other at a distance; the short expression of anger — the longer, deeper, hoarser tone of fear; the murmur almost as deep, but softer, of habitual attachment, and the elevated yet melodious token of sudden recognition. I could carry on a conversation with a dog that I once possessed for several minutes, and one perfectly intelligible to both.

Inflammation of the larynx is a frequent and dangerous complaint. It usually commences with, and can scarcely be distinguished from, catarrh, except that it is attended by cough more violent and painful, and the dog expectorates considerably. Acute laryngitis is not so frequent an occurrence; but there is much danger attending it. Blood must be abstracted to as great an extent as the pulse will bear, or until it becomes evidently affected. To this must follow digitalis, nitre, tartar emetic, and aloes, and to these must be added a powerful blister. A considerable quantity is effused and organized, the membrane is thickened, perhaps permanently so, and the whole of the submucous cellular tissue becomes œdematous.

The dog is subject to sudden attacks of *angina*. It has been imagined, from the appearances that are manifested, that some strange body is arrested in the windpipe or the throat. There is no dread of water or of the usual fluids; the dog will lap once or twice from that fluid which is placed before him, and turns slowly away from it; and this circumstance gives rise to what is called dumb madness. The dog barks in a particular manner, or rather howls like a rabid dog: he is out of spirits, has a strange, anxious, altered countenance, and is alternately cold and hot. Frequently added to this is redness of the buccal and nasal membranes. He refuses all solid food, and either will not drink or finds it difficult to swallow anything. His mouth is generally open, and contains a spumy matter exhaling an offensive smell. His tongue, charged with a great quantity of saliva, protrudes from his mouth, and the submaxillary glands are enlarged. To these appearances are added a yellow tint of the eyes, constipation, and a small quantity of urine, surcharged with a deep yellow colour. At this period the disease has generally reached a considerable degree of virulence. Often the inflammation extends to the back part of the mouth and larynx; and in this last case the respiration is attended by a hoarse, hissing kind of sound.

The progress of the disease is rapid, and, in a few days, it reaches its highest degree of intensity. It is always fatal when it is intense; and, when its influence is widely spread, it is a very dangerous complaint.

Somewhat rarely the subjects of it recover. After death we find great redness and injection in all the affected nervous surfaces, and indications of abscesses in which suppuration was not fully established.

[FOREIGN ARTICLES IN THE THROAT.

When a substance, such as a bone, has become impacted in the throat, the better plan is to attempt to push it downwards into the stomach, as there is but little hope of extracting it.

A portion of sponge may be securely tied on the end of a piece of ratan, whalebone, or other flexible material, and inserted in the mouth, may be carried over the tongue down the throat against the foreign article, which may then be gently pushed before it. If this should not succeed, and the substance appears firmly imbedded in the throat, an incision may be made in the œsophagus and the bone extracted.—L.]

BRONCHOCELE OR GOÎTRE

in the dog is almost daily forced upon our notice. If a spaniel or pug-puppy is mangy, pot-bellied, rickety, or deformed, he seldom fails to have some enlargement of the thyroid gland. The spaniel and the pug are most subject to this disease. The jugular vein passes over the thyroid gland; and, as that substance increases, the vein is sometimes brought into sight, and appears between the gland and the integument, fearfully enlarged, varicose, and almost appearing as if it were bursting. The trachea is pressed upon on either side, and the œsophagus by the left gland, and there is difficulty of swallowing. The poor animal pants distressingly after the least exertion, and I have known absolute suffocation ensue. In a few cases ulceration has followed, and the sloughing has been dreadful, yet the gland has still preserved its characteristic structure. Although numerous abscesses have been formed in the lower part of it, and there has been considerable discharge, viscid or purulent, the upper part has remained as hard and almost as scirrhous as before.

Cause of Goître.—In many cases, this enlargement of the thyroid glands is plainly connected with a debilitated state of the constitution generally, and more particularly with a disposition to rickets. I have rarely seen a puppy that has had mange badly, and especially if mange was closely followed by distemper, that did not soon exhibit goître. Puppies half-starved, and especially if dirtily kept, are thus affected; and it is generally found connected with a loose skin, flabby muscles, enlarged belly, and great stupidity. On the other hand, I have seen hundreds of dogs, to all appearance otherwise healthy, in whom the glands of the neck have suddenly and frightfully enlarged. I have never been able to trace this disease to any particular food, whether solid or liquid; although it is certainly the frequent result of want of nutriment.

Some friends, of whom I particularly inquired, assured me, that it is not to any great extent prevalent in those parts of Derbyshire where goître is oftenest seen in the human being.

It is periodical in the dog. I have seen it under medical treatment, and without medical treatment, perfectly disappear for a while, and soon afterwards, without any assignable cause, return. There is a breed of the Blenheim spaniel, in which this periodical goître is very remarkable; the slightest cold is accompanied by enlargement of the thyroid gland, but the swelling altogether disappears in the course of a fortnight. I am quite assured that it is hereditary; no one that is accustomed to dogs can doubt this for a moment.

Treatment.—I am almost ashamed to confess how many inefficient and cruel methods of treatment I many years ago adopted. I used mercurial friction, external stimulants, and blisters; I have been absurd enough to pass setons through the tumours, and even to extirpate them with the knife. The mercury salivated without any advantage, the stimulants and the blisters aggravated the evil; the setons did so in a tenfold degree, so that many dogs were lost in the irritative fever that was produced; and, although the gland, when dissected out, could not be reproduced, yet I have been puzzled with the complication of vessels around it, and in one case lost my patient by hemorrhage, which I could not arrest.

When the power of iodine in the dispersion of glandular tumours was first spoken of, I eagerly tried it for this disease, and was soon satisfied that it was almost a specific. I scarcely recollect a case in which the glands have not very materially diminished; and, in the decided majority of cases, they have been gradually reduced to their natural size. I first tried an ointment composed of the iodine of potassium and lard, with some, but not a satisfactory result. Next I used the tincture of iodine, in doses of from five to ten drops, and with or without any external local application; but I found, at length, that the simple iodine, made into pills with powdered gum and syrup, effected almost all that I could wish. It is best to commence with the eighth of a grain for a small dog, and rapidly increase it to half a grain, morning and night. A larger dog may take from a quarter of a grain to a grain. In a few instances, loss of appetite and slight emaciation have been produced; but then, the medicine being suspended for a few days, no permanent ill effect has ever followed the exhibition of iodine.

PHLEGMONOUS TUMOUR.

A phlegmonous tumour under the throat, and accompanied by constitutional disturbance, with the exception of there being little or no cough, often appears in the dog. Comparing the size of the animals, these tumours are much larger than in either the horse or ox; but they are situated higher up the face, and do not press so much upon the windpipe, nor is there any apparent danger of suffocation from them. The whole head, however, is sometimes enlarged to a frightful degree, and the eyes are completely closed. More than a pint of fluid has sometimes escaped from a middle-sized dog at the first puncture of the tumour.

The mode of treatment is, to stimulate the part, in order to expedite the suppuration of the tumour, and to lance it freely and deeply, as soon as matter is evidently formed. The wound should be dressed with tincture of aloes, and a thick bandage placed round the neck, to prevent the dog from scratching the part, which often causes dreadful laceration.

These tumours in the throat of the dog are not always of a phlegmonous character. They are cysts, sometimes rapidly formed, and of considerable size, and filled with a serous or gelatinous fluid.

CHAPTER XI.

ANATOMY AND DISEASES OF THE CHEST; THE DIAPHRAGM; THE PERICARDIUM; THE HEART; PLEURISY; PNEUMONIA; SPASMODIC COUGH.

The chest is the superior, or in quadrupeds the anterior, cavity of the trunk of the body: it is divided into two cavities by a membranous partition, termed *mediastinum;* and separated from the abdomen, or cavity which contains the liver, spleen, pancreas, and other abdominal viscera, by the *diaphragm,* which is of a musculo-membranous nature. This membrane may be described, as it is divided, into the main circular muscle, with its central tendinous expansion forming the lower part, and two appendices, or *crura,* as they are termed from their peculiar shape, constituting its superior portion. We trace the fleshy origin of the grand muscle, laterally and inferiorly, commencing from the cartilage of the eighth rib anteriorly, and following somewhat closely, as we proceed backward, the union of the posterior ribs with their cartilages, excepting, however, the two last. The attachment is peculiarly strong. It is denticulated: it encloses the whole of the latter and inferior part of the chest as far as the sternum, where it is connected with the ensiform cartilage.

The diaphragm is the main agent, both in ordinary and extraordinary respiration. In its quiescent state it presents its convex surface towards the thorax, and its concave one towards the abdomen. The anterior convexity abuts upon the lungs; the posterior concavity is occupied by some of the abdominal viscera.

Thus far we have described the diaphragm as found in the horse, ox, and sheep. There is some difference with regard to the dog. The muscular part of the diaphragm is thick and strong in every species of dog, while the aponeurotic expansion is comparatively smaller. From the smaller expanse of the thorax of the dog, and the consequent little expansion of the diaphragm, the action, although occasionally rapid and violent—for he is an animal of speed—is not so extensive, and more muscle and less tendon may be given to him, not only without detriment, but with evident advantage. Therefore, although we have occasional rupture of the heart of the dog, oftener perhaps than in the horse, there is no case of rupture of the diaphragm on record.

The cavity of the thorax is lined by a membrane, termed pleura, which covers the surface of the lungs.

The lungs on either side are enclosed in a separate and perfect bag, and each lung has a distinct pleura. The heart lies under the left lung; and, more perfectly to cut off all injurious connexion or communication of disease between the lungs and the heart, the heart is enclosed in a distinct pleura or bag, termed the *pericardium*. This membrane closely invests the heart, supports it in its situation, prevents too great dilatation when it is gorged with blood, and too violent action when it is sometimes unduly stimulated. Notwithstanding the confinement of the pericardium, the heart, when under circumstances of unusual excitation, beats violently against the ribs, and, were it not thus tied down, would often bruise and injure itself, and cause inflammation in the neighbouring parts.

The *heart* is composed of four cavities; two above, called *auricles*, from their shape, and two below, termed *ventricles*, occupying the bulk of the heart. In point of fact, there are two hearts — the one on the left side propelling the blood through the frame, and the other on the right side conveying it through the pulmonary system; but, united in the manner in which they are, their junction contributes to their mutual strength, and both circulations are carried on at the same time.

The beating of the heart in the dog is best examined behind the elbow on the left side. The hand, applied flat against the ribs, will give the number and character of the pulsations. The pericardium, or outer investing membrane of the heart, is frequently liable to inflammation, indicated by a quickened and irregular respiration, and an action of the heart, bounding at an early period of the disease, but becoming scarcely recognisable as the fluid increases. The patient is then beginning gradually to sink. A thickening of the substance of the heart is occasionally suspected, and, on the other hand, an increased capacity of the cavities of the heart; the parietes being considerably thinner, and the frame of the animal emaciated.

The pulse of the greater part of our domestic animals has been calculated by Mr. Vatel, in his excellent work on Veterinary Pathology, to be nearly as follows:—

In the horse,	from	32	to	38	pulsations in a minute.
" ox or cow,	"	35	"	42	"
" ass,	"	48	"	54	"
" sheep,	"	70	"	79	"

"	goat,	from	72	to	76	pulsations in a minute.
"	dog,	"	90	"	100	"
"	cat,	"	110	"	120	"
"	rabbit	.	.		120	"
"	guinea-pig	.	.		140	"
"	crow	.	.		136	"
"	duck	.	.		136	"
"	hen	.	.		140	"
"	heron	.	.		200	"

The pulse of the dog may be easily ascertained by feeling at the heart or the inside of the knee, and it varies materially, according to the breed, as well as the size of the animal. This is very strikingly the case with some of the sporting dogs, with whom the force as well as the rapidity of the pulse vary materially according to the character and breed of the dog.

There is, occasionally, in the dog as in the human being, an alteration of the quantity, as well as of the quality, of the blood. *Anæmia* is the term used to designate a deficiency in quantity; *plethora* the opposite state of it. M. D'Arbor relates a very curious account of the former:—

Two dogs were sent into the hospital of the veterinary school at Lyons. They did not appear to suffer any considerable pain. Their skin and mucous membranes that were visible had a peculiar appearance. They had also comparatively little power over their limbs; so little, indeed, that they rested continually on one side, without the ability to shift their posture. When they were placed on their feet, their limbs gave way, and they fell the moment they were quitted. In despite of the care that was taken of them, they died on the second day.

Incisions were made through the skin, but in opening them no blood flowed. The venæ cavæ themselves did not contain any—there were only two clots of blood in the cavities of their hearts. One of them, of the size of a small nutmeg, occupied the left ventricle; the other, which was still smaller, was found at the base of the right ventricle. The chest of one of them enclosed a small quantity of serosity; a similar fluid was between the dura mater and the arachnoid membrane, and the same was the case in the larger ventricles of the encephalon. The other viscera did not offer anything remarkable, except the paleness and flaccidity of their tissue. The great fatigues of the chase, and the immersion of these animals in water at the time that they were very much heated, appeared to have been the causes of this singular disease. In the report of the labours of the School of Alfort, in the year 1825, the same anæmia was remarked in two dogs that died there; one of them had lately undergone a considerable hemorrhage, and in the other anæmia had developed itself spontaneously.

It is in fact among dogs that this extreme anæmia has been

principally observed, and is ordinarily fatal. It has been remarked by M. Crusal in a bullock attacked with gastro-enteritis.

This disease, according to M. Vatel, is generally the symptom of a chronic malady, or the instantaneous effect of an excessive hemorrhage. It is rarely primary. The extreme discoloration of the tissues, and of the mucous membrane more particularly, the disappearance of the subcutaneous blood-vessels, and the extreme feebleness of the animal, are the principal symptoms. There also often exists considerable swelling of the limbs.

The following singular case of a wound penetrating into the chest and pericardium of a dog, is recorded by Professor Delafond:—

A mastiff dog fighting with another was stabbed in the chest by the master of his antagonist. Five hours after the accident, the Professor was sent for. On the exterior of the sternum was a laceration an inch and a half in length, covered by a spumy fluid, from the centre of which was heard a gurgling noise, showing that a wound had penetrated into the sac of the pleura. The respiration was quick, and evidently painful; the beating of the heart was also strong and precipitate. The finger being introduced into the wound, penetrated between the fourth and fifth rib on the left side. "Having arrived at the pleuritic sac," says the Professor, "I gently tapped the surface of the lung, in order to assure myself that it was not injured; my finger penetrated into the pericardium, and the point of the heart beat against it."

He bathed the wound with a little diluted wine, and brought the edges of it as near together as he could, and confined them with a suture, administering a mild aperient.

On the following day, the animal walked slowly about, seeking for something to eat; he gave him some milk. On changing the dressing, he tried whether he could again introduce any sound into the wound; but it would only penetrate a very little way; indeed, re-union by adhesion had already taken place.

On the fifth day, the animal was in good spirits; the wound had a healthy red appearance, and all tended to a speedy cure.

On the eighth day he was sent home to his master, a distance of two leagues from his house. He saw the dog eighteen months afterwards, and he was as eager as ever after his game.

The following is a case of rupture of the heart:—A black pointer, of the Scotch breed, had every appearance of good health, except that she frequently fell into a fit after having run a little way, and sometimes even after playing in the yard. She was several times bled during and after these fits. When I examined her, I could plainly perceive considerable and violent spasmodic motion of the heart, and the sounds of the beating of the heart were irregular and convulsive. She was sent to the infirmary, in order to be cured of an attack of mange; but during her stay in the hospital she had these fits several times: the attack almost always followed after she had been playing with other dogs. She appeared as if struck by lightning, and remained motionless for several minutes, her gums losing their natural appearance and assuming a bluish hue. After the lapse of a few minutes, she again arose as if nothing had been the matter. She was bled twice in eight days, and several doses of foxglove were administered to her. The fits appeared to become less frequent; but, playing one day with another dog, she fell and expired immediately.

The *post mortem* examination was made two hours after death. The cavity of the pericardium contained a red clot of blood, which enveloped the whole of the heart; it was thicker in the parts that corresponded with the valve of the heart; and on the left ventricle, and near the base of the left valve of the heart, and on the external part of that viscus, was an irregular rent two inches long. It crossed the wall of the valve of the heart, which was very thin in this place. The size of the heart was very small, considering the height and bulk of the dog. The walls of the ventricles, and particularly of the left ventricle, were very thick. The cavity of the left ventricle was very small; there was evidently a concentric hypertrophy of these ventricles; the left valve of the heart was of great size.

The immediate cause of the rupture of the valve of the heart had evidently been an increase of circulation, brought on by an increase of exercise; but the remote cause consisted in the remarkable thinness of the walls of the valve of the heart. This case is remarkable in more than one respect; first, because examples of rupture of the valve of the heart are very rare; and, secondly, because this rupture had its seat in the left valve of the heart, while, usually, in both the human being and the quadruped, it takes place in the right; and this, without doubt, because the walls and the valves of the right side are thinner.

Diseases of the investing membrane of the lungs, and the pleura of the thoracic cavity, and of the substance of the lungs, are more frequent than those of the heart.

PLEURISY,

or inflammation of the membrane of the chest and the lungs of the dog, is not unfrequent. There are few instances of inflammation of the lungs, or pneumonia, that do not ultimately become connected with or terminate in pleurisy. The tenderness of the sides, the curious twitching that is observed, the obstinate sitting up, and the presence of a short, suppressed, painful cough, which the dog bears with strange impatience, are the symptoms that principally distinguish it from pneumonia. The exploration of the chest by auscultation gives a true picture of it in pleurisy; and, by placing the dog alternately on his chest, his back, or his side, we can readily ascertain the extent to which effusion exists in the thoracic cavity; and, if we think proper, we can get rid of the fluid. It is not a dangerous thing to attempt, although it is very problematical whether much advantage would accrue from the operation. With a favourite dog it may, however, be tried; and, to prevent all accidents, a veterinary surgeon should be entrusted with the case.

PNEUMONIA,

or inflammation of the substance of the lungs, is a complaint of frequent occurrence in the dog, and is singularly marked. The extended head, the protruded tongue, the anxious, bloodshot eye, the painful heaving of the hot breath, the obstinacy with which the animal sits up hour after hour until his feet slip from under him, and the eye closes, and the head droops, through extreme fatigue, yet in a moment being roused again by the feeling of instant suffocation, are symptoms that cannot be mistaken.

Here, from the comparative thinness of the integument and the parietes, we have the progress of the disease brought completely under our view. The exploration of the chest of the dog by auscultation is a beautiful as well as wonderful thing. It at least exhibits to us the actual state of the lungs, if it does not always enable us to arrest the impending evil.

Mr. Blaine and myself used cordially to agree with regard to the treatment of pneumonia, materially different from the opinions of the majority of sportsmen. Epidemic pneumonia was generally fatal, if it was not speedily arrested in its course. The cure was commenced by bleeding, and that to a considerahle extent, when not more than four-and-twenty or six-and thirty hours had passed; for, after that, the progress of the disease could seldom be arrested. Blistering the chest was sometimes resorted to with advantage; and the cantharides ointment and the oil of turpentine formed one of the most convenient as well as one of the most efficacious blisters. A purgative was administered, composed of mutton broth with Epsom salts or castor oil; to which followed the administration of the best sedatives that we have in those cases, namely, nitre, powdered foxglove, and antimonial powder, in the proportion of a scruple of the first, fourgrains of the second, and two grains of the third.

Congestion of the lungs is a frequent termination of pneumonia; and in that congestion the air-cells are easily ruptured and filled with blood. That blood assumes a black pulpy appearance, commonly indicated by the term of *rottenness*, an indication or consequence of the violence of the disease, and the hopelessness of the case. A different consequence of inflammation of the lungs is the formation of tubercles, and, after that, of suppuration and abscess, when, generally speaking, the case is hopeless. A full account of this is given in the work on the Horse.

Two cases of pneumonia will be useful:—

Oct. 22*d*, 1820. A black pointer bitch that had been used to a warm kennel, was made to sleep on flat stones without straw. A violent cough followed, under which she had been getting worse and worse for a fortnight. Yesterday I saw her. The breathing was laborious. The bitch was constantly shifting her position, and, whether she lay down or sat up, was endeavouring to elevate her head. Her usual posture was sitting, and she only lay down for a minute. The eyes were surrounded, and the nose nearly stopped with mucus. V. S. ℥viij. Emet. Fever-ball twice in the day. 23*d*. Breathing not quite so laborious. Will not eat. Medicine as before. Apply a blister on the chest. 24*th*. Nearly the same. V. S. ℥vj., Bol. utheri. 26*th*. Decided amendment. She breathes with much less difficulty. Less discharge both from eyes and nose. Bol. utheri. *Nov.* 7*th*. Sent home well.

A singular and not uninstructive case came before me. A lady in the country wrote to me to say, that her terrier was thin, dull, husking, and perpetually trying to get something from the throat; that her coat stared, and she frequently panted. I replied, that I apprehended she had caught cold; and recommended bleeding to the extent of four ounces, a grain each of calomel and emetic tartar to be given every fourth morning, and a fever-ball, composed of digitalis, nitre, and tartrate of antimony, on each intermediate day.

A few days after this I received another letter from her, saying, that the dog was bled as ordered, and died on the following Thursday. That another veterinary surgeon had been called in, who said that the first one had punctured the *vena cava* in the operation, and that the dog had bled to death internally; and she wished to know my opinion. I replied, that the charge proceeded from ignorance or malice, or both. That in one sense he was right—the jugular, which the other had probably opened, runs into the vena cava, and may, with some latitude, be considered a superior branch of it; therefore, thus far the first man had punctured the vena cava, which I had done many hundred times; but that the point of union of the four principal veins that form the vena cava was too securely seated in the upper part of the thorax for any lancet to reach it. That the rupture of some small arterial vessel might have caused this lingering death, but that the puncture of a vein would either have been speedily fatal, or of no consequence; and that, probably, the animal died of the disease which she had described

SPASMODIC COUGH

is a troublesome disease to manage. Dogs, and especially those considerably petted, are subject to frequent cough, requiring a material difference in the treatment. Sometimes there is a husky cough, not to so great a degree as in distemper, but followed by the same apparent effort to get something from the throat, the same attempt to vomit, and the ejection of mucus, frothy or adhesive, and occasionally discoloured with bile. It proceeds from irritability or obstruction in some of the air-passages, and oftenest of the superior ones. An emetic will clear the fauces, or at least force out a portion of the adhesive matter which is clogging the bronchial tubes.

A cough of this kind, and attended in its early stages by little fever, seldom requires anything more for its cure than the exhibition of a few gentle emetics, consisting of equal portions of calomel and emetic tartar, given in doses varying from half a grain to one grain and a half of each.

A harsh hollow cough is attended by more inflammatory action. The depletive system must be adopted here. A loud and harsh cough will yield only to the lancet and to purgatives, assisted by sedative medicines composed of nitre, antimonial powder, and digitalis, or small doses of syrup of poppies, or more minute doses of the hydrocyanic acid; this last medicine, however, should be carefully watched, and only given under surgical advice.

28*th October*, 1842. A spaniel was apparently well yesterday, but towards evening a violent cough suddenly came on. It was harsh and hollow, and terminated in retching. There was a discharge of water from the eyes; but the nose was cool and moist. Give an emetic, and then two grains of the James's powder. 29*th*. The animal coughed almost the whole of the night. There was more watery discharge from the eyes, which appeared to be red and impatient of light; the nose continued cool, and the dog did not refuse his food. An aperient ball was given; and twice afterwards in the day, the nitre, antimonial powder, and digitalis. 30*th*. The cough is as frequent, but not very loud. Give a mixture of syrup of poppies and prussic acid morning and night, and the ball as yesterday. 31*st*. Nearly in the same state as yesterday, except that he is not so thirsty, and does not eat so well. Give the mixture three times daily. *Nov.* 1*st*. He had an emetic in the morning, which produced a large quantity of phlegm, but the cough is no better. No evacuation during the two last days. Give an aperient ball, and the mixture as before in the evening.

The prussic acid has been fairly tried; it has not in the least mitigated the cough, but begins to make the dog sick, and altogether to destroy his appetite. Give three times in the day a mixture consisting of two-thirds of a drachm of syrup of poppies, and one-third of syrup of buckthorn. The sickness ceased, and the cough remained as before. I then gave twice in the day half a grain of calomel, the same of opium, two each of pulvis antimonialis and digitalis, and four grains of nitre, morning and noon, with six grains of the Dover's powder at night. This was continued on the 3d, 4th and 5th of November, when there were longer intervals of rest, and the dog did not cough so harshly when the fit was on him. On the 6th, however, no medicine was given; but towards evening the dog coughed as much as ever, and a decided mucous discharge commenced from the nose and the eyes, with considerable snorting. An emetic was given, and the balls resorted to as before.

7th. He appeared to be much relieved by the emetic. The cough was better, the dog ate well, and had regained his usual spirits. The ball as before. *9th.* Slight tenesmus now appeared. It quickly became frequent and violent. The dog strained very much; but the discharge was small in quantity, and consisted of adhesive mucus. Give two drachms of castor oil, and the fever-ball with opium. The cough is worse, and the dog still continues to strain, no blood, however, appearing. *11th.* The opium and oil have had their desired effect, and the cough is better. 12th. Except the animal is kept under the influence of opium, the cough is dreadfully troublesome. I have, however, obtained one point. I have been permitted to subtract four ounces of blood; but blood had been mingling with the expectorated mucus before I was permitted to have recourse to the lancet. *13th.* The dog is better, and we again have recourse to the fever mixture, to which, on the *14th,* I added a very small portion of the carbonate of iron, for the dog was evidently getting weak. The sickness has returned, and the cough is decidedly worse. *16th.* Rub a small quantity of rheumatic embrocation, and tincture of cantharides. *17th.* The first application of the blister had not much effect; but this morning it began to act. The dog ran about the house as cross as he could be for more than an hour; there was considerable redness on the throat and chest. The cough, however, was decidedly better. *18th.* The cough is better. Again apply the embrocation. *19th.* The cough and huskiness have returned. Employ an emetic, and continue the embrocation. *20th.* The cough is decidedly worse. Continue the embrocation, and give the fever mixture. *23d.* The embrocation and medicine have been daily used; but the cough is as bad as ever. Balls of assafœtida, squills, and opium were had recourse to. 25th. The second ball produced the most distressing sickness, but the cough was evidently relieved. The assafœtida was discontinued. *28th.* The cough, during the last two days, has been gradually getting worse. It is more laborious and longer, and the intervals between it are shorter Give another emetic and continue the other medicine. 30*th.* The effect of the emetic was temporary, and the cough is again worse.

Dec. 2*d.* Very little change. 5*th.* The cough appears to be stationary. Again have recourse to the antimony, digitalis, and nitre. 8*th.* The cough is certainly better. Try once more the assafœtida. It again produced sickness, but of a very mild character. 12*th.* The assafœtida was again used morning and night. The cough continues evidently to abate. 14*th.* The dog coughs very little, not more than half-a-dozen times in the day. Notwithstanding the quantity of medicine that has been taken, the appetite is excellent, and the spirits good. 16*th.* The cough is still less frequent, but when it occurs it is attended with retching. 19*th.* The cough is daily getting better, and is not heard more than three or four times in the four-and-twenty hours, and then very slight. 30*th.* At length I can say that the cough has ceased. It is seldom that so much trouble would have been taken with a dog. It is the neglect of the medical attendance which is often the cause of death.

Professor Delafond, of Alfort, gives a most interesting and complete table of the usual diagnostic symptoms of pleurisy and pneumonia.

Pleurisy.	Pneumonia.
Commencement of the Inflammation.—Shivering,usually accompanied by slight colicky pains, and followed by general or partial sweating. Inspiration always short, unequal, and interrupted; expiration full; air expired of the natural temperature. Cough unfrequent, faint, short, and without expectoration. Artery full. Pulse quick, small, and wiry.	*Commencement of the Inflammation.*—General shivering, rarely accompanied by colicky pains, followed by partial sweats at the flanks and the inside of the thighs. Inspiration full, expiration short. Air expired hot. Cough frequently followed by slight discharge of red-coloured mucus. Artery full. Pulse accelerated, strong, full, and soft.
Auscultation.—A respiratory murmur, feeble, or accompanied by a slight rubbing through the whole extent of the chest, or in some parts only.	*Auscultation.*—Absence of respiratory murmur in places where the lung is congested; feebleness of that sound in the inflamed parts, with humid crepitating wheezing. The respiratory murmur increased in the sound parts.
Percussion.—Slight, dead, grating sound. Distinct resonance through the whole of the chest, and pain expressed when the sides are tapped or compressed.	*Percussion.*—The dead grating sound confined to the inflamed parts. Distinct resonance at the sound parts; increased sensibility of the walls of the chest slight, or not existing at all.
Terminations.—Delitescence. Cessation of pain; moderate temperature of the skin; sometimes profuse general perspiration. Respiration less ac-	*Terminations.*—Resolution. Temperature of the skin moderate. Sometimes profuse partial sweats. Laborious respiration subsiding; inspira-

PLEURISY.

celerated; inspiration easier and deeper. Pulse fuller and softer. Breath of the natural temperature. Return of the natural respiratory murmur and resonance. The walls of the chest cease to exhibit increased sensibility.

Effusion, false Membranes.—Inspiration more and more full.

Auscultation and Percussion. — Complete absence of the respiratory murmur, with the crepitating wheezing always at the bottom of the chest; sometimes a gurgling noise. Vesicular respiration very strong in the upper region of the chest, or in the sac opposite to the effusion.

Continuance of the Effusion.—Absence of the respiratory murmur gains the middle region of the chest, following the level of the fluid. These symptoms may be found on only one side; a circumstance of frequent occurrence in the dog, but rare in other animals. The respiratory murmur increases in the superior region of the chest, or on the side opposite to the effusion. Inspiration becomes more and more prolonged. Breath always cold. Cough not existing, or rarely, and always suppressed and interrupted. Exercise producing much difficulty of respiration.

Resolution, or Re-absorption of the effused Fluid, and Organization of false Membrane, the conseqnence of Pleurisy. — Slow but progressive reappearance of the respiratory murmur, and disappearance of the sounds produced by the fluid. Diminution of the force of the respiratory murmur in the superior part of the chest, or of the lung opposite to the sac in which the effusion exists. Gradual return of the respiratory murmur to the inferior part of the chest. Inspiration less deep, and returning to its natural state.

Chronic Pleurisy, with Hydrothorax.—Inspiration always deep, expiration short. Cough dry, sometimes with expectoration; frequent or capricious; always absence of complete respiratory murmur in the inferior portion of the chest. Sometimes the

PNEUMONIA.

tion less deep. Artery less full. Pulse yielding. Breath less hot. Gradual and progressive disappearance of the crepitating *râle.* Slow return of the resonance.

Red Hepatization.—Respiration irregular and interrupted.

Auscultation and Percussion.—Circumscribed absence of the respiratory murmur, without any determined place, in one point, or in many distinct parts of the lung. The respiratory murmur increased in one or more of the sound parts of the lungs, or in the sound lung if one is inflamed.

Passage to a State of Gray Induration. — The absence of respiratory murmur indicates extensive hepatization of one lung; a circumstance, however, of rare occurrence. When the induration is of both lungs, and equally so, the respiratory murmur and the inspiration remain the same, except that they become irregular. The cough dry or humid, frequent, and sometimes varying. Exercise accompanied by difficulty of respiration, without dyspnœa.

Resolution or Re-absorption of the Products of Inflammation of the Parenchymatous Substance of the Lungs. —Diminution of the force of the respiratory murmur in the sound parts. Cessation of the crepitating wheezing. Slow return of the respiratory murmur where it had ceased. Respiration ceases to be irregular or interrupted, and returns slowly to its natural state, or it remains interrupted. This indicates the passage from red to gray induration.

Chronic Pneumonia—(*Gray Induration.*)—Inspiration or expiration interrupted. Cough unfrequent; suppressed; rarely with expectoration; always interrupted. Complete absence of respiratory murmur.

(*Softening of the Induration, Ulce

PLEURISY.	PNEUMONIA.
gurgling noise during inspiration and expiration. Strong respiratory murmur in the superior portion. In dogs these symptoms sometimes have existence only on one side of the chest. The mucous membranes are infiltrated; serous infiltration on the lower part of the chest and belly; sometimes of the scrotum or the inferior extremities; generally of the fore legs. The animal lies down frequently, and dies of suffocation.	*rations, Vomicæ, &c.*) — Mucous and wheezing; mucous *râle* in the bronchia; discharge from the nostrils of purulent matter, white, gray, or black, and sometimes fetid. Paleness of the mucous membranes. The animal seldom lies down, and never long at a time. Death by suffocation, when the matter proceeding from the vomicæ, or abscesses, obstructs the bronchial passages, or by the development of an acute inflammation engrafted upon the chronic one.

CHAPTER XII.

ANATOMY OF THE GULLET, STOMACH, AND INTESTINES: TETANUS; ENTERITIS; PERITONITIS; COLIC; CALCULUS IN THE INTESTINES; INTUSSUSCEPTION; DIARRHŒA; DYSENTERY; COSTIVENESS; DROPSY; THE LIVER; JAUNDICE; THE SPLEEN AND PANCREAS; INFLAMMATION OF THE KIDNEY; CALCULUS; INFLAMMATION OF THE BLADDER; RUPTURE OF THE BLADDER; WORMS; FISTULA IN THE ANUS.

THE *œsophagus*, or gullet, of the dog, is constructed in nearly the same manner as that of the horse. It consists of a similar muscular tube passing down the neck and through the chest, and terminating in the stomach, in which the process of digestion is commenced. The orifice by which the gullet enters the stomach is termed the *cardia*, probably on account of its neighbourhood to the heart or its sympathy with it. It is constantly closed, except when the food is passing through it into the stomach.

The *stomach* has three coats: the outermost, which is the common covering of all the intestines, called the peritoneum; the second or muscular coat, consisting of two layers of fibres, by which a constant motion is communicated to the stomach, mingling the food, and preparing it for digestion; and the mucous or villous, where the work of digestion properly commences, the mouths of numerous little vessels opening upon it, which exude the gastric juice, to mix with the food already softened, and to convert it into a fluid called the chyme. It is a simpler apparatus than in the horse or in cattle. It is occasionally the primary seat of inflammation; and it almost invariably sympathises with the affections of the other intestines.

The successive contractions of each portion of the stomach, expose by turns every portion of the alimentary mass to the influence of the gastric juice, and each is gradually discharged into the alimentary canal.

As the chyme is formed, it passes out of the other orifice of the stomach, and enters the first intestine or *duodenum.*

It may be naturally supposed that this process will occasionally be interrupted by a variety of circumstances. Inflammation of the stomach of the dog is very difficult to deal with. It is produced by numerous different causes. There is great and long-continued sickness: even the most harmless medicine is not retained on the stomach. The thirst is excessive; there are evident indications of excessive pain, expressed by the countenance and by groans: there is a singular disposition in the animal to hide himself from all observation; an indication that should never be neglected, nor the frequent change from heat to cold, and from cold to heat.

The mode of treatment is simple, although too often inefficient. The lancet must be immediately resorted to, and the bleeding continued until the animal seems about to fall; and to this should quickly succeed repeated injections. Two or three drops of the croton oil should be injected twice or thrice in the day, until the bowels are thoroughly opened. The animal will be considerably better, or the disease cured, in the course of a couple of days.

There is a singular aptitude in the stomach of the dog to eject a portion of its contents; but, almost immediately afterwards, the food, or a portion if not the whole of it, is swallowed again. This is a matter of daily occurrence. There is a coarse rough grass, the *cynosurus cristatus*, or crested dog's-tail. It is inferior for the purposes of hay, but is admirably suited for permanent pastures. It remains green after most other grasses are burnt by a continuance of dry weather. The dog, if it be in his power, has frequent recourse to it, especially if he live mostly in a town. The dry and stimulating food, which generally falls to his share, produces an irritation of his stomach, from which he is glad to free himself; and for this purpose he has recourse to the sharp leaves of the cynosurus. They irritate the lining membrane of the stomach and intestines, and cause a portion of the food to be occasionally evacuated; acting either as an emetic or a purgative, or both. They seem to be designed by nature to be substituted for the calomel and tartar emetic, and other drugs, which are far too often introduced.

An interesting case of the retention of a sharp instrument in the stomach is related by Mr. Kent of Bristol.

On the 23d of February, Mr. Harford, residing in Bristol, when feeding a pointer-dog, happened to let the fork tumble with the flesh, and the dog swallowed them both. On the following morning, Mr. Kent was desired to see the animal; and, although he could feel the projection of the fork outwardly, which convinced him that the dog had in reality swallowed it, yet, as he appeared well, and exhibited no particular symptoms of pain or fever, Mr. Kent gave it as his opinion that there was a possibility that he might survive the danger, and the animal was sent to him, in order to be more immediately under his care. The treatment he adopted was, to feed him on cow's liver, with a view to keep the stomach distended and the bowels open; and he gave him three times a day half a pint of water, with sufficient sulphuric acid to make it rather strongly sour to the human tongue, with the intention of assisting the stomach in dissolving the iron.

On the following Sunday, the skin, at the projecting point, began to exhibit some indication of ulceration; and on Monday a prong of the fork might be touched with the point of the finger, when pressed on the ulcer. Mr. Kent then determined on making an effort to extract the fork on the following morning, which he accordingly did, and with but little difficulty, assisted by a medical friend of the owner. The dog was still fed on cow's liver; his appetite remained good, and with very little medical treatment the external wound healed. The animal improved rapidly in flesh during the whole time. He left the infirmary in perfect health, and remained so, with one inconvenience only, a very bad cough, and his being obliged to lie at length, being unable to coil himself up in his usual way.

The fork was a three-pronged one, six and a half inches long. The handle, which was of ivory, was digested: it was quite gone; and either the gastric fluid or the acid, or both conjointly, had made a very apparent impression on the iron.

Dogs occasionally swallow various strange and unnatural substances. Considerable quantities of hair are sometimes accumulated in the stomach. Half-masticated pieces of straw are ejected. Straw mingled with dung is a too convincing proof of rabies. Dog-grass is found irritating the stomach, or in too great quantities to be ejected, while collections of earth and dung sometimes threaten suffocation. Pieces of money are occasionally found, and lead, and sponge. Various species of polypus irritate the coats of the stomach. Portions of chalk, or stone, or condensed matters, adhere to each other, and masses of strange consistence and form are collected. The size which they assume increases more and more. M. Galy relates an extraordinary account of a dog. It was about three years old when a tumour began to be perceived in the flank. Some sharp-pointed substance was felt; the veterinary surgeon cut down upon it, and a piece of iron, six inches in length, was drawn out.

The following fact was more extraordinary: it is related by M. Noiret. A hound swallowed a bone, which rested in the superior part of the œsophagus, behind the pharynx, and caused the most violent efforts to get rid of it. The only means by which it could be made to descend into the stomach was by pushing it with the handle of a fork, which, escaping from the hand of the operator, followed the bone into the stomach. Two months afterwards, on examining the stomach, the fork was plainly felt lying in a longitudinal direction, parallel with the position of the body; the owner of the dog wishing mechanically to accelerate the expulsion of this body, endeavoured to push it backwards with his hands. When it was drawn as far back as possible, he inserted two fingers into the anus, and succeeded in getting hold of the handle, which he drew out nearly an inch; but, in order to be enabled fully to effect his object, it was necessary to make an incision into the rectum, and free the substance from every obstacle that could retain it. This he did not venture to do, and he was therefore compelled to allow the fork to pass back into its former position.

About three months after the accident, M. Noiret made an incision, three inches from above to below, and the same from the front backwards. He also made an incision through the muscular tissue. Having arrived at the peritoneum, he made another incision, through which he drew from the abdomen a part of the floating portion of the large intestines, and introduced his fingers into the abdominal cavity. He seized the handle of the fork, which was among the viscera, and free about half-way down, and drew it carefully towards the opening made in the flank. The other half of the fork was found to be closely enveloped by the origin of the mesocolon, which was red, hard, and inflamed. The operator freed it by cutting through the tissues which held the fork, and then drew it easily out. The animal was submitted to a proper course of treatment, and in three weeks afterwards was perfectly cured.

The food, having been converted into chyme by the digestive power of the stomach, soon undergoes another and very important change. It, or a portion of it, is converted into chyle. It is mixed with the bile and a secretion from the pancreas in the duodenum. The white thick liquid is separated, and contains the nutritive part of the food, and a yellow pulpy substance is gradually changed into excrement. As these substances pass on, the separation between them becomes more and more complete. The chyle is gradually taken up by the lacteals, and the excrement alone remains.

The next of the small intestines is the *jejunum*, so called from its being generally empty. It is smaller in bulk than the duodenum, and the chyme passes rapidly through it.

Next in the list is the *ileum;* but it is difficult to say where the jejunum terminates and the ileum commences, except that the latter is usually one-fifth longer than the former.

At the termination of the ileum the *cæcum* makes its appearance, with a kind of valvular opening into it, of such a nature that everything that passes along it having reached the blind or closed end, must return in order to escape; or rather the office of the cæcum is to permit certain alimentary matters and all fluids to pass from the ileum, but to oppose their return.

The *colon* is an intestine of very large size, being one of the most capacious, as well as one of the longest, of the large intestines. It commences at the cæcum caput coli, and soon expands into a cavity of greater dimensions than even that of the stomach itself. Having attained this singular bulk, it begins to contract, and continues to do so during its course round the cæcum, until it has completed its second flexure, where it grows so small as scarcely to exceed in calibre one of the small intestines; and though, from about the middle of this turn, it again swells out by degrees, it never afterwards acquires its former capaciousness; indeed, previously to its junction with the rectum, it once more materially differs in size.

At the upper part of the margin of the pelvis the colon terminates in the *rectum,* which differs from the cæcum and colon by possessing only a partial peritoneal covering, and being destitute of bands and cells. It enlarges towards its posterior extremity, and is furnished with a circular muscle, the sphincter ani, adapted to preserve the anus closed, and to retain the feculent matter until so much of it is accumulated in the rectum as to excite a desire to discharge it.

TETANUS,

a disease of great fatality, often depends upon the condition of the stomach; but it is not frequent in dogs.

Why the dog is so little subject to *tetanus,* or lock-jaw, I am unable to explain. Sportsmen say that it sometimes attacks him when, being heated in the chase, he plunges into the water after the stag. The French give it the name of *mal de cerf,* from stags being supposed to be attacked in a similar way, and from the same cause. In the course of nearly forty years' practice, I have seen but four cases of it. The first arose from a wound in the foot. The cause of the second I could not learn. In both the spasmodic action was dreadful as well as universal. The dogs lay on their sides, the neck and legs stretched out, and the upper legs kept some inches from the ground by the intensity of the spasm. They might be taken up by either leg, and not a portion of the frame change its direction. At the same time, in their countenances, and by their hoarse cries, they indicated the torture which they endured.

In the third case, which occurred 12th June, 1822, the head was drawn permanently on one side, and the whole body formed a kind of bow, the dog walking curiously sideways, often falling as it walked, and frequently screaming violently. I ordered him to be well rubbed with an ammoniacal liniment, and balls of tonic and purging medicine to be given twice in the day. The dog gradually recovered, and was dismissed cured on the 20th.

On the 16th November, in the same year, a bull-terrier had a similar complaint. He had been tried in the pit a fortnight before, and severely injured, and the pain and stiffness of his joints were increasing. The head was now permanently drawn on one side. The dog was unable to stand even for a moment, and the eyes were in a state of spasmodic motion. He was a most savage brute; but I attempted to manage him, and, by the assistance of the owner, contrived to bleed him, and to give him a physic-ball. At the same time I advised that he should be destroyed.

His master would not consent to this; and, as the dog occasionally ate a little, we contrived to give a grain each of calomel and opium every sixth hour. In the course of three days he was materially recovered. He could stand, but was exceedingly weak. I ordered the calomel to be omitted, but the opium to be continued. Three days afterwards he was sent into the country, and, as I heard, perfectly recovered.

The following is a very interesting case of tetanus, detailed by M. Debeaux, of the Royal French Chasseurs:

A favourite dog was missing. Four days had passed, and no intelligence could be obtained with regard to him until he returned home, fatigued and half-starved. He had probably been stolen. In the excess of their joy, the owners crammed him with meat until he became strangely ill. His throat was filled with froth, the pupils of his eyes were dilated, the conjunctiva was strongly injected, his neck was spasmodically contracted, and the spine of the back was bowed, and most highly sensible to the touch. M. Debeaux was sent for; it was an hour before he could attend. The dog was lying on his belly; the four limbs were extended and stiff. He uttered the most dreadful and prolonged howling every two or three minutes. The surgeon ordered the application of a dozen leeches to the chest and belly; laxative medicines were given, and embrocations applied to the spine and back.

Three days passed, and the symptoms evidently augmented. The excrement was dark and fetid, and the conjunctiva had a strong yellow tint. Leeches were again employed; emollient lotions and aperient medicines were resorted to. The sensibility of the spine and back was worse than ever; the animal lay on his belly, stretching out his four limbs, his neck fixed, his jaws immovable, his voice hoarse, and he was utterly unable to move.

The bathings, lotions, and aperients were continued, with very few intermissions, until the 14th day, when the muscles began to be a little relaxed; but he cried whenever he was touched. On the 15th, for the first time, he began to eat a little, and his natural voice returned; still, however, the spasms occasionally appeared, but very much mitigated, and on the 20th the pain had entirely ceased.

On the 5th of the next month he travelled two leagues with his master. It was cold, and the snow fell. On his reaching home, all the horrible spasms returned, and it was eleven days before he was completely cured.[a]

Mr. Blaine gives the following account of his experience of this disease: "It is remarkable, that although dogs are subject to various spasmodic affections, yet they are so little subject to lock-jaw that I never met with more than three cases of it among many thousands of diseased dogs. Two of these cases were *idiopathic;* one being apparently occasioned by exposure to cold air all night; in the other the cause was obscure. The third was of that kind called *sympathetic,* and arose from extreme injury done to one of the feet. In each of these cases the convulsive spasm was extreme, and the rigidity universal but not intense. In one case the jaw was only partially locked. Both warm and cold bathings were tried. Large doses of opium and camphor were given by the mouth, and also thrown up in clysters. The spine of one was blistered. Stimulating frictions were applied to all, but in neither case with any salutary effect."[b]

ENTERITIS.

Enteritis, or inflammation of the intestines, is a disease to which dogs are very liable. It may be produced by the action of several causes. The intestines of the dog are peculiarly irritable, and subject to take on inflammatory action, and this tendency is often much increased by the artificial life which they lead. It is a very frequent complaint among those dogs that are much petted. A cold temperature is also a common cause of disease in these dogs.

I was consulted with regard to a dog who was hiding himself in a cold, dark corner, paved with stone. Every now and then he lifted his head and uttered a howl closely resembling that of a rabid dog. He fixed his gaze intently upon me, with a peculiarity of expression which many would have mistaken for rabid. They,

[a] Tetanus observed on a Dog, by M. Debeaux.—Pract. Méd. Vét. 1829, p. 543.
[b] Blaine's Canine Pathology, p. 151.

however, who have had the opportunity of seeing many of these cases, will readily perceive the difference. The conjunctiva is not so red, the pupil is not so dilated, and the dog appears to implore pity and not to menace evil.

In this state, if the dog is approached, he will not permit himself to be touched until he be convinced that no harm is intended. A peculiar slowness attends each motion; his cries are frequent and piteous; his belly hot and tender; two cords, in many cases, seem to run longitudinally from the chest to the pubis, and on these he cannot bear the slightest pressure. He abhors all food; but his thirst for water, and particularly cold water, is extreme; he frequently looks round at his flanks, and the lingering gaze is terminated by a cry or groan. In the majority of cases there is considerable costiveness; but, in others, the bowels are freely opened from the beginning.

The peritoneal inflammation is sometimes pure, but oftener involves the muscular coat of the intestines. Its prevailing cause is exposure to cold, especially after fatigue, or lying on the wet stones or grass. Now and then it is the result of neglected rheumatism, especially in old and petted dogs.

The treatment is simple. Bleed until the pulse falters, put the animal in a warm bath, and let the belly be gently rubbed while the dog is in the water, and well fomented afterwards: the drink should consist of warm broth, or warm milk and water. The bleeding should be repeated, if little or unsatisfactory relief is obtained; and the examination of the rectum with the finger, and the removal of any hardened fæces that may have accumulated there, and the cautious use of enemata, neither too stimulating nor too forcibly injected, should be resorted to. No medicine should be employed until the most urgent symptoms are abated. Castor oil, the mildest of our purgatives — syrup of buckthorn assisting the purgative property of the oil, and containing in its composition as much stimulating power as is safe—and the spirit of white poppies — the most convenient anodyne to mingle with the other medicines — will generally be successful in allaying the irritation already existing, and preventing the development of more. Even this must not be given in too large quantities, and the effect must be assisted by a repetition of the enemata every fifth or sixth hour. On examination after death the nature of the disease is sufficiently evident: the peritoneum, or portions of it, is highly injected with blood, the veins are turgid, the muscular membrane corrugated and hardened, while often the mucous membrane displays not a trace of disease. In violent cases, however, the whole of the intestines exhibit evidence of inflammation.

I was much gratified a few years ago in witnessing the decided manner in which Professor Spooner expressed himself with regard to the treatment of enteritis in the dog. "I should deem it advisable," said he, "to administer a purgative; but of what would that consist? Calomel? Certainly not. I was surprised to hear one gentleman assert that he should administer it to the extent of from five to ten grains, and another to say that he should not hesitate to exhibit a scruple of calomel to a dog, and to all carnivorous animals. I should never think of exhibiting it as a cathartic. I should only administer it in small doses, and for the purpose of producing its specific effect on the liver, which is the peculiar property of this drug. Given in larger doses it would not be retained, and if it got into the intestines it would act as a powerful drastic purgative."[a]

In our treatment of the horse we have got rid of a great proportion of the destructive urine-balls and drastic purgatives of the farrier. The cow is no longer drenched with half-a-dozen deleterious stimulants. A most desirable change has been effected in the medical treatment of these animals. Let us not, with regard to the dog, continue to pursue the destructive course of the keeper or the huntsman.

The following case of enteritis, with rupture of the colon, may be useful:—

On March 15, 1840, I was requested to attend a large dog of the bull breed, three years old, who had not appeared to be well during the last four or five days.

I had scarcely arrived ere I recognised it to be a case of enteritis. He had a dreadful shivering fit, to which succeeded heat of the skin and restlessness. The muzzle was dry and hot, as also was the tongue. The eyes were sunken and redder than usual; the breathing was accelerated, but not very laborious; the extremities were cold, while the surface of the body was hot and painful to the touch. The bowels were constipated, and had been so during the last week; some dung however was evacuated, but it was hard and dry, and in small quantities. The pulse was quick, but full; and there was a slight pain and considerable irritation in the rectum. I took from him ʒx. of blood before the desired effect was produced, and then gave him tinct. opii gr.xiv., et spt. ether. nit. gutt. viij., cum ol. ricini ʒiij., and an opiate enema to allay the irritation of the rectum. This was about 8 o'clock, A. M.

11 A.M.—The bowels have not been moved, and the pain is more intense; his countenance expresses great anxiety; he frequently lies on his stomach, and the pulse is small but quick. I gave him a little broth, and ordered the abdomen to be fomented with hot flannels.

---

[a] Proceedings of the Veterinary Medical Association, 1839–40.

2 P.M.—He has had distressing sickness, and is extremely anxious for water. I introduced my finger into the rectum, but could not discover any hardened fæces. Enemata, composed of mag. sulphas and warm water, were frequently thrown into the intestines; as soon as one came away another was thrown up.

4 P.M.—No better: gave him pulv. aloes ℨj.; calomel, gr. vj. et pulv. opii gr. viij. The fomentations to be continued, and the abdomen rubbed with a lin. terebinthinæ.

5 P.M.—A great change has taken place within the last hour; the hind extremities are paralysed; the mouth and ears are cold; the pulse is more hurried and irregular, and almost imperceptible; the respiration is laborious and irregular, as is the pulse; and the dog is frequently sick. To be kept quiet.

6 P.M.—Another change: he lies panting and groaning piteously; his limbs are bathed in sweat, with convulsive struggles. At twenty minutes past six he died.

A post-mortem examination presented general marks of inflammation; the small intestines were extremely red, while the large ones were in a gangrenous state and most offensive, with a rupture of the colon. I did not expect to meet with the rupture, and am at a loss to account for it. The liver was of a pale ashen colour, and very light. I put a piece of it into some water, and it floated on the surface. The other contents of the abdomen did not show the slightest appearance of disease.

September 2d, **1843.**—A black pug-bitch, 18 months old, was yesterday taken violently sick; the vomiting continued at intervals the greater part of the day, and she had not eaten during the last **24** hours. I could not possibly get at her, on account of her ferocity: as she had not had the distemper, and as I was misled by her age and the watery discharge from her eyes, and as she had had several motions yesterday, I imagined that the attack might be the beginning of that disease. Learning that she was fond of sweet things, I prepared an emetic containing a grain of calomel and a grain of tartar emetic: she took it readily, and I promised to call on the following day.

Sept. 3.—The weakness at the eyes had disappeared, but there had been no motion. On getting at her by main force I found her belly very tense and rather hot: she had again been sick, was very eager for water, and still refused to eat. The disease was now evident. As she appeared too unmanageable for anything else, I produced a physic-ball, in giving which I was bitten.

Six hours afterwards I again went: no fæces had passed: I administered two enemas, the second of which was returned with a small quantity of hardened fæces and an intolerable smell. I ordered the water to be removed, and broth to be substituted.

Sept. 4.—The dog is in good spirits, has eaten heartily, and had no motion, probably because it was habitually cleanly, and had not been taken out of doors. Her owner considered her as quite well, and dismissed me. Three days afterwards a servant came to say that all was going on very well.

PERITONITIS.

Chronic inflammation of the *peritoneal membrane* is a frequent disease among dogs. The animal loses his appetite and spirits; he sometimes eats a little and sometimes not; he becomes thin, his belly is tucked up, and when we closely examine him we find it contracted and hard, and those longitudinal columns of which I have already spoken are peculiarly dense and almost unyielding. He now and then utters a half-suppressed whine, and he occasionally seeks to hide himself. In the greater number of cases he after a while recovers; but he too often pines away and dies. On examination after death the case is plain enough. There is inflammation of the peritoneal membrane, more indicated by undue congestion of the bowels than by the general blush of the membrane. The inflammation has now spread to the muscular coat, and the whole of the intestine is corrugated and thickened.

There is another peritoneal affection, aggravated by combination with a rheumatic tendency, to which the dog is more disposed than any other domesticated animal. It has its most frequent origin in cold, or being too much fed on stimulating and acrid food, and probably from other causes which have not yet been sufficiently developed.

Here also no drastic purgative is to be admitted; it would be adding fuel to fire: not a grain of calomel should be used, if the life of the animal is valued. The castor oil mixture will afford the most certain relief, a drop or two of the oil of peppermint being added to it.

COLIC.

The dog is also subject to fits of *colic*, principally to be traced to improper food, or a sudden change of food, or exposure to cold. This is particularly the case with puppies. There is no redness of the eye, no heat of the mouth, no quickened respiration; but the animal labours under fits of pain. He is not quiet for a minute. He gets into one corner and another, curling himself closely up, but he does not lie there more than a minute or two; another fit of pain comes on; he utters his peculiar yelp, and seeks some new place in which he may possibly find rest.

It is with considerable diffidence that I offer an opinion on this subject contrary to that of Mr. Blaine. He states that the treatment of this species of colic is seldom successful, and that which has seemed the most efficacious has been mercurial purgatives;

namely, calomel one grain, aloes a scruple, and opium a quarter of a grain, until the bowels are opened. I have seldom found much difficulty in relieving the patient suffering under this affection; and I gave no aloes nor calomel, but the oleaginous mixture to which I have so often referred. I should not so much object to the aloes, for they constitute an excellent purgative for the dog; nor to a dog that I was preparing for work, or that was suffering from worms, should I object to two or three grains of calomel intimately mixed with the aloes: from the combined effect of the two, some good might be obtained.

CALCULUS IN THE INTESTINES.

Many persons have a very foolish custom of throwing stones, that their dogs may dive or run after them, and bring them to their owner's feet: the consequence is, that their teeth are soon worn down, and there are too many cases on record in which the stone has been swallowed. It has been impeded in its progress through the intestinal canal, inflammation has ensued, and the animal has been lost, after having suffered the most dreadful torture.

Professor Simonds relates a case in which a dog was thus destroyed. The animal for some days previous to his admission into the hospital had refused his food, and there was obstinate constipation of the bowels, to remove which aperient medicine had been given. The pulse was accelerated, there was distension of the abdomen with evident tenderness on pressure, the extremities were cold, no fæces were voided, and he occasionally vomited. Some aperient medicine was given, which was retained on the stomach, and enemas and external stimulants were resorted to, but two days afterwards he died.

The intestines were examined, and the offending body was found to be a common pebble. The dog had long been accustomed to fetch stones out of the water. One of these stones had passed through the stomach into the intestines, and, after proceeding some distance along them, had been impacted there. The inflammation was most intense so far as the stone had gone; but in the part of the intestine to which it had not reached there was not any. This was an interesting and instructive case, and should make its due impression.

Another account of the strange contents of the intestines of a bitch may be here introduced.

A valuable pointer-bitch was sent to the infirmary of Mr. Godwin of Litchfield. She presented a very emaciated appearance, and had done so for four or five months. Her evacuations for a day or two were very thin and copious, and afterwards for several days nothing was passed. When pressing the abdomen with both hands, a hard substance was distinctly felt in the inferior part of the umbilical region. She was destroyed, and, upon *post-mortem* examination, a calculus was discovered in the ileum about the size and shape of a hen's egg, the nucleus of which was a portion of hair. The coats of the intestines were considerably thickened and enlarged, so as to form a kind of sac for its retention. Anterior to this was another substance, consisting of a ball of hair, covered with a layer of earthy matter about the eighth of an inch thick, and next to this another ball of hair of less dimensions, intermixed with a gritty substance. The stomach contained a large quantity of hair, and a portion of the omentum, about the size of a crown piece, was thickly studded with small white calculi, the largest about the size of a pea, and exceedingly hard.

INTUSSUSCEPTION.

If *peritonitis*—inflammation—is neglected, or drastic purgatives are too often and too plentifully administered, a peculiar contraction of the muscular membrane of the intestine takes place, and one portion of the bowel is received within another—there is *intussusception*. In most cases, a portion of the anterior intestine is received into that which is posterior to it. Few of us have opened a dog that had been labouring under this peculiar affection without being struck with the collapsed state of the canal in various parts, and in some much more than in others. Immediately posterior to this collapsed portion, it is widened to a considerable extent. The peristaltic motion of the intestine goes on, and the consequence is, that the constricted portion is received into that which is widened, the anterior portion is invaginated in the posterior: obstruction of the intestinal passage is the necessary consequence, and the animal dies, either from the general disturbance of the system which ensues, or the inflammation which is set up in the invaginated part.

I will say nothing of medical treatment in this case; for I do not know the symptoms of intussusception, or how it is to be distinguished from acute inflammation of the bowels. Acute inflammation will not long exist without producing it; and, if its existence should be strongly suspected, the treatment would be the same as for inflammation.

The domesticated dog, from the nature of his food, more than from any constitutional tendency, is liable to constipation. This should never be neglected. If two or three days should pass without an evacuation, the case should be taken in hand; otherwise inflammation will be very soon established. In order to procure an evacuation, the aloetic ball, with one or two grains of calomel, should be given. Beyond that, however, I should not dare to go; but, if the constipation continued, I should have recourse to the castor-oil mixture. I should previously examine and empty the rectum, and have frequent recourse to the enema-syringe; and I should continue both. It would be my object to evacuate the intestinal canal with as little increased action as possible.

DIARRHŒA

is the discharge of fæces more frequently than usual, and thinner than their natural consistence, but otherwise not materially altered in quality; and the mucous coat of the intestines being somewhat congested, if not inflamed. It is the consequence of over-feeding, or the use of improper food. Sometimes it is of very short continuance, and disappears without any bad consequence; the health being unaffected, and the character of the fæces no otherwise altered than by assuming a fluid character. It may not be bad practice to wait a day, or possibly two, as it is desirable for the action of the intestines to be restored without the aid of art. I should by no means give a physic-ball, or a grain of calomel, in simple diarrhœa. I should fear the establishment of that species of purging which is next to be described. The castor-oil mixture usually affords the best hope of success.

Habitual diarrhœa is not an unfrequent disease in petted dogs: in some it is constitutional, in others it is the effect of neglected constipation. A state of chronic inflammation is induced, which has become part of the constitution of the dog; and, if repressed in the intestines, it will appear under a more dangerous form in some other place.

DYSENTERY

is a far more serious complaint. In most cases a considerable degree of inflammation of the mucous coat exists, and the mucus is separated from the membrane beneath, and discharged per anum. The mucus thus separated from the intestinal membrane assumes an acrid character. It not only produces inflammation of the membrane, dangerous and difficult to treat, but it excoriates the anus and neighbouring parts, and produces pain and tenesmus.

This disease has sometimes been fatally misunderstood. A great deal of irritation exists in the intestinal membrane generally, and in the lower part of the rectum particularly. The fæces passing over this denuded surface cause a considerable degree of pain, and there is much straining, and a very small bit or portion of fæces is evacuated. This has often been seen by the careless observer; and, as he has taken it as an indication of costiveness, some drastic purgative has been administered, and the animal quickly killed.

No one that had ascertained the real nature of the disease would administer calomel in any form or combination; but the anodyne mixture as an enema, and also administered by the mouth, is the only medicine from which benefit can be expected.

COSTIVENESS

is a disease when it becomes habitual. It is connected with disease of the intestinal canal. Many dogs have a dry constipated habit, often greatly increased by the bones on which they are too frequently fed. This favours the disposition to mange and to many diseases depending on morbid secretions. It produces indigestion, encourages worms, blackens the teeth, and causes fetid breath. The food often accumulates in the intestines, and the consequence is inflammation of these organs. A dog should never be suffered to remain costive more than a couple of days. An aloetic ball or some Epsom salts should then be administered; and this failing to produce the desired effect, the castor-oil mixture, with spirits of buckthorn and white poppies, should be administered, and the use of the clyster-pipe resorted to. It may be necessary to introduce the finger or the handle of a spoon when the fæcal matter is more than usually hard, and it is with difficulty broken down: small doses of castor-oil should be afterwards resorted to, and recourse be occasionally had to boiled liver, which the dog will rarely refuse. The best means, however, of preventing costiveness in dogs, as well as in men, is regular exercise. A dog who is kept chained up in a kennel should be taken out and have a certain quantity of exercise once in the twenty-four hours. When this cannot be done, the food should consist chiefly of well-boiled farinaceous matter.

DROPSY.

Another disease, which is not confined to the abdominal cavity, is dropsy: but, as in the dog it most commonly assumes that form which is termed ascites, or dropsy of the abdomen, it may be noticed in this place. It is seldom an idiopathic or primary affection, but is generally the consequence of some other disease, most commonly of an inflammatory kind.

Dropsy is a collection of fluid in some part of the frame, either from increased exhalation, or from diminished absorption, the consequence of inflammation. The divisions of dropsy are into active and passive, or acute and chronic. The causes are also very pro perly arranged as predisposing and exciting. The diseases on which dropsy most frequently supervenes are fevers and visceral inflammations and obstructions. The dog is peculiarly subject to *ascites* or *dropsy of the belly*, and the quantity of fluid contained in the abdomen is sometimes almost incredible. It is usually accompanied or characterised by a weak, unequal, small, and frequent pulse—paleness of the lips, tongue, and gums—flaccidity of the muscles, hurried breathing on the least exertion, feebleness of the joints, swellings of the lower limbs, effusion of fluid into the integuments or among the muscles, before there is any considerable effusion into the thorax or the abdomen, and an unhealthy appearance of the cutaneous surface. The urine seldom coagulates. This form of dropsy is usually seated in the abdomen or cellular tissue.

The treatment of ascites is seldom perfectly successful. The great extent of the peritoneum, the number and importance of the viscera with which it is connected, and of the absorbent glands which it encloses, the number and weakness of the veins which transmit their blood to the portal vessels, and the absence of valves, in some measure account for the frequent accumulation of fluid in this cavity. It appears in both sexes from the usual causes of inflammatory disease. Unwholesome diet, the drastic operation of purgatives, external injuries, the suppression of accustomed secretions and discharges, all are exciting causes of dropsy.

The animal has suffered materially from mange, which has been apparently cured: the itchiness and eruption altogether disappear, but many weeks do not elapse ere ascites begins to be seen, and the abdomen is gradually distended with fluid. When this appears in young and healthy animals, it may be conquered; but when there has been previous disease of almost any kind, comparatively few patients permanently recover. Irritability of the stomach, and a small and accelerated pulse, are unfavourable. If the operation of tapping has taken place, at all times there is danger; but, if there is a thick, brown, albuminous or fetid discharge, it is very unlikely that any permanent advantage will result from the operation.

We will introduce a few cases as they occur in our clinical records.

November 7th, 1821.—A spaniel, nine years old, had been, during four months, alternately asthmatic or mangy, or both. Within the last few days she had apparently increased in size. I was sent for. The first touch of the abdomen betrayed considerable fluctuation. She likewise had piles, sore and swelled. I ordered an alterative ball to be given morning and night. *8th.* One of the balls has been given, and two doses of castor oil; but no effect has been produced. An injection was administered. *9th.* A small evacuation of water has been produced, and the bowels have been slightly opened. Give a dose of the castor-oil mixture. *10th.* The obstruction has been removed; the enlargement is somewhat diminished; much water has passed. Give an alterative ball every morning *14th.* The alteratives have been continued, and there is a slow but evident decrease of the abdomen. 18*th.* I cannot detect any effusion in the abdomen. Give a pill every alternate day for a fortnight. At the expiration of this period the dog was apparently well.

April 23*d*, 1822.—A terrier, ten years old, had cough and mange, which ceased. The belly for the first time began to enlarge, and on feeling the dog considerable fluctuation was evident. He would not eat, but he drank immoderately. Give daily a ball consisting of tonic and physic mist., with powdered digitalis and tartrate of iron. *May* 6*th.*—He is in better spirits, feeds tolerably well, but is rather increased in size. Give daily a ball of tartrate of iron, digitalis, ginger, and a grain of calomel. 22*d.* Much thinner, the belly very considerably diminished: a slight fluctuation is still to be perceived. Continue medicine, with a half-grain only of calomel. *July* 17*th.*—The medicine has been regularly given, and the water of the abdomen has rapidly disappeared, until a fortnight ago: since that time it has been once more filling. The medicine was ordered to be repeated. *August* 6*th.*—The medicine has once more produced its proper effect, and the fluid has disappeared. On the 16*th*, however, the fluctuation was again too plainly felt, and the owner determined to have nothing more to do with the case. The animal was never brought again, nor could I trace it. The dog might have been saved if the owner had done it justice.

As soon as dropsy appears to be established, proper medicines must be resorted to. Foxglove, nitre, and ginger should be first tried in the proportional doses of one, ten, and eight grains, given morning and night. If this does not succeed, iodine from half-a-grain to a grain may be given morning and night, and a weak solution of iodine rubbed on the belly.

This being ineffectual, recourse may be had to tapping, taking care that the trocar is not plunged sufficiently deep to wound the intestines. The place for the operation is directly on the *linea alba*, or middle line of the belly, and about midway between the pubis and the navel. The whole of the intestinal fluid may be suffered to escape. A bandage should then be applied round the belly, and retained there a week or more.

Mr. Blaine very properly states, that the difference between fatness and dropsy is, that the belly hangs pendulous in dropsy, while the back bone stands up, and the hips are protruded through the skin; while the hair is rough, and the feeling of the coat is peculiarly harsh. It may be distinguished from pregnancy by the teats enlarging, in the latter case, as gestation advances, and the young ones may occasionally be felt to move. In addition to this it may be stated, that the presence of water is readily and unerringly detected. If the right hand is laid on one side of the belly, and the other side is gently struck with the left hand, an undulating motion will be readily perceived.

In old dogs, dropsy, under the title of "anasarca," is an unfrequent but occasional accompaniment of ascites. If pressure is made on any particular parts, they yield and continue depressed for a longer or shorter period of time, and slowly and by degrees regain their natural form. The skin is dry and distended, and with no natural action; the circulation is languid and small, the muscular powers are diminished, the animal is unquiet, the thirst is great, the tongue is pale, the appetite diminished, and the limbs are swelled. The best mode of treatment is the infliction of some very small punctures in the distended skin, and the application of gentle friction. The majority of cases of this kind are usually fatal, and so is almost every case of encysted dropsy.

A dog had cough in February, 1825. Various medicines were administered, and at length the cough almost suddenly ceased, and evident ascites appeared. The thirst was insatiable, the dog would not touch food, and he was unable to lie down more than two minutes at a time. Digitalis, cream of tartar, and hydrarg. submur. were given on the 9th April. On the 13th he was much worse, and apparently dying. He had been unable to rise for the last twelve hours, and lay panting. I punctured the abdomen, and four quarts of fluid were evacuated. *14th.* The panting continues. The dog will not eat, but he can lie down in any posture. *15th.* The panting is diminished, the appetite is returning, and water continues to ooze from the wound. *17th.* The wound healed on the night of the 15th, and already the fluid begins to collect. The medicine still continued. *20th.* The spirits good, and strength improving; but the belly is evidently filling, and matter is discharged from both the nose and eyes. *26th.* The swelling a little diminished, respiration easy, and the dog walking comfortably about, and feeding well. *May 13th.*—The swelling, which for some days past diminished, is now again increasing; but the dog is strong and breathes easily. Medicine as before. *24th.* The dog is thinner, weaker, filling fast, and the thirst excessive. ℞ Crem. tart., ferri tart. ʒij., pulv. flor. anthemid. ʒiiij., conser. ros. q. s.: divide in bol. xii.: cap. in dies. *27th.* During two days he has been unable to lie down more than a minute at a time. Again tapped: fully as much fluid was evacuated as before; but there is now blood mingling with it. *30th.* Much relieved by the tapping, and breathes with perfect ease; but, now that the enormous belly is reduced, the dog is very thin. Bol. continued. *June 8th.* Within the last three days the animal has filled again with extraordinary rapidity. ℞ Ferr. tart. ℈j., opii. gr. ¼, pulv. gentianæ ℈j., cons. ros. q. s.: f. bol. capiend. in dies. *13th.* Is again strangely distended; I advised, or rather solicited, that it might be destroyed;

but this not being granted, I once more tapped him. At least a gallon of dark-coloured fluid was evacuated. *22d.* Again rapidly filling, but not losing either flesh or strength. *July 4th.*—Once more punctured, and a gallon of dark-coloured fluid evacuated. *12th.* Again filling and rapidly losing flesh and strength. *26th.* Once more tapped: immediately after which he appeared to be revived, but almost immediately began again to fill. *Aug. 2d.*—He had eaten tolerably; appeared to have nothing more than usual the matter with him, when, being missed for an hour, he was found dead. No examination was permitted.

In 1824 a spaniel, six years old, was brought to the infirmary. It had had an asthmatic cough, which had left it. It was now hollow in the flanks, the belly pendulous, and an evident fluctuation of water. The owner would not consent to any operation. An aloetic physic-ball, however, was given every fifth day, and a ball, composed of tartrate of iron, digitalis, nitre, and antimonial powder, on every intermediate morning and night. The water evidently accumulated; the dog was sent for, and died in the course of a week.

There are a few medicines that may be useful in arresting the effusion of the fluid; but they too often fail in producing any considerable benefit. The fox-glove is, perhaps, possessed of the greatest power, combined with nitre, squills, and bitartrate of potash. At other times chamomile, squills, and spirit of nitrous ether, may be tried.

The following case, treated by the administration of iodine, by Professor Dick, is important:—

A black and tan coloured retriever was sent to me labouring under ascites. He was tapped, and two quarts of fluid abstracted. Tonics, combined with diuretics were given, but the fluid continued to accumulate, and in three weeks he was again tapped, and another two quarts drawn away. The disease still went on, and a fortnight afterwards a similar quantity was withdrawn. Various remedies were tried in order to check the power of the disease, but without effect, and the abdomen again became as much distended with the effused serum as before.

He was then put under a course of iodine, which soon began to show its beneficial influence by speedily allaying his excessive thirst; and in about a month the whole of the effused fluid was absorbed, although from the size of the abdomen it must have amounted to a similar quantity to that drawn off on the previous occasions. The dog's appetite soon returned; he gained flesh rapidly, and has continued quite well, and, from being a perfect skeleton, soon became overloaded with fat.

Induced by the great benefit derived in this case from the iodine, I took the opportunity of trying it on a Newfoundland dog similarly affected. He was put on a course of iodine, and the quantity of the drug was gradually increased. As absorption rapidly commenced, the fluid was completely taken up; but, partly in consequence of pushing the medicine too far, and partly from extensive disease in the liver, unfavourable symptoms took place, and he sunk rather unexpectedly. Still, however, from the obvious and decided advantage derived from the medicine, I have no doubt that iodine will be found one of the most efficient remedies in dropsy in dogs.

Iodine is a truly valuable drug. When first introduced into veterinary practice it was observed that it readily accomplished the reduction of the enlarged glands that frequently remain after catarrh; but it was presently evident that it reduced almost every kind of tumour, even the growth of tubercles in the lungs. Professor Morton, in his Manual of Pharmacy, has admirably described the different combinations of iodine.

THE LIVER

of the dog seems to follow a law of comparative anatomy, that its bulk shall be in an inverse proportion of that of the lungs. The latter are necessarily capacious; for they need a large supply of arterial blood, in order to answer to their rapid expenditure when the utmost exertion of strength and speed is required. The liver is, therefore, restricted in its size and growth. Nevertheless, it has an important duty to fulfil, namely, to receive the blood that is returned from the intestines, to separate from the blood, or to secrete, by means of it, the bile; and then to transmit the remaining portion of it to the lungs, where it undergoes the usual process of purification, and is changed to arterial blood. In the performance of this office, the liver often undergoes a state of inflammation, and disease ensues, inveterate, and setting at defiance every means of cure. Both the skin and the urine become tinged with a yellow effusion. The animal is dull, and gradually wastes away.

In a few days the yellow hue becomes more intense, and particularly on the cuticle, the conjunctiva, the iris, the gums, and the lips. A state of fever becomes more and more perceptible, and there are alternations of cold and heat. The pulse varies from 80 to 120; the dry tongue hangs from the mouth; the appetite ceases, but the animal is peculiarly desirous of cold water. The dog becomes restless; he seeks to hide himself; and he groans, if the parts in the neighbourhood of the liver are pressed upon.

Frequent vomitings now appear, slimy, and evidently containing gall. The animal becomes visibly thinner, obstinately refuses all solid food, and only manifests thirst. He begins to stagger as he walks; he withdraws himself from observation; he anxiously seeks some dark place where he may lay himself with his chest and belly resting on the cold ground, his fore legs stretched out before him, and his hind legs almost as far behind him. The fever increases, the skin becomes of a dark yellow colour, the mucous membrane of the mouth and conjunctiva is of a dirty red, the expired air is evidently hot, the gaze is anxious, the urine is of a saffron yellow, or even darker: in short, there now appears every symptom of inflammation of the liver, with jaundice.

As the disease proceeds the animal begins to vomit masses of a yellowish green substance, occasionally mixed with blood. He wastes away to a skeleton, he totters in his walk, he is half unconscious, the pulse becomes weak and interrupted, the temperature sinks, and death ensues.

The duration and course of the disease are deceptive. It occasionally proceeds so insidiously that several days are suffered to pass before the owner perceives any marks of disease, or seeks any aid. The duration of the disease is usually from ten to twelve days. It terminates in congestion of blood in the liver, or a gradual restoration to health. The latter can only take place in cases where the inflammation has proceeded very slowly; where the commencement and progress of the disease could be discovered by debility and slight yellowness of the skin, and especially where speedy recourse has been had to medical aid.

The predisposing causes of this disease are often difficult to discover. The dog, in warm climates, seems to have a natural disposition to it. As exciting causes, atmospheric influence may be reckoned, sultry days, cold nights, and damp weather. Other occasional causes may be found in violent falls, bruises, and overfeeding. Fat petted dogs that are easily overheated by exertion are often attacked by this disease. The result of the disease depends on its duration, course, and complication. If it is attended to early, it can generally be cured. If it has existed for several days, and the fever has taken on a typhoid character—if the yellow hue is perceptible—the appetite failing, and vomiting ensuing, the cure is doubtful; and, if inflammation of the stomach has taken place, with high fever, vomiting of blood, wasting away, and fits occurring, there is no chance of cure.

When simple jaundice alone is visible, a moderate laxative of sulphate of magnesia and tartaric acid, in conjunction with some aromatic and mucilaginous fluid, or, quite in the beginning of the disease, an emetic, will be found of considerable service; but, when the yellow colour has become more intense, and the animal will no longer eat, and the fever and weakness are increased, it is necessary to give calomel, tartar-emetic, camphor, and opium, in the form of pills, and to rub some strong liniment on the region of the liver: the doses of calomel, however, must be very small. If inflammation of the stomach appears, mucilaginous fluids only must be given. Bleeding may be of service in the commencement of the disease, but afterward it is hurtful.

This is an account of hepatitis as it occasionally appears, and particularly on the Continent; but it does not often assume so virulent a character in our country. There is often restlessness, thirst, and sickness, accompanied by much prostration of strength; or general heat and tenderness. Occasionally there is purging; but much oftener constipation, that bids defiance to almost every medicine. The principal or almost only hope of cure consists in bleeding, physicking, and blistering on the right side.

Of bilious disease, assuming the character of inflammation, we have too many cases. It may be spontaneous or brought on by the agency of other affections. Long-continued and inveterate mange will produce it. It is often connected with, or produced by, distemper, or a dull inflammatory disease of the liver, and it is generally accompanied by pustular eruption on the belly. The skin is usually tinged of a yellow hue, and the urine is almost invariably impregnated with bile. The suffusion which takes place is recognised among sportsmen by the term "yellows." The remedy should be some mercurial, with gentian and aloes given twice in the day, and mercurial ointment well rubbed in once in the day. If this treatment is steadily pursued, and a slight soreness induced in the mouth, the treatment will usually be successful. Mr. Blaine observes, "A moderate soreness of the mouth is to be encouraged and kept up. I have never succeeded in removing the complaint without it."

JAUNDICE.

M. W. Leblanc, of Paris, has given an interesting account of the causes and treatment of *jaundice* in the dog.

The prevailing symptom of this disease in the dog is a yellow discoloration of the skin and the mucous membranes of greater or less intensity. It generally announces the existence of very serious disease, as inflammation of the liver and its excretory ducts, or of the gall-bladder, or the stomach, or small intestines, or contraction or obliteration of the excretory ducts of the liver, in consequence of inflammation of these vessels, or the presence of concrete substances formed from the bile. The dogs in which he found the most decided traces of this disease laboured under diarrhœa, with stools of a reddish brown or black colour for one, two, or three days.

The causes of jaundice are chiefly over-fatigue (thus, greyhounds are more subject to it than pointers), immersions in water, fighting, emetics or purgatives administered in over-doses, the repeated use of poisonous substances not sufficiently strong at once to destroy the animal, the swallowing of great quantities of indigestible food, and contusions of the abdominal viscera, especially about the region of the liver. The most serious, if not the most common cause, is cold after violent and long-continued exercise; and especially when the owners of dogs, seeing them refuse their food after a long chase, give them powerful purgatives or emetics.

The treatment should have strict relation to the real or supposed cause of jaundice, and its most evident concomitant circumstances. Some of these symptoms are constant and others variable. Among the first, whatever be the cause of the disease, we reckon acceleration of the pulse; fever, with paroxysms of occasional intensity; and a yellow or reddish-yellow discoloration of the urine. Among the second are constipation, diarrhœa, the absence or increase of colour in the fæcal matter, whether solid or fluid. When they are solid, they are usually void of much colour; when, on the contrary, there is diarrhœa, the fæces are generally mingled with blood more or less changed. Sometimes the dejections are nearly black, mixed with mucus. It is not unusual for a chest affection to be complicated with the lesions of the digestive organs, which are the cause of jaundice.

With these leading symptoms there are often others connected that are common to many diseases; such as dryness and heat of the mouth, a fetid smell, a staggering gait, roughness of the hair, and particularly of that of the back; an insatiable thirst, accompanied by the refusal of all food; loss of flesh, which occasionally proceeds with astonishing rapidity; a tucked-up flank, with hardness and tenderness of the anterior part of the belly.

The jaundice which is not accompanied with fever, nor indeed with any morbid change but the colour of the skin, will require very little treatment. It will usually disappear in a reasonable time, and M. Leblanc has not found that any kind of treatment would hasten that disappearance.

When any new symptom becomes superadded to jaundice, it must be immediately combated. Fever, injection of the vessels of the conjunctiva, constipation, diarrhœa, or the discoloration of the urine, require one bleeding at least, with some mucilaginous drinks. Purgatives are always injurious at the commencement of the disease. "I consider," says M. Leblanc, "this fact to be of the utmost importance. Almost the whole of the dogs that have been brought to me seriously ill with jaundice, have been purged once or more; and either kitchen salt, or tobacco, or jalap, or syrup of buckthorn, or emetic tartar, or some unknown purgative powders, have been administered.

"Bleeding should be resorted to, and repeated if the fever continues, or the animal coughs, or the respiration be accelerated

When the pulse is subdued, and the number of pulsations are below the natural standard — if the excrements are still void of their natural colour — if the constipation continues, or the animal refuses to feed — an ounce of manna dissolved in warm water should be given, and the dog often drenched with linseed tea. If watery diarrhœa should supervene, and the belly is not hot nor tender, a drachm or more, according to the size of the dog, of the sulphate of magnesia or soda should be administered, and this medicine should be repeated if the purging continues; more especially should this aperient be had recourse to when the fæces are more or less bloody, there being no fever nor peculiar tenderness of the belly.

"When the liquid excrement contains much blood, and that blood is of a deep colour, all medicines given by the mouth should be suspended, and frequent injections should be thrown up, consisting of thin starch, with a few drops of laudanum. Too much cold water should not be allowed in this stage of the disease. Injections, and drinks composed of starch and opium, are the means most likely to succeed in the black diarrhœa, which is so frequent and so fatal, and which almost always precedes the fatal termination of all the diseases connected with jaundice.

"In simple cases of jaundice the neutral salts have seldom produced much good effect; but I have obtained considerable success from the diascordium, in doses of half a drachm to a drachm.

"Great care should be taken with regard to the diet of the dog that has had jaundice, with bloody or black diarrhœa; for the cases of relapse are frequent and serious, and almost always caused by improper or too abundant food. A panada of bread, with a little butter, will constitute the best nourishment when the dog begins to recover his appetite. From this he may be gradually permitted to return to his former food. Most especially should the animal not be suffered to take cold, or to be left in a low or damp situation. This attention to the food of the convalescent dog may be thought to be pushed a little too far; but experience has taught me to consider it of the utmost importance, and it is neither expensive nor troublesome."

THE SPLEEN AND PANCREAS.

The spleen is generally regarded as an appendage to the absorbent system. Tiedemann and Gmelin consider that its specific function is to secrete from the blood a fluid which possesses the property of coagulation, and which is carried to the thoracic duct, and then, being united with the chyle, converts it into blood, and causes an actual communication between the arterial and absorbent systems. According, however, to Dr. Bostock, there is a fatal objection to this, namely, that animals have been known to live an indefinite length of time after the removal of the spleen, without any obvious injury to their functions, which could not have been the case if the spleen had been essentially necessary for so important a process.

A knowledge of the diseases of the spleen in the dog appears to be less advanced than in any other animal. In the cases that I have seen, the earliest indications were frequent vomiting, and the discharge of a yellow, frothy mucus. The animal appeared uneasy, shivering, the ears cold, the eyes unnaturally protuberant, the nostrils dilated, the flanks agitated, the respiration accelerated, and the mucous membranes pale. The best treatment I know is the administration, twice in the day, of a ball composed of a grain of calomel and the same quantity of aloes, and five grains of ginger. The dog frequently cries out, both when he is moved and when he lies on his bed. In the course of three days the yellow mucus is generally disappearing, and the expression of pain is materially diminished.

If the bowels are much constipated after two days have passed, two scruples of aloes may be given, and a grain of calomel; frequent injections may also be administered.

We are almost totally ignorant of the functions of the *pancreas.* It probably is concerned in assimilating the food, and converting the chyme of the stomach into chyle.

INFLAMMATION OF THE KIDNEY

is a serious and dangerous malady. This organ is essentially vascular in its texture; and although it is small in volume, yet, on account of the quantity of blood which it contains, and the rapidity with which its secretions are performed, it is disposed to frequent and dangerous inflammation. The immediate causes of inflammatory action in this viscus are blows and contusions in the lumbar region; hard work long continued, and the imprudent use of stimulating substances employed as aphrodisiacs; the presence of calculi in the kidney, and the arrest of the urine in the bladder. The whole of the kidney may be affected with anæmia or defect of blood, or this may be confined to the cortical substance, or even to the tubular. The kidneys are occasionally much larger than usual, without any other change of structure; or simple hypertrophy may affect but one of them. They are subject to atrophy, which may be either general or partial; or one of the kidneys may be completely wanting, and this evidently the consequence of violence or disease.

Hydatids, though seldom met with in the human kidney, are not unfrequently found in that of the dog. All these are circumstances that have not received sufficient attention.

CALCULOUS CONCRETIONS

are of more frequent occurrence than is generally imagined, but they are not confined to the kidneys; there is scarcely a portion of the frame in which they have not been found, particularly in the brain, the glandular substance, and the coats of the intestines.

I cannot say with Mr. Blaine that I have seen not less than 40 or 50 calculi in my museum; but I have seen too many fearful examples of the complaint. There has been usually great difficulty in the urinary evacuation; and at length one of the calculi enters the urethra, and so blocks up the flow of the urine that mortification ensues.

M. Lautour relates a case of renal calculus in a dog. He had occasionally voided his urine with some difficulty, and had walked slowly and with evident pain. August 20, 1827, a sudden exacerbation came on, and the dog was dreadfully agitated. He barked and rolled himself on the ground almost every minute; he made frequent attempts to void his urine, which came from him drop by drop. When compelled to walk, his hind and fore legs seemed to mingle together, and his loins were bent into a perfect curve; his flanks were drawn in; he could scarcely be induced to eat; and he evidently suffered much in voiding his fæces. Mild and demulcent liquids were his only food. Warm baths and injections were applied almost unceasingly, and in eight days he seemed to have perfectly gained his health.

In March, in the following year, the symptoms returned with greater intensity. His hind limbs were dragged after him; he rapidly lost flesh, and his howlings were fearful and continuous. The same mode of treatment was adopted without any good effect, and, his cries continuing, he was destroyed.

The stomach and intestines were healthy. The bladder was enlarged from the thickness and induration of its parietes; the mucous membrane of it was covered with ecchymoses; the kidneys were three or four times their natural size; and the pelvis contained a calculus weighing 126 grains, composed of 58 grains of uric acid and 58 of ammonia, with 10 grains of phosphate of lime.

Of the nature and causes of urinary calculi in the bladder we know very little. We only know that some solid body finds its way or is formed there, gradually increases in size, and at length partially or entirely occupies the bladder. Boerhaave has given a singular and undeniable proof of this. He introduced a small round pebble into the bladder of a dog. The wound perfectly healed. A few months afterwards the animal was killed, and there was found a calculus of considerable size, of which the pebble was the nucleus.

Occasionally the pressure of the bladder on the calculus which it contains is exceedingly great, so much so, indeed, as to crush the calculus. A small calculus may sometimes be forcibly extracted, or cut down upon and removed; but when the calculus is large, a catheter or bougie must be passed up the penis as far as the curve in the urethra, and then somewhat firmly held with the left hand, and pressing against the urethra. A scalpel should be taken, and an incision made into the urethra. The catheter being now withdrawn, and the finger or a pair of forceps introduced into the bladder, the calculus may be grasped and extracted.

There are some instances in which as many as 20 or 30 small calculi have been taken from the bladder of a dog. Twice I have seen calculi absolutely crushed in the bladder of a dog; and Mr. Blaine says that he found no fewer than 40 or 50 in the bladder of a Newfoundland dog. One of them had passed out into the urethra, and had so blocked up the passage that the flow of urine was prevented, and the animal died of mortification.

With much pleasure I refer to the details of Mr. Blaine with regard to the management of *vesical calculi.* "When a small calculus," says he, "obstructs the urethra, and can be felt, it may be attempted to be forced forward through the urethra to the point of the penis, whence it may be extracted by a pair of forceps. If it cannot be so moved, it may be cut down upon and removed with safety; but when one or more stones are within the bladder, we must attempt lithotomy, after having fully satisfied ourselves of their existence there by the introduction of the sound; to do which it must be remembered that the urethra of the dog in passing the bladder proceeds nearly in a direct line backwards, and then, making an acute angle, it passes again forwards to the bladder. It must be therefore evident, that when it becomes necessary to introduce a catheter, sound, or bougie, it must first be passed up the penis to the extremity of this angle; the point of the instrument must then be cut down upon, and from this opening the instrument may be readily passed forward into the bladder. The examination made, and a stone detected, it may, if a very small one, be attempted to be pushed forward by means of a finger passed up the anus into the urethra; but, as this could be practicable only where the dog happened to be a large one, it is most probable that nothing short of the operation of lithotomy would succeed. To this end, the sound being introduced, pass a very small gorget, or otherwise a bistoury, along its groove into the bladder, to effect an opening sufficient to admit of the introduction of a fine pair of forceps, by which the stone may be laid up and extracted."—***Blaine's Canine Pathology***, p. 180.

INFLAMMATION OF THE BLADDER

is of frequent occurrence in the dog; it is also occasionally observed in the horse and the ox. It sometimes appears as an epizootic. It is generally announced by anxiety, agitation, trembling of the hinder limbs, frequent attempts to urine, vain efforts to accomplish it, the evacuation small in quantity, sometimes clear and aqueous, and at other times mucous, laden with sediment, thick and bloody, escaping by jets, painfully and with great difficulty, and then suddenly rushing out in great quantity. To this list of symptoms colic may often be added. The animal drinks with avidity, but seldom eats much, unless at the commencement of the complaint. The skin is hard and dry, he looks at his flanks, and his back and flanks are tender when pressed upon.

During the latter portion of my connexion with Mr. Blaine, this disease assumed an epidemic character. There was a great drought through almost every part of the country. The disease was characterised by general uneasiness; continual shifting of the posture; a tucked-up appearance; an anxious countenance; a quick and noisy pulse; continued panting; the urine voided in small quantities, sometimes discharged drop by drop, or complete stoppage of it. The belly hot, swelled, and tender to the touch; the dog becoming strangely irritable, and ready to bite even his master.

1st May, 1824.—Two dogs had been making ineffectual attempts to void their urine for nearly two days. The first was a terrier, and the other a Newfoundland. The terrier was bled, placed in a warm bath, and an aloetic ball, with calomel, administered. He was bled a second time in the evening, and a few drops of water were discharged. On the following day, the urine slowly passed involuntarily from him; but when he attempted to void any, his efforts were totally ineffectual. Balls composed of camphor, pulv. uva ursi, tinct. ferri mur., mass purg., and pulv. lini. et gum. arab., were administered morning, noon, and night. On the 5th the urine still passed involuntarily. Cold lotions were employed, and tonic and astringent medicines administered, with castor oil. He gradually got well, and no trace of the disease remained until June the 6th, when he again became thin and weak, and discharged much bloody urine, but apparently without pain. The uva ursi, oak bark, and powdered gum-arabic were employed. On the 12th he had become much better, and so continued until the 1st of July, when he again exhibited the same complaint more violently than before. He was exceedingly tender on the loins, and screamed when he was touched. He was bled, returned to his uva ursi and powdered gum, and recovered. I saw him two years afterwards apparently well.

The Newfoundland dog exhibited a similar complaint, with

nearly the same accompaniments. *May* 1.—He was disinclined to move; his belly was hard and hot, and he was supposed to be costive. Gave an aloetic ball with iron. 2*d*. He has endeavoured, in vain, several times to void his urine. He walks stiffly with his back bound. Subtract eight ounces of blood; give another physic-ball, and apply cold affusion to the loins. 3*d*. He frequently attempts to stale, and passes a little urine at each time; he still walks and stands with his back bound. Syr. papav. et rhamni, with tinct. ferr. mur., a large spoonful being given morning and night. 4*th*. He again tries, ineffectually, to void his urine. Mist. et pulv. 5*th*. Unable to void a drop of urine; nose hot; tongue hangs down; pants considerably; will not eat; the countenance has an anxious character. Bleed to twelve ounces; apply cold affusion. Medicine as before, with cold affusion. 6*th*. Appears to be in very great pain; not a drop of water has passed from him. Medicine and other treatment as before. In the evening he lay down quietly. On the next morning he was found dead. All the viscera were sound except the bladder, which was ruptured; the abdomen contained two quarts of bloody fluid. The mucous membrane of the bladder appeared to be in the highest state of inflammation. It was almost black with extravasated blood. On the neck of the bladder was an enlargement of the size of a goose's egg, and almost filling the cavity of the pelvis. On cutting into it, more than two ounces of pus escaped.

On June 29, 1833, a poodle was brought to me. He had not been observed to pass any urine for two days. He made frequent attempts to void it, and cried dreadfully. The bladder could be felt distended in the abdomen. I put him into a warm bath, and took from him a pound of blood. He seemed to be a little relieved. I did not leave him until after midnight, but was soon roused by his loud screams, and the dog was also retching violently. The cries and retching gradually abated, and he died. The bladder had burst, and the parietes were in a dreadful state of inflammation.

A dog had laboured under incontinence of urine more than two months. The water was continually dropping from him. The servant told me that, three months before, he had been shut into a room two days, and, being a cleanly animal, would not stale until he was liberated. Soon after that the incontinence of urine was observed. I gave the usual tonic balls, with a small portion of opium, night and morning, and ordered cold water to be frequently dashed on the perinæum. A month afterwards he was quite well.

Comparatively speaking, *profuse staling* is not a common disease, except when it is the consequence of bad food, or strong diuretics, or actual inflammation. The cause and the result of the treatment are often obscure. Bleeding, purging, and counter irritation, would be indicated to a certain extent, but the lowering system must not be carried too far. The medicine would probably be catechu, uva ursi, and opium.

At times blood mingles with the urine, with or without coagulation. The cause and the source of it may or may not be determined. Generally speaking it is the result of some strain or blow.

A terrier bitch, in January, 1820, had incontinence of urine. No swelling or injury could be detected. I used with her the simple tonic balls. *10th January.*—She is now considerably better, and only a few drops are observed. *2d February.*—The disease which had seemingly been conquered began again to reappear; the medicine had been neglected. Again have recourse to it. *4th March.*—The disease now appears to be quite checked by the cold lotion and the balls.

A CASE OF RUPTURE OF THE BLADDER.

This is a singular account, and stands almost alone.

The patient was a valuable spaniel belonging to that breed known as "The Duke of Norfolk's," and now possessed in its full perfection by the Earl of Albemarle. Professor Simonds shall give his own account:—I was informed that almost from a puppy to the time when he was two years old, the dog had always been delicate in his appearance, and was observed to void his urine with difficulty; but there were not sufficient indications of disease for the owner to suppose that medical attendance was necessary until within a few days of his death, and then, finding that the act of staling was effected with increased difficulty, and accompanied with extreme pain; that the dog refused his food, was feverish; that at length there were frequent or ineffective efforts to expel the urine, the dog crying out from extremity of pain, and it was sufficiently evident that great mischief was going on, he was placed under my care; and even then he was walked a mile and a half to my infirmary.

My attention was immediately directed to him; the man who brought him informing me that he seemed much easier since he left home. On examination, I at once pronounced that he could not recover; in fact, that he was rapidly sinking; but, from his then state, I could give no opinion with regard to the precise nature or extent of his disease. He was placed upon a bed in an appropriate apartment, with directions not to be disturbed, and in a few hours he died.

The *post-mortem* appearances were the abdomen containing from four to five pints of fluid, having much the character of, but more bloody than, that found in cases of ascites. The peritoneum seemed to be dyed from its immersion in this fluid, as it showed a general red hue, not apparently deeper in some parts than in others. There was an absence, to a great extent, of that beautiful appearance and well-marked course of the minute blood-vessels which accompany many cases of original peritonitis. Extending the examination, I found the bladder to be ruptured, and that the fluid of which I have spoken was to a large extent composed of urine, mingled with some other secretion from the peritoneal investure of the abdomen and its viscera, probably produced from the presence of an irritant, the urine being brought into direct contact with the membrane. Farther research showed that this rupture of the bladder was caused in the manner which I have stated. The *post-mortem* examination displayed a chronic enlargement of the prostate gland of a considerable size, causing by its pressure a mechanical obstruction to the passage of the urine. Death in this instance was not immediately brought about by the abnormal state of the original organ affected; but the prostate gland, having early in the life of the animal become diseased, and, being gradually increased in size, became a cause of still more serious disease, attacking more important organs.

WORMS.

There are various kinds of worms to which the dog is subject; they have occasionally been confounded with each other; but they are essentially different in the situations which they occupy, and the effects which they produce.

The *ascarides* are small thread-like worms, generally not more than six or ten lines in length, of a white colour, the head obtuse, and the tail terminating in a transparent prolongation. They are principally found in the rectum. They seem to possess considerable agility; and the itching which they set up is sometimes absolutely intolerable. To relieve this, the dog often drags the fundament along the ground.

All the domesticated animals are subject to the annoyance which these worms occasion. They roll themselves into balls as large as a nut, and become entangled so much with each other that it is difficult to separate them. Sometimes they appear in the stomach, and in such large masses that it is almost impossible to remove them by the act of vomiting. It has been said that packets of ascarides have been collected in the stomach containing more than one hundred worms. These collections are rarely or never got entirely rid of. Enormous doses of medicine may be given, and the worms may not be seen again for several weeks; but, at length, they reappear as numerous as ever.

Young dogs are exceedingly subject to them, and are with great difficulty perfectly freed from their attacks.

Another species of worm is the *teres*. It would resemble the earth-worm in its appearance, were it not white instead of a red colour. They are very common among dogs, especially young dogs, in whom they are often attended by fits. Occasionally they crawl into the stomach, and there produce a great deal of irritation.

Another, and the most injurious of the intestinal worms, is the *tænia*, or *tape-worm*. It is many inches in length, almost flat in the greater part of its extent, and its two extremities are nearly or quite equal. Tape-worms associate in groups like the others, but they are not so numerous; they chiefly frequent the small intestines. They are sometimes apt to coil themselves, and form a mechanical obstruction which is fatal to the dog.

The presence of all these worms is readily detected. There is generally a dry, short cough, a staring coat, a hot and fetid breath, a voracious appetite, and a peculiar state of the bowels; alternately constipated to a great degree, or peculiarly loose and griping. In young dogs the emaciated appearance, stinted growth, fetid breath, and frequent fits, are indications not to be mistaken.

At other times, however, the dog is filled with worms with scarcely any indication of their presence. Mr. Blaine very properly remarks that it does not follow, because no worms are seen to pass away, that there are none: neither when they are not seen does it follow even that none pass; for, if they remain long in the intestines after they are dead, they become digested like other animal matter.

The means of expelling or destroying worms in the intestines of the dog are twofold: the first and apparently the most natural mode of proceeding, is the administration of purgatives, and usually of drastic ones; but there is much danger connected with this; not merely the fæces will be expelled, but a greater or less portion of the mucus that lines the intestinal canal. The consequence of this will be griping and inflammation to a very dangerous extent. Frequent doses of Epsom salts have been given; but not always with success, and frequently with griping. Mercurial medicines have been tried; but they have not always succeeded, and have often produced salivation. One method of expelling the worm has been adopted which has rarely failed, without the slightest mischief—the administration of glass finely powdered. Not a particle of it penetrates through the mucus that lines the bowels, while it destroys every intestinal worm. The powdered glass is made into a ball with lard and ginger.

The following account of the symptoms caused by tænia may be interesting. A dog used to be cheerful, and particularly fond of his master; but gradually his countenance became haggard, his eyes were red, his throat was continually filled with a frothy spume, and he stalked about with an expression of constant inquietude and suffering. These circumstances naturally excited considerable fear with regard to the nature of his disease, and he was shut up in a court, with the intention of his being destroyed. Thus shut up, he furiously threw himself upon every surrounding object, and tore them with his teeth whenever he could seize them. He retired into one of the corners of the court, and there he was continually rubbing his nose, as it were to extract some foreign body; sometimes he bit and tore up the earth, barking and howling violently; his hair stood on end, and his flanks were hollow.

During the whole of his disease he continued to recognise his master. He ran to him at the slightest word. He refused nothing to drink; but he would not eat. He was killed on account of the fear excited among the neighbours.

The veterinary surgeon who attended him suspected that there was some affection of the head, on account of the strange manner in which he had rubbed and beaten it. The superior part of the nose was opened, and two tæniæ lanceolatæ were found: it was plain enough that they were the cause of all the mischief.

The proprietor of the dog nevertheless believed that it was a case of rabies; he had the caustic applied to his hands, and could not persuade himself that he was safe until he had been at the baths of Bourbonne.[a]

There is a worm inhabiting the stomach of young dogs, the *Ascaris Marginata*, a frequent source of sickness, and occasionally of spasmodic colic, by rolling itself into knots. It seems occasionally to take a dislike to its assigned residence, and wanders into the œsophagus, but rarely into the larger intestines. A dog had a severe cough, which could not be subdued by bleeding or physic, or sedative or opiate medicines. He was destroyed, and one of these ascarides was found in the trachea. Others find their way into the nasal cavity; and a dreadful source of irritation they are when they are endeavouring to escape, in order to undergo one of the changes of form to which they are destined, or when they have been forced into the nostril in the act of vomiting.

I once had a dog as a patient, whose case, I confess, I did not understand. He would sneeze and snort, and rub his head and nose along the carpet. I happened to say that the symptoms in some respects resembled those of rabies, and yet, that I could not satisfy myself that the dog was rabid. The mention of rabies was sufficient, and in defiance of my remonstrances the animal was destroyed.

The previous symptoms led me to examine the nasal cavity, and I found two of these ascarides, one concealed in the middle and

[a] Prat. Méd. Vét. 1824, p. 14.

the other in the upper meatus, through neither of which could any strong current of air be forced, and from which the ascarides could not be dislodged.

Worms may be the cause of sudden death in a dog. The following case, communicated by Professor Dick, illustrates this fact:—I lately had the body of a dog sent to me: his owner sent the following letter by the same conveyance. "My keeper went out shooting yesterday morning with the dog which I now send to you. He was quite lively, and apparently well, during the former part of the day; but towards evening he was seized with violent vomiting. When he came home he refused to eat, and this morning about eight o'clock he died. As I have lost all my best dogs rather suddenly, I will thank you to have him examined, and the contents of his stomach analyzed; and have the kindness to inform me whether he has been poisoned, or what was the cause of his death."

On opening the abdomen, the viscera appeared quite healthy: the stomach was removed, and the contents were found to be more decidedly acid than usual. The acids were the muriatic and acetic: the finding of an increased quantity of these is far from being unusual. There was not a trace of arsenical, mercurial, nor any other metallic poison present. Of the vegetable poisons, I can only say there was not the slightest trace of the morbid effects of any of them. The pericardium and the left side of the thorax contained a small quantity of bloody serous fluid, and the heart was full of black blood. The left lung was a little inflamed. The trachea contained some frothy yellow mucous matter, similar to the contents of the stomach. In the larynx was found one of those worms occasionally inhabiting the cavities of the nose, and which had probably escaped from the nose while the dog had been hunting; and, lodging in the larynx, had destroyed the animal by producing spasms of the larynx. The worm was about one inch and a half in length, and had partly penetrated through the rima glottidis. Another worm about the same size was found in the left bronchia, and a still smaller one among the mucus of the trachea: there were also four others in the nose.

Some years ago I found some worms of the filacia species in the right ventricle of the heart of a dog, which had produced sudden death by interrupting the action of the valves.

The following is a curious case of tape-worm, by Mr. Reynold:—

On an estate where a great quantity of rabbits are annually destroyed in the month of November, we have observed that several dogs that were previously in good health and condition soon became weak, listless, and excessively emaciated, frequently passing large portions of the tape-worm. This induced us to examine the intestines of several hares and rabbits; and, with very few exceptions, we found each to contain a perfect tape-worm from three to four feet in length. We then caused two of the dogs whose cases appeared the worst to be separated from the others, feeding them on potatoes, &c.; and, in eight or ten days, after voiding several feet of the worms, they were perfectly restored to their former strength and appearance. The worm disease, hitherto so formidable to the spaniel and pointer, may in a great measure be fairly attributed to the custom of giving them the intestines of their game, under the technical appellation of "the paunch." The facts above stated, in explaining the cause of the disease, at the same time suggest the remedy.

A worm in the urethra of a dog.—M. Séon, veterinary surgeon of the Lancers of the Body Guard, was requested to examine a dog who strained in vain to void his urine, often uttering dreadful cries, and then eagerly licking his penis. M. Séon, after having tried in vain to abate the irritation, endeavoured to pass an elastic bougie. He perceived a conical body half an inch long protruding from the urethra with each effort of the dog to void his urine, and immediately afterwards returning into the urethra. He crushed it with a pair of forceps, and drew it out. It proved to be a worm resembling a strongylus, four and a half inches long. It was living, and moving about. M. Séon could not ascertain its species. The worm being extracted, the urine flowed, and the dog soon recovered.[a]

FISTULA IN THE ANUS.

This is a too frequent consequence of piles. It is often the result of the stagnation of hardened fæces in the rectum, which produces inflammation and ulceration, and frequently leaves a fistulous opening. If we may judge what the quadruped suffers by the sufferings of human beings, it is a sadly painful affair, whether the fistula is external or internal. Whether it may be cured by a mild stimulant daily inserted to the bottom of the abscess, or whether there is a communication with the opening of the rectum which buries itself in the cellular tissues around it, and requires an operation for its cure, it will require the assistance of a skilful surgeon to effect a cure in this case.

---

[a] Prat. Méd. Vét., Fév. 1828.

CHAPTER XIII.

BLEEDING; TORSION; CASTRATION; PARTURITION; AND SOME DISEASES CONNECTED WITH THE ORGANS OF GENERATION.

BLEEDING.

This operation is exceedingly useful in many accidents and diseases. It is, in fact, as in the horse, the sheet-anchor of the practitioner in the majority of cases of an inflammatory character. There is some difference, however, in the instrument to be used. The lancet is the preferable instrument in the performance of this operation. The fleam should be banished from among the instruments of the veterinary surgeon.

A ligature being passed round the lower part of the neck, and the head being held up a little on one side, the vein will protrude on either side of the windpipe. It will usually be advisable to cut away a little of the hair over the spot designed to be punctured. When a sufficient quantity of blood is abstracted, it will generally be necessary, and especially if the dog is large, to pass a pin through both edges of the orifice, and secure it with a little tow.

When no lancet is at hand, the inside of the flap of the ear may be punctured with a pen-knife, the course of a vein being selected for this purpose. In somewhat desperate cases a small portion of the tail may be amputated.

The *superficial brachial vein*, the *cephalic* vein of the human subject, and the *plat* vein of the farrier, may be resorted to in all lamenesses of the fore limb, and especially in all shoulder-wrenches, strains of the loins, and of the thigh and the leg, and muscular and ligamentous extensions of any part of the hind limbs; the *vena saphena major*, and the *anterior tibial* vein may be punctured in such cases.

The quantity of blood to be abstracted must be regulated according to the size and strength of the dog and the degree of inflammation.

One or two ounces may be sufficient for a very small dog, and seven or eight for a large one.

TORSION.

To M. Amusat, of Paris, we are indebted for the introduction of the artery-forceps for the arresting of hemorrhage. I shall do but justice to him by describing his mode of proceeding. He seizes the divided vessel with a pair of torsion-forceps in such a manner as to hold and close the mouth of the vessel in its teeth.

The slide of the forceps then shuts its blade, and the artery is held fast. The artery is then drawn from out of the tissues surrounding it, to the extent of a few lines, and freed, with another forceps, from its cellular envelope, so as to lay bare its external coat. The index and thumb of the left hand are then applied above the forceps, in order to press back the blood in the vessel. He then begins to twist the artery. One of the methods consists in continuing the torsion until the part held in the forceps is detached. When, however, the operator does not intend to produce that effect, he ceases, after from four to six revolutions of the vessel on its axis for the small arteries, and from eight to twelve for the large ones. The hemorrhage instantly stops. The vessel which had been drawn out is then replaced, as the surrounding parts give support to the knot which has been formed at its extremities. The knot becomes further concealed by the retraction of the artery, and this retraction will be proportionate to the shortening which takes place by the effect of the twisting, so that it will be scarcely visible on the surface of the stump. It is of the utmost importance to seize the artery perfectly, and to make the stated number of twists, as otherwise the security against the danger of consecutive hemorrhage will not be perfect.

Mr. W. B. Costello, of London, was present when the operation was performed at Paris. He brought back a full account of it as performed there, and availed himself of an early opportunity of putting it to the test before some of our metropolitan surgeons. A dog was placed on the table, the forceps were applied, and the operation perfectly succeeded.

A few days afterwards a pointer bitch was brought to my infirmary, with a large scirrhous tumour near the anterior teat on the left side. It had been gradually increasing during the last five months. It was becoming more irregular in its form, and on one of its tuberculous prominences was a reddish spot, soft and somewhat tender, indicating that the process of suppuration was about to commence.

I had often, or almost uniformly, experienced the power of iodine in dispersing glandular enlargements in the neck of the dog, and also those indurated tumours of various kinds which form about the joints of some domesticated animals, particularly of cattle; but frequent disappointment had convinced me that it was, if not inert, yet very uncertain in its effect in causing absorption of tumours about the mammæ of the bitch. Having also been taught that the ultimate success of the excision of these enlargements depended on their removal before suppuration had taken place, and the neighbouring parts had been inoculated by the virus which so plentifully flowed from the ulcer, I determined on an immediate operation; and, as the tumour was large, and she was in high condition, I thought it a good case for *the first trial of torsion.* She was well physicked, and on the third day was produced before my class and properly secured. I had not provided myself with the *torsion forceps*, but relied on the hold I should have on the vessel by means of a pair of common artery forceps; and the effect of these imperfect instruments beautifully established the power of torsion in arresting hemorrhage.

Two elliptical incisions were made on the face of the tumour, and prolonged anteriorly and posteriorly about an inch from it. The portion of integument that could be spared was thus enclosed, while the opposed edges of the wound could be neatly and effectually brought together after the operation. The dissection of the integument from the remaining part of the face of the tumour was somewhat slow and difficult, for it was in a manner identified with the hardened mass beneath; but the operation soon proceeded more quickly, and we very soon had the scirrhus exposed, and adhering to the thorax by its base. About two ounces of venous blood had now been lost.

I was convinced that I should find the principal artery, by which the excrescence was fed, at its anterior extremity, and not far from the spot where the suppuration seemed to be preparing: therefore, beginning posteriorly, I very rapidly cut through the cellular texture, elevating the tumour and turning it back, until I arrived at the inner and anterior point, and there was the only source of supply; the artery was plainly to be seen. In order to give the experiment a fair chance, I would not enclose it in the forceps, but I cut through it. A jet of blood spirted out. I then seized the vessel as quickly as I could, and began to turn the forceps, but before I could effect more than a turn and a half I lost my hold on the artery. I was vexed, and paused, waiting for the renewed gush of blood that I might seize the vessel again; but to my surprise not a drop more blood came from the arterial trunk. That turn and a half, considerable pressure having been used, had completely arrested the hemorrhage. I can safely say that not more than four drachms of arterial blood were lost.

The wound was sponged clean: there remained only a very slight oozing from two or three points; the flaps were brought together, secured by the ordinary sutures, and the proper bandages applied. The weight of the tumour was twenty-two ounces; there was no after-bleeding, no unpleasant occurrences; but the wound, which had been nearly six inches in length, was closed in little more than three weeks.

He will essentially promote the cause of science, and the cause of humanity, who will avail himself of the opportunity which country practice affords of putting the effect of torsion to the test;

and few things will be more gratifying than the consciousness of rescuing our patients from the unnecessary infliction of torture.

In docking, it will be found perfectly practicable: our patients will escape much torture, and tetanus will often be avoided. The principal danger from castration has arisen from the severity with which the iron has been employed. The colt, the sheep, and the dog will be fair subjects for experiment. The cautery, as it regards the first, and the brutal violence too frequently resorted to in operating upon the others, have destroyed thousands of animals.

CASTRATION.

This operation is performed on a great portion of our domestic animals. It renders them more docile, and gives them a disposition to fatten. It is followed by fewest serious accidents when it is performed on young animals. The autumn or spring should, if possible, be chosen for the operation, for the temperature of the atmosphere is then generally uniform and moderate. It should be previously ascertained that the animal is in perfect health; and he should be prepared by a mash diet and bleeding, if he is in a plethoric state, or possessed of considerable determination. If it is a young animal that is to be operated upon, an incision may be made into the scrotum, the testicle may be protruded, and the cord cut without much precaution, for the blood will soon be stayed; but for older animals it will be advisable to use a ligature, applied moderately tightly round the spermatic cord a little more than an inch beyond its insertion into the testicle: the scalpel is then used, and a separation effected between the ligature and the testis. The vas derens needs not to be included; a great deal of pain will then be spared to the animal.

The ordinary consequences of castration are pain, inflammation, engorgement, and suppuration. The pain and suppuration are inevitable, but generally yield to emollient applications. The engorgement is often considerable at first, but soon subsides, and the suppuration usually abates in the course of a few days. It has been said that the castrated dog is more attached and faithful to his master than he who has not been deprived of his genital powers: this, however, is to be much doubted. He has, generally speaking, lost a considerable portion of his courage, his energy, and his strength. He is apt to become idle, and is disposed to accumulate fat more rapidly. His power of scent is also very considera bly diminished, and he is less qualified for the sports of the field. Of this there can be no doubt. It has been said that he is more submissive: I very much doubt the accuracy of that opinion. He may not be so savage as in his perfect state; he may not be so eager in his feeding; but there is not the devotion to his master, and the quickness of comprehension which belongs to the perfect dog.

The removal of the ovaries, or spaying of the female, used to be often practised, and packs of spayed bitches were, and still are, occasionally kept. In performing this operation, an opening is made into the flank on one side, and the finger introduced — one of the ovaries is laid hold of and drawn a little out of the belly; a ligature is then applied round it, just above the bifurcation of the womb, and it is cut through, the end of the ligature being left hanging out of the wound. The other ovary is then felt for and drawn out, and excised and secured by a ligature. The wound is then sewed up, and a bandage is placed over the incision. Some farriers do not apply any ligature, but simply sew up the wound, and in the majority of cases the edges adhere, and no harm comes of the operation, except that the general character of the animal is essentially changed. She accumulates a vast quantity of fat, becomes listless and idle, and is almost invariably short-lived.

The female dog, therefore, should always be allowed to breed. Breeding is a necessary process; and the female prevented from it is sure to be affected with disease sooner or later; enormous collections and indurations will form, that will inevitably terminate in scirrhus or ulceration.

A troublesome process often occurs when the female is not permitted to have young ones; namely, the accumulation of milk in the teats, especially if at any previous time, however distant, she may have had puppies once. The foundation is laid for many unpleasant and unmanageable complaints. If she is suffered to bring up one litter after another, she will have better health than those that are debarred from intercourse with the male.

The temporary union which takes place between the male and female at the period at which they are brought together is a very singular one. The corpora cavernosa of the male and the clitoris of the female being suddenly distended with blood, it is impossible to withdraw either of them until the turgescence of the parts has entirely ceased.

PARTURITION.

The pupping usually takes place from the sixty-second to the sixty-fourth day; and the process having commenced, from a quarter to three quarters of an hour generally takes place between the production of each puppy.

Great numbers of bitches are lost every year in the act of parturition: there seems to be a propensity in the females to associate with dogs larger than themselves, and they pay for it with their lives. The most neglected circumstance during the period of pregnancy is the little exercise which the mother is permitted to take, while, in point of fact, nothing tends more to safe and easy parturition than her being permitted or compelled to take a fair quantity of exercise.

When the time of parturition has arrived, and there is evident difficulty in producing the fœtus, recourse should be had to the ergot of rye, which should be given every hour or half hour, according to circumstances. If after a certain time some, although little, progress has been made, the ergot must be continued in smaller doses, or perhaps suspended for a while; but, if all progress is evidently suspended, recourse must be had to the hook or the forceps. By gentle but continued manipulation much may be done, especially when the muzzle of the puppy can be brought into the passage. As little force as possible must be used, and especially the fœtus little broken. Many a valuable animal is destroyed by the undue application of force.

If the animal seems to be losing strength, a small quantity of laudanum and ether may be administered. "The patience of bitches in labour is extreme," says Mr. Blaine; "and their distress, if not removed, is most striking and affecting. Their look is at such time particularly expressive and apparently imploring." When the pupping is protracted, and the young ones are evidently dead, the mother may be saved, if none of the puppies have been broken. In process of time the different puppies may, one after another, be extracted; but when violence has been used at the commencement, or almost at any part of the process, death will assuredly follow.

June 15, 1832.—A spaniel bitch was brought to my infirmary to-day, who has been in great and constant pain since yesterday, making repeated but fruitless efforts to expel her puppies. She is in a very plethoric habit of body; her bowels are much confined, and she exhibits some general symptoms of febrile derangement, arising, doubtless, from her protracted labour. This is her first litter. Upon examination, no young could be distinctly felt.

Place her in a warm bath, and give her a dose of castor oil, morning and evening.

June 16.—The bitch appears in the same state as yesterday, except that the medicine has operated freely upon the bowels, and the febrile symptoms have somewhat decreased. Her strainings are as frequent and distressing as ever. Take two scruples of the ergot of rye, and divide into six doses, of which let one be given every half hour.

In about ten minutes after the exhibition of the last dose of this medicine, she brought forth, with great difficulty, one dead puppy, upon taking which away from her, she became so uneasy that I was induced to return it to her. In about a quarter of an hour after this I paid her another visit; the puppy could not now be found; but a suspicious appearance in the mother's eye betrayed at once that she had devoured it. I immediately administered an emetic; and in a very short time the whole fœtus was returned in five distinct parts, viz., the four quarters and the head. After this, the bitch began to amend very fast; she produced no other puppy; and as her supply of milk was small, she was soon convalescent.

Twelve months afterwards she was again taken in labour, about eleven o'clock in the morning, and after very great difficulty, one puppy was produced. After this the bitch appeared in great pain, but did not succeed in expelling another fœtus, in consequence of which I was sent for about three o'clock, P. M. I found her very uneasy, breathing laboriously; the mouth hot, and the bowels costive; but I could not discover any trace of another fœtus. She was put into a warm bath, and a dose of opening medicine was administered.

About five o'clock she got rid of one dead and two living puppies.

2d. She is still very ill; she evinces great pain when pressed upon the abdomen; and it is manifest that she has another fœtus within her. I ordered a dose of the ergot, and in about twenty minutes a large puppy was produced, nearly dying. She survived with due care.

I cannot refrain from inserting the following case at considerable length.

Sept. 4, 1820.—A very diminutive terrier, weighing not 5 lbs., was sent to my hospital in order to lie in. She was already restless and panting. About eight o'clock at night the labour pains commenced; but until eleven scarcely any progress was made. The *os uteri* would not admit my finger, although I frequently attempted it.

At half-past eleven, the membranes began to protrude; at one the head had descended into the pelvis and the puppy was dead. In a previous labour she had been unable to produce her young, although the ergot of rye had been freely used. I was obliged to use considerable force, and she fought terribly with me throughout the whole process. At half-past one, and after applying considerable force, I brought away a large fœtus, compared with her own size. On passing my finger as high as possible, I felt another fœtus living, but the night passed and the whole of the following day, and she ate and drank, and did not appear to be much injured.

Several times in the day I gave her some strong soup and the ergot. Some slight pains now returned, and by pressing on the belly the nose of the fœtus was brought to the superior edge of the pelvis. The pains again ceased, the pudenda began to swell from frequent examination, the bitch began to stagger, and made frequent attempts to void her urine, with extreme difficulty in accomplishing it. I now resorted to the crotchet; and after many unsuccessful attempts, in which the superior part of the vagina must have been considerably bruised, I fixed it sufficiently firmly to draw the head into the cavity of the pelvis. Here for a while the shoulder resisted every attempt which I could make without the danger of detruncating the fœtus. At length by working at the side of the head until my nails were soft and my fingers sore, I extracted one fore leg. The other was soon brought down; another large puppy was produced, but destroyed by the means necessary for its production. This was the fruit of two hours' hard work.

She was completely exhausted, and scarcely able to stand. When placed on the ground she staggered and fell at almost every step. Her efforts to void her urine were frequent and ineffectual.

At four o'clock I again examined her; the external pudenda were sore and swelled, and beginning to assume a black hue. It was with considerable difficulty that I could introduce my finger. A third fœtus irregularly presented was detected. I could just feel one of the hind legs. No time was to be lost. I introduced a small pair of forceps by the side of my finger, and succeeded in laying hold of the leg without much difficulty, and, with two or three weak efforts from the mother,—I could scarcely call them pains,—I brought the leg down until it was in the cavity of the pelvis. I solicited it forward with my finger, and, by forcibly pressing back the *labia pudendi*, I could just grasp it with the finger and thumb of the right hand. Holding it there, I introduced the finger of the right hand, and continued to get down the other leg, and then found little difficulty until the head was brought to the superior edge of the pelvis. After a long interval, and with considerable force, this was brought into the pelvis, and another puppy extracted. This fully occupied two hours.

The bitch now appeared almost lifeless. As she was unable to stand, and seemed unconscious of every thing around her, I concluded that she was lost: I gave her one or two drops of warm brandy and water, covered her up closely, and put her to bed.

To my surprise, on the following morning, she was curled round in her basket; she licked my hands, and ate a bit of bread and butter; but when put on her legs staggered and fell. The pudendum was dreadfully swollen, and literally black. In the afternoon she again took a little food: she came voluntarily from her basket, wagged her tail when spoken to, and on the following day she was taken in her basket a journey of 70 miles, and afterwards did well; no one could be more rejoiced than was her master, who was present at, and superintended the greater part of the proceedings.

The beneficial effect of Ergot of Rye in difficult Parturition.— The following case is from the pen of Professor Dick:—On the 10th instant, a pointer bitch produced two puppies; and it was thought by the person having her in charge that she had no more. She was put into a comfortable box, and with a little care was expected to do well. On the next morning, however, she was sick and breathed heavily, and continued rather uneasy all the day.

On the forenoon of the following day I was requested to see her. I found her with her nose dry, breath hot, respiration frequent, mouth hot and parched, coat staring, back roached, pulse 120, and a black fetid discharge from the vagina. Pressure on the abdomen gave pain. A pup could be obscurely felt; the secretion of milk was suppressed, and the skin had lost its natural elasticity.

Tepid water with a little soap dissolved in it was immediately injected into the uterus, which in a considerable degree excited its action; and this injection was repeated two or three times with the same effect.

After waiting for half an hour, the fœtus was not discharged nor brought forward; therefore a scruple of the ergot of rye was then made into an infusion with two ounces of water, and one-third of it given as a dose; in half an hour, another one-third of it; the injections of warm water and soap being also continued. Soon after the second dose of the infusion, a dead puppy was expelled; the bitch rapidly recovered, and, with the exception of deficiency of milk, is now quite well.

This case would seem to prove the great power of the ergot of rye over the uterus; but, until more experiments are made, it is necessary to be cautious in ascribing powers to medicines which have not been much tried in our practice. It is not improbable that the warm water and soap might have roused the uterus into action without the aid of the ergot; and it is therefore necessary that those who repeat this experiment should try the effects of the medicine unaided by the auxiliary.

The Professor adds, that the great power which this drug is said to have on the human being, and the apparent effect in the case just given, suggest the propriety of instituting a further trial of it, and of our extending our observations to cattle, amongst which difficult cases of calving so frequently occur.

Mr. Simpson thus concludes some remarks on ergot in difficult parturition. This medicine possesses a very great power over the uterus, rousing its dormant or debilitated contractility, and stimulating it to an extra performance of this necessary function after its natural energy has been in some measure destroyed by forcible but useless action. The direct utility of the ergot was manifested in cases where the uterus appeared quite exhausted by its repeated efforts; and certainly it is but fair to ascribe the decidedly augmented power of the organ to the stimulus of the ergot, for no other means were resorted to in order to procure the desired effect. Its action, too, is prompt. Within ten minutes of the administration of a second or third dose, when nature has been nearly exhausted, the parturition has been safely effected.

Puerperal Fits.—Nature proportions the power and resources of the mother to the wants of her offspring. In her wild undomesticated state she is able to suckle her progeny to the full time; but, in the artificial state in which we have placed her, we shorten the interval between each period of parturition, we increase the number of her young ones at each birth, we diminish her natural powers of affording them nutriment, and we give her a degree of irritability which renders her whole system liable to be excited and deranged by causes that would otherwise be harmless: therefore it happens that, when the petted bitch is permitted to suckle the whole of her litter, her supply of nutriment soon becomes exhausted, and the continued drain upon her produces a great degree of irritability. She gets rapidly thin; she staggers, is half unconscious, neglects her puppies, and suddenly falls into a fit of a very peculiar character. It begins with, and is sometimes confined to, the respiratory apparatus: she lies on her side and pants violently, and the sound of her laboured breathing may be heard at the distance of twenty yards. Sometimes spasms steal over her limbs; at other times the diaphragm and respiratory muscles alone are convulsed. In a few hours she is certainly lost; or, if there are moments of remission, they are speedily succeeded by increased heavings.

The practitioner unaccustomed to this fearful state of excitation, and forgetful or unaware of its cause, proceeds to bleed her, and he seals her fate. Although one system is thus convulsively labouring, it is because others are suddenly and perfectly exhausted; and by abstraction of the vital current he reduces this last hold of life to the helpless condition of the rest. There is not a more common or fatal error than this.

The veterinary practitioner is unable to apply the tepid bath to his larger patients, in order to quiet the erythism of certain parts of the system, and produce an equable diffusion of nervous influence and action; and he often forgets it when he has it in his power to save the smaller ones. Let the bitch in a fit be put into a bath, temperature 96° Fahrenheit, and covered with the water, her head excepted. It will be surprising to see how soon the simple application of this equable temperament will quiet down the erythism of the excited system. In ten minutes, or a quarter of an hour, she may be taken out of the bath evidently relieved, and then, a hasty and not very accurate drying having taken place, she is wrapped in a blanket and placed in some warm situation, a good dose of physic having been previously administered. She soon breaks out in a profuse perspiration. Everything becomes gradually quiet, and she falls into a deep and long sleep, and at length awakes somewhat weak, but to a certain degree restored.

If, then, all her puppies except one or two are taken from her, and her food is, for a day or two, somewhat restricted, and after that given again of its usual quantity and kind, she will live and do well; but a bleeding at the time of her fit, or suffering all her puppies to return to her, will inevitably destroy her.

A bitch that was often brought to my house was suckling a litter of puppies. She was foolishly taken up and thrown into the Serpentine in the month of April. The suppression of milk was immediate and complete. There was also a determination to the head, and attacks resembling epilepsy. The puppies that were suffered to remain with the mother, were very soon as epileptic as she was, and were destroyed. A seton was inserted on each side of her neck. Ipecacuanha was administered; and that having sufficiently worked, a small quantity of diluted sulphuric acid was given. A fortnight afterwards she was perfectly well.

Inversion of the Uterus in a Bull Bitch after Pupping. Extirpation and Cure. By M. Cross, M. V., Milan.—In July, 1829, I was desired to attend a small bull bitch six years old, and who had had puppies four times. The uterus was completely inverted, and rested all its weight on the vaginal orifice of the urethra, preventing the discharge of the urine, and thus being the cause of great pain when the animal endeavoured to void it, or the fæcal matter. The uterus was become of almost a black colour, swelled, softened, and exhaling an insupportable odour. Judging from this that the preservation of the uterus was impossible, and reckoning much on the good constitution of the patient, I warned the proprietor of the danger of its reduction, even supposing that it was practicable, and proposed to him the complete extirpation of the uterus as the only means that remained of saving the bitch.

Armed with his consent, I passed a ligature round the neck of the uterus, at the bottom of the vagina, and drew it as tight as I possibly could. On the following day I again tightened the ligature, in order to complete the mortification of the part, and the separation of the womb. On the third day I extirpated the womb entirely, close to the haunch. There was very slight loss of blood, but there ran from the walls of the vagina a small quantity of ichorous fluid, with a strong fetid smell. The operation was scarcely completed ere she voided a considerable quantity of urine, and then searched about for something to eat and to drink.

The portion of the uterus that was removed weighed fourteen ounces. The mucous membrane by which it was lined was in a highly disorganized state. From time to time injections of a slight infusion of aromatic plants were introduced into the vagina, and the animal was nourished with liquid food of easy digestion.

The first day passed without the animal being in the slightest degree affected; but, on the following day, in despite of all our care, an ichorous fluid was discharged, which the dog would lick notwithstanding all our efforts to prevent it. The general health of the animal did not seem to be in the slightest degree affected. We continued our aromatic infusion and our regimen.

On the fourth day after the operation, the cords that had served as a ligature fell off, and all suppuration from the part gradually ceased.

October 20th.—Three months have passed since the operation, and she is perfectly well.

CHAPTER XIV.

THE DISTEMPER.

By this singular name is distinguished a prevalent disease now about to come under our consideration, which was first observed on the continent. The rapidity with which it spread, the strange protean appearances which it assumed, and its too frequent fatal termination, surprised and puzzled the veterinary surgeons; and they called it "la maladie des chiens," the disease or distemper in dogs.

It is comparatively a new disease. It was imported from France about one hundred years since, although some French authors have strangely affirmed that it is of British origin. Having once gained footing among us, it has established itself in our country, to the vexation and loss of the sportsman, and the annoyance of the veterinary surgeon. However keepers, or even men of education, may boast of their specifics, it is a sadly fatal disease, and destroys fully one-third of the canine race.

Dogs of all ages are subject to its attack. Many, nine and ten years old, have died of pure distemper; and I have seen puppies of only three weeks fall victims to it; but it oftenest appears between the sixth and twelfth month of the animal's life. If it occurs at an early period, it proves fatal in the great majority of cases; and, if the dog is more than four years old, it generally goes hard with him. It is undeniably highly contagious, yet it is

30

frequently generated. In this it bears an analogy to mange, and to farcy and glanders in the horse.

One attack of the disease, and even a severe one, is no absolute security against its return; although the dog that has once laboured under distemper possesses a certain degree of immunity; or, if he is attacked a second time, the malady usually assumes a milder type. I have, however, known it occur three times in the same animal, and at last destroy him.

Violent catarrh will often terminate in distemper; and low and insufficient feeding will produce it. It frequently follows mange, and especially if mercury has been used in the cure of the malady. When we see a puppy with mange, and that peculiar disease in which the skin becomes corrugated, and more especially if it is a spaniel, and pot-bellied or rickety, we generally say that we can cure the mange, but it will not be long before the animal dies of distemper; and so it happens in three cases out of four. Whatever debilitates the constitution predisposes it for the reception or the generation of distemper. It, however, frequently occurs without any apparent exciting cause.

That it is highly contagious cannot admit of doubt. A healthy dog can seldom, for many days, be kept with another that labours under distemper without becoming affected; and the disease is communicated by the slightest momentary contact. There is, however, a great deal of caprice about this. I have more than once kept a dog in the foul-yard of my hospital for several successive weeks, and he has not become diseased. Inoculation with the matter that flows from the nose, either limpid or purulent, and in an early or advanced stage of the distemper, will, with few exceptions, produce the disease; yet I have failed to communicate it even by this method. Inoculation used to be recommended as producing a milder and less fatal disease. So far as my experience goes, the contrary has been the result.

Distemper is also epidemic. It occurs more frequently in the spring and autumn than in the winter and summer. If one or two dogs in a certain district are affected, we may be assured that it will soon extensively prevail there; and where the disease could not possibly be communicated by contagion. Sometimes it rages all over the country. At other times it is endemic, and confined to some particular district.

Not only is the disease epidemic or endemic, but the form which it assumes is so. In one season, almost every dog with distemper has violent fits; at another, in the majority of cases, there will be considerable chest affection, running on to pneumonia; a few months afterwards, a great proportion of the distempered dogs will be worn down by diarrhœa, which no medicine will arrest; and presently it will be scarcely distinguishable from mild catarrh.

It varies much with different breeds. The shepherd's dog, generally speaking, cares little about it; he is scarcely ill a day. The cur is not often seriously affected. The terrier has it more severely, especially the white terrier. The hound comes next in the order of severity; and after him the setter. With the small spaniel it is more dangerous; and still more so with the pointer, especially if he has the disease early. Next in the order of fatality comes the pug; and it is most fatal of all with the Newfoundland dog. Should a foreign dog be affected, he almost certainly dies. The greater part of the northern dogs brought by Captain Parry did not survive a twelvemonth; and the delicate Italian greyhound has little chance, when imported from abroad.

Not only does it thus differ in different species of dogs, but in different breeds of the same species. I have known several gentlemen who have laboured in vain for many years, to rear particular and valuable breeds of pointers and greyhounds. The distemper would uniformly carry off five out of six. Other sportsmen laugh at the supposed danger of distemper, and declare that they seldom lose a dog. This hereditary predisposition to certain kinds of disease cannot be denied, and is not sufficiently attended to. When a peculiar fatality has often followed a certain breed, the owner should cross it from another kennel, and especially from the kennel of one who boasts of his success in the treatment of distemper. This has occasionally succeeded far beyond expectation.

It is time to proceed to the symptoms of this disease; but here there is very considerable difficulty, for it is a truly protean malady, and it is impossible to fix on any symptom that will invariably characterise it.

An early and frequent symptom is a gradual loss of appetite, spirits, and condition: the dog is less obedient to his master, and takes less notice of him. The eyes appear weak and watery; and there will be a very slight limpid discharge from the nose. In the morning there will, perhaps, be a little indurated mucus at the inner corner of the eye. This may continue two or three weeks without serious or scarcely recognisable illness. Then a peculiar husky cough is heard, altogether different from the sonorous cough of catarrh, or the wheezing of asthma. It is an apparent attempt to get something from the fauces or throat. By degrees the discharge from the eyes and nose, and particularly the former, will increase. More mucus will collect in the corners of the eye; and the eye will sometimes be closed in the morning. The conjunctiva, and particularly that portion which covers the sclerotica, will be considerably injected, but there will not be the usual intense redness of inflammation. The vessels will be large and turgid rather than numerous, and frequently of a darkish hue.

Occasionally, however, the inflammation of the conjunctiva will be exceedingly intense, the membrane vividly red, and the eye impatient of light. An opacity spreads over the cornea, and this is quickly succeeded by ulceration. The first spot of ulceration is generally found precisely in the centre of the cornea, and is perfectly circular; this will distinguish it from a scratch or other injury. The ulcer widens and deepens, and sometimes eats through the cornea, and the aqueous humour escapes. Fungous granulations spring from it, protrude through the lids, and the animal evidently suffers extreme torture.

A remarkable peculiarity attends this affection of the eye. However violent may be the inflammation, and by whatever disorganization it may be accompanied, if we can cure the distemper, the granulations will disappear, the ulcer will heal, the opacity will clear away, and the eye will not eventually suffer in the slightest degree. One-fourth part of the mischief in other cases, unconnected with distemper, would inevitably terminate in blindness; but permanent blindness is rarely the consequence of distemper.

It may not be improper here shortly to revert to the different appearance of the eye in rabies. In the early stage of this malady there is an unnatural and often terrific brightness of the eye; but the cornea in distemper is from the first rather clouded. In rabies there is frequent strabismus, with the axis of the eye distorted outwards. The apparent squinting of the eye in distemper is caused by the probably unequal protrusion of the membrana nictitans over a portion of the eye at the inner canthus, in order to protect it from the light. In rabies, the white cloudiness which I have described, and the occasional ulceration with very little cloudiness, and the ulceration, are confined to the cornea; but a dense green opacity comes on, speedily followed by ulceration and disorganization of every part of the eye.

The dog will, at this stage of distemper, be evidently feverish, and will shiver and creep to the fire. He will more evidently and rapidly lose flesh. The huskiness will be more frequent and troublesome, and the discharge from the nose will have greater consistence. It will be often and violently sneezed out, and will gradually become more or less purulent. It will stick about the nostrils and plug them up, and thus afford a considerable mechanical obstruction to the breathing.

The progress of the disease is now uncertain. Sometimes fits come on, speedily following intense inflammation of the eye; or the inflammation of the nasal cavity appears to be communicated, by proximity, to the membrane of the brain. One fit is a serious thing. If it is followed by a second within a day or two, the chances of cure are diminished; and if they rapidly succeed each other, the dog is almost always lost. These fits seldom appear without warning; and, if their approach is carefully watched, they may possibly be prevented.

However indisposed to eat the dog may previously have been, the appetite returns when the fits are at hand, and the animal becomes absolutely voracious. Nature seems to be providing for the great expenditure of power which epilepsy will soon occasion. The mucus almost entirely disappears from the eyes, although the discharge from the nose may continue unabated; and for an hour or more before the fit there will be a champing of the lower jaw, frothing at the mouth, and discharge of saliva. The champing of the lower jaw will be seen at least twelve hours before the first fit, and will a little while precede every other. There will also be twitchings of some part of the frame, and usually of the mouth, cheek, or eyelid. It is of some consequence to attend to these, as enabling us to distinguish between fits of distemper and those of teething, worms, or unusual excitement. The latter come on suddenly. The dog is apparently well, and racing about full of spirits, and without a moment's warning he falls into violent convulsions.

We may here, likewise, be enabled to distinguish between rabies and distemper. When a person, unacquainted with dogs, sees a dog struggling in a fit, or running along unconscious of every surrounding object, or snapping at everything in his way, whether it be a human being or a stone, he raises the cry of "mad dog," and the poor brute is often sacrificed. The very existence of a fit is proof positive that the dog is not mad. No epilepsy accompanies rabies in any stage of that disease.

The inflammation of the membrane of the nose and fauces is sometimes propagated along that of the windpipe, and the dog exhibits unequivocal proofs of chest affection, or decided pneumonia.

At other times the bowels become affected, and a violent purging comes on. The fæces vary from white with a slight tinge of gray, to a dark slate or olive colour. By degrees mucus begins to mingle with the fæcal discharge, and then streaks of blood. The fæcal matter rapidly lessens, and the whole seems to consist of mingled mucus and blood; and, from first to last, the stools are insufferably offensive. When the mingled blood and mucus appear, so much inflammation exists in the intestinal canal that the case is almost hopeless.

The discharge from the nose becomes decidedly purulent. While it is white and without smell, and the dog is not too much emaciated, the termination may be favourable; but when it becomes of a darker colour, and mingled with blood, and offensive, the ethmoid or turbinated bones are becoming carious, and death supervenes. This will particularly be the case if the mouth and lips swell, and ulcers begin to appear on them, and the gums ulcerate, and a sanious and highly offensive discharge proceeds from the mouth. A singular, half-fetid smell arising from the dog, is the almost invariable precursor of death.

When the disease first visited the continent, it was regarded as a humoral disease. Duhamel, who was one of the earliest to study the character of the malady, contended that the biliary sac contained the cause of the complaint; the bile assumed a concrete form, and its superabundance was the cause of disease. Barrier, one of the earliest writers on the subject, described it as a violent irregular bilious fever. Others regarded it as a mucous discharge, or a depurative; and others, as a salutary crisis, removing from the constitution that which oppressed the different organs. Others had recourse to inoculation, in order to give it a more benign character; and others, and among them Chabert, considered that it possessed a character of peculiar malignity, and he gave it a name expressive of its nature and situation—*nasal catarrh*. It exhibited the ordinary symptoms of coryza: it was a catarrhal affection in its early stage; but it afterwards degenerated into a species of palsy. The causes were unknown. By some, they were attributed to the natural voracity of the dog; by others, to his occasional lasciviousness; by others, to his frequent feeding on carrion, or the refuse of fat and soups.

There is no doubt that nasal catarrh is, to a very considerable degree, contagious on the continent. It often spreads over a wide extent of country, and includes numerous animals of various descriptions. It is complicated with various diseases; and particularly, at an early stage, with ophthalmia. It may be interesting to the reader to trace the progress of the disease among our continental neighbours. It commences with a certain depression of spirits; a diminution of appetite; a heaviness of the head; a heat of the mouth; an attempt to get something from the throat; an insatiable thirst; an elevated temperature of the body; a dry and painful suffocating cough; and all these circumstances continue from twenty to thirty days, until at length the dog droops and dies.

The duration of distemper is uncertain. It sometimes runs its course in five or six days; or it may linger on two or three months. In some cases the emaciation is rapid and extreme: danger is then to be apprehended. When the muscles of the loins are much attenuated, or almost wasted, there is little hope; and, although otner symptoms may remit, and the dog may be apparently recovering, yet, if he continues to lose flesh, we may be perfectly assured that he will not live. On the other hand, let the discharge from the nose be copious, and the purging violent, and every other symptom threatening, yet if the animal gains a little flesh, we may confidently predict his recovery.

When the dog is much reduced in strength and flesh, a spasmodic affection or twitching of the muscles will sometimes be observed. It is usually confined at first to one limb; but the most decisive treatment is required, or these spasms will spread until the animal is altogether unable to stand; and while he lies every limb will be in motion, travelling, as it were, at the rate of twenty miles an hour, until the animal is worn out, and dies of absolute exhaustion. When these spasms become universal and violent, they are accompanied by constant and dreadful moans and cries.

In the pointer and the hound, and particularly when there is little discharge from the eyes or nose, an intense yellowness often suddenly appears all over the dog. He falls away more in twenty-four hours than it would be thought possible; his bowels are obstinately constipated; he will neither eat nor move; and in two or three days he is dead.

In the pointer, hound, and greyhound, there sometimes appears on the whole of the chest and belly a pustular eruption, which peels off in large scales. The result is usually unfavourable. A more general eruption, however, either wearing the usual form of mange, or accompanied by minute pustules, may be regarded as a favourable symptom. The disease is leaving the vital parts, and expending its last energy on the integument.

The *post-mortem* appearances are exceedingly unsatisfactory: they do not correspond with the original character of the disease, but with its strangely varying symptoms. If the dog has died in fits, we have inflammation of the brain or its membranes, and particularly at the base of the brain, with considerable effusion of a serous or bloody fluid. If the prevailing symptoms have led our attention to the lungs, we find inflammation of the bronchial passages, or, in a few instances, of the substance of the lungs, or the submucous tissue of the cells. We rarely have inflammation of the pulmonary pleura, and never to any extent of the intercostal pleura. In a few lingering cases, tubercles and vomicæ of the lungs have been found.

If the bowels have been chiefly attacked, we have intense inflammation of the mucous membrane, and, generally speaking, the small intestines are almost filled with worms. If the dog has gradually wasted away, which is often the case when purging to any considerable extent has been encouraged or produced, we have contraction of the whole canal, including even the stomach, and sometimes considerable enlargement of the mesenteric glands.[a]

[a] The following is a very frequent and unexaggerated history of distemper, when calomel has been given in too powerful doses:—

The membrane of the nose will always exhibit marks of in flammation, and particularly in the frontal sinuses and ethmoidal cells; and I have observed the portion of membrane on the septum, or cartilaginous division of the nostrils, between the frontal sinuses and ethmoidal cells, to be studded with small miliary tubercles. In advanced stages of the disease, attended with much defluxion from the nose, the cells of the ethmoidal bone and the frontal sinuses are filled with pus.

Ulceration is sometimes found on the membrane of the nose, oftenest on the spot to which I have referred — occasionally confined to that; and now and then spreading over the whole of the septum, and even corroding and eating through it; generally equal on both sides of the septum; in a few instances extending into the fauces; seldom found in the larynx, but occasionally seen in the bronchial passages. The other viscera rarely present any remarkable morbid appearance.

The distemper is clearly a disease of the mucous membranes, usually commencing in the membrane of the nose, and resembling nasal catarrh. In the early stage it is *coryza*, or nasal catarrh; but the affection rapidly extends, and seems to attack the mucous membranes generally, determined to some particular one, either by atmospheric influence or accidental causes, or constitutional predisposition. The fits arise from general disturbance of the system, or from the proximity of the brain to the early seat of inflammation.

This account of the nature and treatment of distemper will, perhaps, be unsatisfactory to some readers. One thing, however, is clear, that for a disease which assumes such a variety of forms, there can be no specific; yet there is not a keeper who is not in possession of some supposed infallible nostrum. Nothing can be more absurd. A disease attacking so many organs, and presenting so many and such different symptoms, must require a mode of treatment varying with the organ attacked and the symptom

August 30, 1828. — A spaniel, six months old, has been ailing a fortnight, and three doses of calomel have been given by the owner. He has violent purging, with tenesmus and blood. Half an ounce of castor-oil administered.—31*st*. Astringents, morning, noon, and night. — *Sept.* 6. The astringents have little effect, or, if the purging is restrained one day, it returns with increased violence on the following day. Getting rapidly thin. Begins to husk. Astringents continued.—10*th*. The purging is at last overcome, but the huskiness has rapidly increased, accompanied by laborious and hurried respiration.—Bleed to the extent of three ounces. —11*th*. The breathing relieved, but he obstinately refuses to eat, and is forced several times in the day with arrow-root or strong soup.—18*th*. He had become much thinner and weaker, and died in the evening. No appearance of inflammation on the thoracic viscera, nor in any part of the alimentary canal. The intestines are contracted through their whole extent.—Veterinarian, ii. 290.

prevailing. The faith in these boasted specifics is principally founded on two circumstances—atmospheric influence and peculiarity of breed. There are some seasons when we can scarcely save a dog; there are others when we must almost wilfully destroy him in order to lose him. There are some breeds in which, generation after generation, five out of six die of distemper, while there are others in which not one out of a dozen dies. When the season is favourable, and the animal, by hereditary influence, is not disposed to assume the virulent type of the disease, these two important agents are overlooked, and the immunity from any fatal result is attributed to medicine. The circumstances most conducive to success will be the recollection that it is a disease of the mucous surfaces, and that we must not carry the depleting and lowering system too far. Keeping this in view, we must accommodate ourselves to the symptoms as they arise.

The natural medicine of the dog seems to be an emetic. The act of vomiting is very easily excited in him, and, feeling the slightest ailment, he flies to the dog-grass, unloads his stomach, and is at once well. In distemper, whatever be the form which it assumes, an emetic is the first thing to be given. Common salt will do when nothing else is at hand; but the best emetic, and particularly in distemper, consists of equal parts of calomel and tartar emetic. From half a grain to a grain and a half of each will constitute the dose.

This will act first as an emetic, and afterwards as a gentle purgative. Then, if the cough is urgent, and there is heaving at the flanks, and the nose is hot, a moderate quantity of blood may be taken—from three to twelve ounces — and this, if there has been previous constipation, may be followed by a dose of sulphate of magnesia, from two to six drachms.

In slight cases this will often be sufficient to effect a cure: but, if the dog still droops, and particularly if there is much huskiness, the antimonial or James's powder, nitre and digitalis, in the proportion of from half a grain to a grain of digitalis, from two to five grains of the James's powder, and from a scruple to a drachm of nitre, should be administered twice or thrice in a day. If on the third or fourth day the huskiness is not quite removed, the emetic should be repeated.

In these affections of the mucous membranes, it is absolutely necessary to avoid or to get rid of every source of irritation, and worms will generally be found a very considerable one in young dogs. If we can speedily get rid of them, distemper will often rapidly disappear; but, if they are suffered to remain, diarrhœa or fits are apt to supervene: therefore some worm medicine should be administered.

I have said that vomiting is very easily excited in the dog; and that for this reason we are precluded from the use of a great many medicines in our treatment of him. Calomel, aloes, jalap, scammony, and gamboge will generally produce sickness. We are, therefore, driven to some mechanical vermifuge; and a very effectual one, and that will rarely fail of expelling even the tape-worm, is tin filings or powdered glass. From half a drachm to a drachm of either may be advantageously given twice in the day. There may generally be added to them digitalis, James's powder, and nitre, made into balls with palm oil and a little linseed meal. This course should be pursued in usual cases until two or three emetics have been given, and a ball morning and night on the intermediate days. Should the huskiness not diminish after the first two or three days, if the dog has not rapidly lost flesh, I should be disposed to take a little more blood, and to put a seton in the poll. It should be inserted between the ears, and reaching from ear to ear.

When there is fever and huskiness, and the dog is not much emaciated, a seton is an excellent remedy; but, if it is used indiscriminately, and when the animal is already losing ground, and is violently purging, we shall only hasten his doom, or rather make it more sure.

It is now, if ever, that pneumonia will be perceived. The symptoms of inflammation in the lungs of the dog can scarcely be mistaken. The quick and laborious breathing, the disinclination or inability to lie down, the elevated position of the head, and the projection of the muzzle, will clearly mark it. More blood must be subtracted, a seton inserted, the bowels opened with Epsom salts, and the digitalis, nitre, and James's powder given more frequently and in larger doses than before.

Little aid is to be derived from observation of the pulse of the dog; it differs materially in the breed, and size, and age of the animal. Many years' practice have failed in enabling me to draw any certain conclusion from it. The best place to feel the pulse of the dog is at the side. We may possibly learn from it whether digitalis is producing an intermittent pulse, which it frequently will do, and which we wish that it should do: it should then be given a little more cautiously, and in smaller quantities.

If the pneumonia is evidently conquered, or we have proceeded thus far without any considerable inflammatory affection of the chest, we must begin to change our plan of treatment. If the huskiness continues, and the discharge from the nose is increased and thicker, and the animal is losing flesh and becoming weak, we must give only half the quantity of the sedative and diuretic medicine, and add some mild tonic, as gentian, chamomile, and ginger, with occasional emetics, taking care to keep the bowels in a laxative but not purging state. The dog should likewise be urged to eat; and, if he obstinately refuses all food, he should be forced with strong beef jelly, for a very great degree of debility will now ensue.

We have thus far considered the treatment of distemper from its commencement; but it may have existed several days before we were consulted, and the dog may be thin and husky, and refusing to eat. In such case we should give an emetic, and then a dose of salts, and after that proceed to the tonic and fever balls.

Should the strength of the animal continue to decline, and the discharge from the nose become purulent and offensive, the fever medicine must be omitted, and the tonic balls, with carbonate of iron, administered. Some veterinary surgeons are very fond of gum resins and balsams. Mr. Blaine, in his excellent treatise on the distemper in his Canine Pathology, recommends myrrh and benjamin, and balsam of Peru and camphor. I much doubt the efficacy of these drugs. They are beginning to get into disrepute in the practice of human medicine; and I believe that if they were all banished from the veterinary Materia Medica we should experience no loss. When the dog begins to recover, although not so rapidly as we could wish, the tonic balls, without the iron, may be advantageously given, with now and then an emetic, if huskiness should threaten to return; but mild and wholesome food, and country or good air, will be the best tonics.

If the discharge from the nose become very offensive, the lips swelled and ulcerated, and the breath fetid, half an ounce of yeast may be administered every noon, and the tonics morning and night; and the mouth should be frequently washed with a solution of chloride of lime.

At this period of the disease the sub-maxillary glands are sometimes very much enlarged, and a tumour or abscess is formed, which, if not timely opened, breaks, and a ragged, ill-conditioned ulcer is formed, very liable to spread, and very difficult to heal. It is prudent to puncture this tumour as soon as it begins to point, for it will never disperse. After the opening, a poultice should be applied to cleanse the ulcer; after which it should be daily washed with the compound tincture of benjamin, and dressed with calamine ointment. Some balls should be given, and the animal liberally fed.

Should the fits appear in an early stage, give a strong emetic; then bleed, and open the bowels with five or six grains of calomel and a quarter of a grain of opium: after this insert a seton, and then commence the tonic balls.

The progress of fits in the early stages of the disease may thus be arrested. The occurrence of two or three should not make us despair; but, if they occur at a later period, and when the dog is much reduced, there is little hope. This additional expenditure of animal power will probably soon carry him off. All that is to be done, is to administer a strong emetic, obviate costiveness by castor oil, and give the tonic balls with opium.

Of the treatment of the yellow disease little can be said; we shall not succeed in one case in twenty. When good effect has been produced, it has been by one large bleeding, opening the bowels well with Epsom salts, and then giving grain doses of calomel twice a day in a tonic ball.

While it is prudent to obviate costiveness, we should recollect that there is nothing more to be dreaded, in every stage of distemper, than diarrhœa. The purging of distemper will often bid defiance to the most powerful astringents. This shows the folly of giving violent cathartics in distemper; and, when I have heard of the ten, and twenty, and thirty grains of calomel that are sometimes given, I have thought it fortunate that the stomach of the dog is so irritable. The greater part of these kill-or-cure doses is ejected, otherwise the patient would soon be carried off by super-purgation. There is an irritability about the whole of the mucous membrane that may be easily excited, but cannot be so readily allayed; and, therefore, except in the earliest stage of distemper, or in fits, or limiting ourselves to the small portion of calomel which enters into our emetic, I would never give a stronger purgative than castor-oil or Epsom salts. It is of the utmost consequence that the purging of distemper should be checked as soon as possible.

In some diseases a sudden purging, and even one of considerable violence, constitutes what is called the crisis. It is hailed as a favourable symptom, and from that moment the animal begins to recover; but this is never the case in distemper: it is a morbid action which is then going on, and which produces a dangerous degree of debility.

The proper treatment of purging in cases of distemper, is first to give a good dose of Epsom salts, in order to carry away anything that may offend, and then to ply the animal with mingled absorbents and astringents. A scruple of powdered chalk, ten grains of catechu, and five of ginger, with a quarter of a grain of opium, made into a ball with palm oil, may be given to a middle-sized dog twice or thrice every day. To this may be added injections of gruel, with the compound chalk mixture and opium.

When the twitchings which I have described begin to appear, a seton is necessary, whatever may be the degree to which the animal is reduced. Some stimulating embrocation, such as tincture of cantharides, may be rubbed along the whole course of the spine; and the medicine which has oftenest, but not always, succeeded, is castor-oil, syrup of buckthorn, and syrup of white poppies, given morning and night, and a tonic ball at noon. If the dog will not now feed, he should be forced with strong soup. As soon, however, as the spasms spread over him, accompanied by a moaning that increases to a cry, humanity demands that we put an end to that which we cannot cure. Until this happens I would not despair; for many dogs have been saved that have lain several days perfectly helpless.

As to the chorea which I have mentioned as an occasional sequel of distemper, if the dog is in tolerable condition, and especially if he is gaining flesh, and the spring or summer is approaching, there is a chance of his doing well. A seton is the first thing; the bowels should be preserved from constipation; and the nitrate of silver, in doses of one-eighth of a grain, made into a pill with linseed meal, and increased to a quarter of a grain, should be given morning and night.

We should never make too sure of the recovery of a distempered dog, nor commit ourselves by too early a prognosis. It is a treacherous disease; the medicines should be continued until every symptom has fairly disappeared; and for a month at least.

It may be interesting to add the following account of the distemper in dogs, by Dr. Jenner. Several of our modern writers have copied very closely from him.

"That disease among dogs which has familiarly been called the 'distemper,' has not hitherto, I believe, been much noticed by medical men. My situation in the country favouring my wishes to make some observations on this singular malady, I availed myself of it, during several successive years, among a large number of foxhounds belonging to the Earl of Berkeley; and, from observing how frequently it has been confounded with hydrophobia, I am induced to lay the result of my inquiries before the Medical and Chirurgical Society. It may be difficult, perhaps, precisely to ascertain the period of its first appearance in Britain. In this and the neighbouring counties, I have not been able to trace it back beyond the middle of the last century; but it has since spread universally. I knew a gentleman who, about forty-five years ago, destroyed the greater part of his hounds, from supposing them mad, when the distemper first broke out among them; so little was it then known by those most conversant with dogs. On the continent I find it has been known for a much longer period; it is as contagious among dogs as the small-pox, measles, or scarlet fever among the human species; and the contagious miasmata, like those arising from the diseases just mentioned, retain their infectious properties a long time after separation from the distempered animal. Young hounds, for example, brought in a state of health into a kennel, where others have gone through the distemper, seldom escape it. I have endeavoured to destroy the contagion by ordering every part of a kennel to be carefully washed with water, then whitewashed, and finally to be repeatedly fumigated with the vapour of marine acid, but without any good result.

"The dogs generally sicken early in the second week after exposure to the contagion: it is more commonly a violent disease than otherwise, and cuts off at least one in three that are attacked by it. It commences with inflammation of the substance of the lungs, and generally of the mucous membrane of the bronchi. The inflammation at the same time seizes on the membranes of the nostrils, and those lining the bones of the nose, particularly the nasal portion of the ethmoid bone. These membranes are often inflamed to such a degree as to occasion extravasation of blood, which I have observed coagulated on their surface. The breathing is short and quick, and the breath is often fetid; the teeth are covered with a dark mucus. There is frequently a vomiting of a glairy fluid. The dog commonly refuses food, but his thirst seems insatiable, and nothing cheers him like the sight of water. The bowels, although generally constipated as the disease advances, are frequently affected with diarrhœa at its commencement. The eyes are inflamed, and the sight is often obscured by mucus secreted from the eyelids, or by opacity of the cornea. The brain is often affected as early as the second day after the attack; the animal becomes stupid, and his general habits are changed. In this state, if not prevented by loss of strength, he sometimes wanders from his home. He is frequently endeavouring to expel by forcible expirations the mucus from the trachea and fauces, with a peculiar rattling noise. His jaws are generally smeared with it, and it sometimes flows out in a frothy state, from his frequent champing.

"During the progress of the disease, especially in its advanced stages, he is disposed to bite and gnaw anything within his reach; he has sometimes epileptic fits, and a quick succession of general though slight convulsive spasms of the muscles. If the dog survive, this affection of the muscles continues through life. He is often attacked with fits of a different description; he first staggers, then tumbles, rolls, cries as if whipped, and tears up the ground with his teeth and fore feet: he then lies down senseless and exhausted. On recovering, he gets up, moves his tail, looks placid, comes to a whistle, and appears in every respect much better than before the attack. The eyes, during this paroxysm, look bright, and, unless previously rendered dim by mucus, or opacity of the cornea, seem as if they were starting from their sockets. He becomes emaciated, and totters from feebleness in attempting to walk, or from a partial paralysis of the hind legs. In this state he sometimes lingers on till the third or fourth week, and then either begins to show signs of returning health (which seldom happens when the symptoms have continued with this degree of violence), or expires. During convalescence, he has sometimes, though rarely, profuse hæmorrhage from the nose.

"When the inflammation of the lungs is very severe, he frequently dies on the third day. I know one instance of a dog dying within twenty-four hours after the seizure; and in that short space of time the greater portion of the lungs was, from exudation, converted into a substance nearly as solid as the liver of a sound animal. In this case the liver itself was considerably inflamed, and the eyes and flesh universally were tinged yellow, though I did not observe anything obstructing the biliary ducts. In other instances I have also observed the eyes looking yellow.

"The above is a description of the disease in its several forms; but in this, as in the diseases of the human body, there is every gradation in its violence.

"There is also another affinity to some human diseases, viz., that the animal which has once gone through it very rarely meets with a second attack. Fortunately this distemper is not communicable to man. Neither the effluvia from the diseased dog nor the bite have proved in any instance infectious; but, as it has often been confounded with canine madness, as I have before observed, it is to be wished that it were more generally understood; for those who are bitten by a dog in this state are sometimes thrown into such perturbation that hydrophobic symptoms have actually arisen from the workings of the imagination. Mr. John Hunter used to speak of a case somewhat of this description in his lectures.

"A gentleman who received a severe bite from a dog, soon after fancied the animal was mad. He felt a horror at the sight of liquids, and was actually convulsed on attempting to swallow them. So uncontrollable were his prepossessions, that Mr. Hunter conceived he would have died had not the dog which inflicted the wound been found and brought into his room in perfect health. This soon restored his mind to a state of tranquillity. The sight of water no longer afflicted him, and he quickly recovered."[a]

Palsy, more or less complete, is sometimes the termination of the distemper in dogs.

It is usually accompanied by chorea, and it is then, in the majority of cases, hopeless. Setons should be inserted in the poll, being then, as nearly as possible, at the commencement of the spinal cord. They should be well stimulated and worn a considerable time. If they fail, a plaster composed of common pitch, with a very small quantity of yellow wax and some powdered cantharides, spread on sheep's-skin, should be placed over the whole of the lumbar and sacral regions, extending half-way down the thigh

[a] Medico-Chirurgical Transactions, 21st March, 1809.

on either side. The bowels should be kept open by mild aperients, in order that every source of irritation may be removed from the intestinal canal. Some mild and general tonic will likewise be useful, such as gentian and ginger.

CHAPTER XV.

SMALL-POX; MANGE; WARTS; CANCER; FUNGUS HÆMATODES; SORE FEET.

SMALL-POX.

In 1809, there was observed, at the Royal Veterinary School at Lyons, an eruptive malady among the dogs, to which they gave the name of *small-pox.* It appeared to be propagated from dog to dog by contagion. It was not difficult of cure; and it quickly disappeared when no other remedies were employed than mild aperients and diaphoretics. A sheep was inoculated from one of these dogs. There was a slight eruption of pustules formed on the place of inoculation, but nowhere else; nor was there the least fever.

At another time, also, at the school at Lyons, a sheep died of the regular sheep-pox. A part of the skin was fastened, during four-and-twenty hours, on a healthy sheep, and the other part of it on a dog, both of them being in apparent good health. No effect was produced on the dog, but the sheep died of confluent sheep-pox.

The essential symptoms of small-pox in dogs succeed each other in the following order: the skin of the belly, the groin, and the inside of the fore arm, becomes of a redder colour than in its natural state, and sprinkled with small red spots irregularly rounded. They are sometimes isolated, sometimes clustered together. The near approach of this eruption is announced by an increase of fever.

On the second day the spots are larger, and the integument is slightly tumefied at the centre of each.

On the third day the spots are generally enlarged, and the skin is still more prominent at the centre.

On the fourth day the summit of the tumour is yet more prominent. Towards the end of that day, the redness of the centre begins to assume a somewhat gray colour. On the following days, the pustules take on their peculiar characteristic appearance, and cannot be confounded with any other eruption. On the summit is a white circular point, corresponding with a certain quantity of nearly transparent fluid which it contains, and covered by a thin and transparent pellicle. This fluid becomes less and less transparent, until it acquires the colour and consistence of pus. The pustule, during its serous state, is of a rounded form. It is flattened when the fluid acquires a purulent character, and even slightly depressed towards the close of the period of suppuration, and when that of desiccation is about to commence, which ordinarily happens towards the ninth or tenth day of the eruption. The desiccation and the desquamation occupy an exceedingly variable length of time; and so, indeed, do all the different periods of the disease. What is the least inconstant, is the duration of the serous eruption, which is about four days, if it has been distinctly produced and guarded from all friction. If the general character of the pustules is considered, it will be observed, that, while some of them are in a state of serous secretion, others will only have begun to appear.

The eruption terminates when desiccation commences in the first pustules; and, if some red spots show themselves at that period of the malady, they disappear without being followed by the development of pustules. They are a species of abortive pustules. After the desiccation, the skin remains covered by brown spots, which, by degrees, die away. There remains no trace of the disease, except a few superficial cicatrices on which the hair does not grow.

The causes which produce the greatest variation in the periods of the eruption are, the age of the dog, and the temperature of the situation and of the season. The eruption runs through its different stages with much more rapidity in dogs from one to five months old than in those of greater age. I have never seen it in dogs more than eighteen months old. An elevated temperature singularly favours the eruption, and also renders it confluent and of a serous character. A cold atmosphere is unfavourable to the eruption, or even prevents it altogether. Death is almost constantly the result of the exposure of dogs having small-pox to any considerable degree of cold. A moderate temperature is most favourable to the recovery of the animal. A frequent renewal or change of air, the temperature remaining nearly the same, is highly favourable to the patient; consequently close boxes or kennels should be altogether avoided.

I have often observed, that the perspiration or breath of dogs labouring under variola emits a very unpleasant odour. This smell is particularly observed at the commencement of the desiccation of the pustules, and when the animals are lying upon dry straw; for the friction of the bed against the pustules destroys their pellicles, and permits the purulent matter to escape; and the influence of this purulent matter is most pernicious. The fever is increased, and also the unpleasant smell from the mouth, and that of the fæces. In this state there is a disposition which is rapidly developed in the lungs to assume the character of pneumonia. This last complication is a most serious one, and almost always terminates fatally. It has a peculiar character. It shows itself suddenly, and with all its alarming symptoms. It is almost immediately accompanied by a purulent secretion from the bronchi, and the second day does not pass without the characters of pneumonia being completely developed. The respiration is accompanied by a mucous *râle* which often becomes sibilant. The nasal cavities are filled with a purulent fluid. The dog that coughs violently at the commencement of the disease, employs himself, probably, on the following day, in ejecting, by a forcible expulsion from the nostrils, the purulent secretion which is soon and plentifully developed. When he is lying quiet, and even when he seems to be asleep, there is a loud, stertorous, guttural breathing.

MANGE.

The existence of certain insects found burrowing under the skin of the human being, and of various tribes of animals, has been acknowledged from the 12th century. In the 17th century, correct engravings of these insects were produced. On the other hand many doubted their existence, because it had not been their lot to see them. In 1812, Galés, a pupil in the hospital of St. Louis, pretended to have found some of them. They were put into the hands of M. Raspail, of Paris, who proved that they were nothing more than the common cheese-mites; and substituted by Galés for those seen by Bonomo.

Professor Hertwig, of Berlin, has given a graphic sketch of these insects (Veterinarian, vol. xi. pp. 373, 489).

Mr. Holthouse states that, "placed on the skin of a healthy individual, they excite a disease in the part to which they were confined, having all the characters of scabies; that insects taken from mangy sheep, horses, and dogs, and transplanted to healthy individuals of the same species, produce in them a disease analogous to that in the animals from which they were taken; and that there are too many well-attested cases on record to permit us to doubt of scabies having been communicated from animals to man.

Mange may in some degree be considered as an hereditary disease. A mangy dog is liable to produce mangy puppies, and the progeny of a mangy bitch will certainly become affected sooner or later. In many cases a propensity to the disease will be speedily produced. If the puppies are numerous, and confined in close situations, the effluvia of their transpiration and fæcal discharges will often be productive of mange very difficult to be removed. Close confinement, salted food, and little exercise, are frequent causes of mange.

The Scabby Mange is a frequent form which this disease assumes. It assumes a pustular and scabby form in the red mange, particularly in white-haired dogs, when there is much and painful inflammation. A peculiar eruption, termed surfeit, which resembles mange, is sometimes the consequence of exposure to cold after a hot sultry day. Large blotches appear, from which the hair falls and leaves the skin bare and rough. Acute mange sometimes takes on the character of erysipelas; at other times there is considerable inflammation. The animal exhibits heat and restlessness, and ulcerations of different kinds appear in various parts, superficial but extensive. Bleeding, aperient and cooling medicines are indicated, and also applications of the subacetate of lead, or spermaceti ointment. A weak infusion of tobacco may be resorted to when other things fail, but it must be used with much caution. The same may be said of all mercurial preparations. The tanner's pit has little efficacy, except in slight cases. Slight bleedings may be serviceable, and especially in full habits; setons may be resorted to in obstinate cases. A change in the mode of feeding will often be useful. Mild purgatives, and especially Epsom salts, are often beneficial, and also mercurial alteratives, as Æthiop's mineral with cream of tartar and nitre. The external applications require considerable caution. If mercury is used, care must be taken that the dog does not lick it. The diarrhœa produced by mercury often has a fatal effect.

Unguents are useful, but considerable care must be taken in their application. They must be applied to the actual skin, not over the hair. In old and bad cases much time and patience will be requisite. Mr. Blaine had a favourite setter who had virulent mange five years. He was ordered to be dressed every day, or every second day, before the disease was completely conquered.

Cutaneous affections have lately been prevalent to an extent altogether unprecedented on this and on the other side of the channel. In the latter part of 1843 the disease assumed a character which had not been known among us for many years. The common mange, which we used to think we could easily grapple with, was now little seen: even the usual red mange with the fox-coloured stain was not of more frequent occurrence than usual, but an intolerable itchiness with comparatively little redness of skin, and rarely sufficient to account for the torture which the animal seemed to endure, and often with not the slightest discoloration of the integument, came before us almost every day, and under its influence the dog became ill-tempered, dispirited, and emaciated, until he sunk under its influence. All unguents were thrown away here

Lotions of corrosive sublimate, decoction of bark, infusion of digitalis or tobacco, effected some little good; but the persevering use of the iodine of potassium, purgatives, and the abstraction of blood very generally succeeded.

The sudden appearance of redness of the skin, and exudation from it, and actual sores attending the falling off of the hair, and itching, that seemed to be intolerable, have also been prevalent to an unprecedented extent. This mange, however, is to a certain degree manageable. A dose or two of physic should be given, with an application of a calamine powder, and the administration of the iodide of potassium.

Mr. Blaine gives a most valuable account of mange in the dog, part of which I shall quote somewhat at length. Mange exerts a morbid constitutional action on the skin; it is infectious from various miasmata, and it is contagious from personal communication. In some animals it may be produced by momentary contact: it descends to other animals of various descriptions; there is no doubt that it is occasionally hereditary: it is generated by effluvia of many various kinds; almost every kind of rancid or stimulating food is the parent of it. High living with little exercise is a frequent cause of it, and the near approach of starvation is not unfavourable to it. The scabby mange is the common form under which it generally appears. In red mange the whole integument is in a state of acute inflammation; surfeit, or blotches, a kind of cuticular eruption breaks out on particular parts of the body without the slightest notice, and, worse than all, a direct febrile attack, with swelling and ulceration, occurs, under which the dog evidently suffers peculiar heat and pain. Last of all comes local mange. Almost every eruptive disease, whether arising from the eye, the ear, the scrotum, or the feet, is injurious to the quality as well as the health of every sporting dog: the scent invariably becomes diseased, and the general powers are impaired.

There are several accounts of persons who, having handled mangy dogs, have been affected with an eruption very similar to the mange. A gentleman and his wife who had been in the habit of fondling a mangy pug dog, were almost covered with an eruption resembling mange. Several of my servants in the dog-hospital have experienced a similar attack; and the disease was once communicated to a horse by a cat that was accustomed to lie on his back as he stood in the stall.

WARTS.

These are often unpleasant things to have to do with. A Newfoundland dog had the whole of the inside of his mouth lined with warts. I applied the following caustic:—Hyd. suc-corrosivi ʒj., acidi mur. ʒ, alcoholis ℥iiij., aquæ ℥ij. The warts were touched twice every day, and in less than a fortnight they had all disappeared.

Another dog had its mouth filled with warts, and the above solution was applied. In four days considerable salivation came on, and lasted a week, but at the expiration of that time the warts had vanished. The owner of the dog had applied the solution with the tip of her finger; she experienced some salivation, which she attributed to this cause.

The skin of the dog, from the feebleness of its perspiratory functions, is little sensible to the influence of diaphoretics: therefore we trust so much to external applications for the cure of diseases of the skin of that animal.

CANCER.

This is a disease too frequent among females of the dog tribe, and occasionally seen in the male. Its symptoms, local and general, are various. They are usually very obscure in their commencement; they increase without any limit; they are exasperated by irritants of any kind; and in the majority of cases their reproduction is almost constant, and perfectly incurable.

With regard to the female, it is mostly connected with the secretion of milk. Two or three years may pass, and at almost every return of the period of œstrum, there will be some degree of enlargement or inflammation of the teats. Some degree of fever also appears; but, after a few weeks have passed away, and one or two physic balls have been administered, everything goes on well. In process of time, however, the period of œstrum is attended by a greater degree of fever and enlargement of the teats, and at length some diminutive hardened nuclei, not exceeding in size the tip of a finger, are felt within one of the teats. By degrees they increase in size; they become hard, hot, and tender. A considerable degree of redness begins to appear. Some small enlargements are visible. The animal evidently exhibits considerable pain when these enlargements are pressed upon. They rapidly increase, they become more hot and red, various shining protuberances appear about the projection, and at length the tumour ulcerates. A considerable degree of sanious matter flows from the aperture.

The tumours, however, after a while diminish in size; the heat and redness diminish; the ulcer partly or entirely closes, but, after a while, and especially when the next period of œstrum arrives, the tumour again increases, and with far greater rapidity than before, and then comes the necessity of the removal of the tumour, or if not, the destruction of the animal. In the great majority of cases, the removal of the cancer does not destroy the dog, but lessens its torture. The knife and the forceps must usually be resorted to, and in the hands of a skilful surgeon the life of the animal will be saved.

When the cancer is attached to the neighbouring parts by cellular substance alone, no difficulty will be experienced in detaching the whole of it. The operation will be speedily performed, and there will be an end of the matter; but, if the tumour has been neglected, and the muscular, the cellular, or even the superficial parts have been attacked, the utmost caution is requisite that every diseased portion shall be removed. Mr. Blaine adds to this that "it must also be taken into the account, that, although in the canine cancer ulceration does not often reappear in the intermediate part, when the operation has been judiciously performed, yet, when the constitution has been long affected with this ulcerative action, it is very apt to show itself in some neighbouring part soon after."

FUNGUS HÆMATODES.

In the month of March, 1836, a valuable pointer dog was sent to Mr. Adam of Beaufort, quite emaciated, with total loss of appetite, and with a large fungus hæmatodes about the middle of the right side of his neck. It had begun to appear about five months before, and was not at first larger than a pea. Mr. Adam gave him a purgative of Barbadoes aloes, which caused the discharge of much fetid matter from the intestines. At the expiration of three days he removed the tumour with the knife. There was a full discharge of healthy matter from the wound. During the period of its healing the animal was well fed, and ferruginous tonics were given. In a little more than three weeks the wound had completely filled up with healthy granulations, and the dog was sent home to all appearance quite well.

At the expiration of three months another tumour made its appearance near the situation of the former one, growing fast; it had attained nearly the size of the other. Mr. Adam removed it immediately, ordering a system of nutritive feeding and tonics. It appeared at first to go on favourably; but, five days after the removal of the second one, a third made its appearance.

This was removed at the expiration of another five days; but the animal was totally unable to walk, with very laborious breathing and cold extremities. A cathartic was given and the legs bandaged; but the wounds made no progress towards healing, and at the end of three days he died. On exposing the cavity of the thorax it was almost covered with variously formed tumours, from the size of a pigeon's egg to that of a small pea. The intercostal muscles had many of these adhering to them, and a few small ones were developed on the heart. There were three on the diaphragm, in the centre of which matter was formed. The blood-vessels, kidneys, &c., were free from disease. These tumours were white, or nearly so, rather hard, and of a glandular substance. The external ones were soft, red, and almost destitute of blood-vessels, except the first, which bled considerably. There was dropsy of the abdomen.

SORE FEET

constitute a frequent and troublesome complaint. It consists of inflammation of the vascular substance, between the epidermis and the parts beneath. It is the result of numerous slight contusions, produced by long travelling in dry weather, or hunting over a hard and rough country, or one covered with frost and snow. The irritation with which it commences continues to increase, and a certain portion of fluid is determined to the feet, and tubercles are formed, hard, hot, and tender, until the whole foot is in a diseased state, considerably enlarged. The animal sadly suffers, and is scarcely able to stand up for a minute. Sometimes the ardour of the chase will make him for a while forget all this; but on his return, and when he endeavours to repose himself, it is with difficulty that he can be got up again. The toes become enlarged, the skin red and tender, and the horny sole becomes detached and drops. Local fever, and that to a considerable extent, becomes established; it reacts on the general economy of the animal, who scarcely moves from his bed, and at length refuses all food. At other times a separation takes place between the dermis and the epidermis, which is a perfect mass of serosity.

Still, however, it is only when all this has much increased, or has been neglected, that any permanently dangerous consequences take place. When violent inflammation has set in, the feet must be carefully attended to, or the dog may be lamed for life. One or two physic-balls may be given; all salted meat should be removed, and the animal supplied with food without being compelled to move from his bed. The feet should be bathed with warm water, and a poultice of linseed meal applied to them twice in the day. If, as is too often the case, he should tear this off, the feet should be often fomented. It is bad practice in any master of dogs to suffer them to be at all neglected when there are any tokens of inflammation of the feet. The neglect of even a few days may render a dog a cripple for life. If there are evident appearances of pus collecting about the claws, or any part of the feet, the abscess should be opened, well bathed with warm water, and friar's balsam applied to the feet.

When the feet have been neglected, the nail is apt to grow very rapidly, and curve round and penetrate into the foot. The forceps should be applied, and the claws reduced to their proper size.

If there are any indications of fever, or if the dog should be continually lying down, or he should hold up his feet, and keep them apart as much as he can, scarifications or poultices, or both, should be resorted to.

When the feet of a dog become sore in travelling, the foolish habit of washing them with brine should never be permitted, although it is very commonly resorted to. Warm fomentations, or warm pot-liquor, or poultices of linseed meal should be applied, or, if matter is apparently forming, the lancet may be resorted to.

Dogs are frequently sent to the hospital with considerable redness between the toes, and ichorous discharge, and the toes thickened round the base of the nails, as if they were inclined to drop off. The common alterative medicine should be given, and a lotion composed of hydrarg. oxym. gr. vi., alcohol ℥j., et aq. calcis ℥iiij., should be applied to the feet three times every day. Leathern gloves should be sewn on them. These cases are often very obstinate.

Generally speaking, the dog has five toes on the fore feet, and four on the hind feet, with a mere rudiment of a fifth metatarsal bone in some feet; but, in others, the fifth bone is long and well proportioned, and advances as far as the origin of the first phalanx of the neighbouring toe.

[The editor begs leave to add a more detailed and systematic treatise of the affections generally attacking the feet and limbs of our dogs.

DISEASES OF THE FEET.

SORE FEET.

Inflammation of the feet, a disease somewhat analogous to founder in horses, and often attended with equally bad results, particularly in the English kennels, is comparatively rare with us, although there are few sportsmen but have met with some cases among their dogs. The feet become tender, swollen, and hot, violent inflammatory action sets in, the toes become sore, the claws diseased, and the balls very painful, and often suppurate.

The animal is thus speedily rendered useless; not being able to support his body, owing to the intense pain, he remains in his house, and employs the most of his time in temporarily assuaging his sufferings by constantly licking the diseased members.

Causes.—Running long distances over frozen or stony grounds, hunting over a rough and ill-cleaned country, over-feeding, confinement, and lazy habits, are all conducive in some measure to this affection.

This form of disease is not uncommon among those dogs used in toling ducks on the Chesapeake bay, these animals being obliged to run incessantly to and fro over the gravel shores, in their efforts to attract the canvass-back. We have seen many dogs that have been made cripples by this arduous work, and rendered prematurely old while yet in their prime. It would certainly be wise and humane on the part of those who pursue this sport either for pleasure or gain, to provide suitable boots for these sagacious animals, who in return would repay such kindness by increased ardour and length of service. These articles might be made of leather, or some other durable substance, in such a manner that they could be laced on every morning before commencing their labours.

The claws should be allowed to project through openings in the boot, as this arrangement will give much more freedom to the feet, and the boot itself will not be destroyed so soon by the penetration of the toes through its substance. Boots thus neatly made will neither interfere with his locomotive nor swimming powers, but add greatly to the comfort of the animal, and secure his services for many years.

Treatment.—No stimulating applications to the feet are to be used, such as salt water, ley, fish brine, or urine, but rather emollient poultices and cooling washes. These last-mentioned remedies should be carefully applied, and the dog confined to his house as much as possible: in fact, there is little difficulty in restraining him in this respect, as he has but little inclination or ability to move about.

Purging balls should be administered every night, and blood abstracted if there be much fever, as indicated in the heat, swelling, and pain of the limbs.

If the balls continue to swell, and there is a collection of pus within them, they may be opened by the lancet, and the contents evacuated, after which apply a linseed poultice. When the inflammation has subsided, simple dressings of melted butter or fresh lard will generally effect a cure.

PUSTULAR AFFECTION OF THE FEET.

Dogs frequently have a pustular eruption between the toes, either accompanying mange or some other skin disease, or entirely independent of any other affection.

Causes.—Want of cleanliness, bad housing, improper food, vermin, and depraved constitution.

Treatment.—Frequent washing with castile soap and water will correct this disease; the feet and legs after washing should be rubbed dry, particularly between the toes. When the pustules are large, they may be opened with the lancet and a poultice applied. If the disease appears complicated with mange, or dependent upon other general causes, the primary affection must be removed by the proper remedies, which generally carries off with it the second ary disease.

SPRAINS.

It is not an uncommon occurrence for dogs, while running, climbing fences, or jumping ditches, to sprain themselves very severely in the knee, or more frequently in the shoulder-joint; and if not properly attended to, will remain cripples for life, owing to enlargement of the tendon and deposition of matter.

We once had a fine, large, powerful bull-dog, that sprained himself in the shoulder while running very violently in the street after another dog, and in some way, owing to his great eagerness to overtake the other, tripped up when at the top of his speed, fell on his chest, and when he arose commenced limping, and evidently suffered from considerable pain. On taking him home, we examined his feet, limbs, and chest very particularly, expecting to find a luxation or fracture of some of the bones of the leg or feet, or perhaps the presence of a piece of glass or other article deeply imbedded in the ball. None of the above accidents, however, being brought to light by our examination, or that of a medical friend who expressed a wish to see our patient, we concluded that a simple sprain of some of the tendons had taken place.

On the following day there was slight swelling and tenderness of the shoulder-joint, accompanied by great unwillingness to put the foot to the ground, owing to the pain that seemed to be produced by the extension of the leg. The limb was fomented, and the dog confined for several days, till the swelling and tenderness disappeared; but, greatly to our astonishment and that of others, he still remained lame as before.

This lameness continued for several months, when we parted with him, sending him to a relative in the country, who informed us that he never recovered the use of his limb, but that it became shrivelled and deformed for want of use.

The cause of lameness in this dog is as unaccountable as some cases of lameness we see in horses. We are convinced that there was neither fracture nor luxation, nor any other unnatural displacement of the parts, and can attribute it to nothing but enlargement of one of the tendons of the shoulder-joint, resulting from inflammation. If it had been in our power, we should have liked to have examined this animal after death.

Treatment. — Hot fomentations to the part affected, together with purging balls and bleeding, if there be great tenderness and swelling of the limb. When the inflammation and tumefaction have disappeared, rub the parts with opodeldoc, or other stimulating mixtures.

WOUNDS OF THE FEET.

Dogs are apt to cut their feet by stepping upon sharp tools, bits of oyster-shell, old iron, &c., or by the introduction of thorns, burrs, nails, bits of glass, and other articles, into their balls.

Treatment.—If the cut be very deep, or divides the ball, the foot must be washed in tepid water, and the edges of the wound drawn together and retained in their position by a couple of sutures or a strap or two of adhesive plaster, and the animal confined.

Where thorns or sand-burrs have pierced the foot, diligent search should be made to extract them, or the wound will suppurate, and the dog continue lame for a long time. This caution is particularly necessary when minute particles of glass have entered the foot. A poultice in such cases should be applied, after removing every particle within our reach, and the foot be wrapped up, or, what is better, enclosed in a boot of some kind, sufficiently strong to protect it from the dirt or other small particles which otherwise would enter the wound and prevent its healing. In a case of great emergency, one of our friends hunted a setter dog three successive days in a leather boot, which we instructed a country cobbler to put on him to protect his foot from a recent and deep cut, that he had received from treading upon some farming utensils. The boot was taken off every night, the foot nicely cleaned, the leather oiled and replaced ready for the following day. The wound afterwards healed up, and no trace of the incision now remains. The boot should be made of stout, flexible leather, and extend beyond the first joint; the seam must be in front, so as not to interfere with the dog's tread. There should be openings for the claws, and the sole large enough to allow the expansion of the ball pads when in motion: a small layer of tow had better be laid on the bottom of the foot before putting on the boot.

It is often very difficult to tell the exact spot where a briar or thorn has entered the foot, owing to its penetrating so far into the substance of the ball as to be entirely concealed under the skin, or by the swelling of the parts surrounding it. In all such cases the bottom of the foot should be gently pressed by the thumb, and the point where the dog exhibits symptoms of most pain should be particularly examined, and, if necessary, cut down upon to extract the extraneous substance, no matter what it may be.

LONG NAILS OR CLAWS.

The nails of some dogs require occasional cutting, otherwise they grow so long and fast that they turn in and penetrate the ball of the foot. If we cut them, a strong, sharp knife is necessary for the purpose; filing them off we consider far preferable.

LAMENESS.

Dogs, as well as horses, become lame from stiff joints, splints, and sprains. Stiff joints are occasioned by anchylosis, or the deposit of calcareous or osseous matter within the ligament or around the head of the bone, which latter defect is known as ring-bone in the horse.

Treatment.—Stimulating friction to the parts, such as spirits of camphor, or camphorated liniment, mercurial ointment, tincture of iodine, opodeldoc, blistering, &c.—L.]

CHAPTER XVI.

FRACTURES.

These are of not unfrequent occurrence in the dog; and I once had five cases in my hospital at the same time.

In the human subject, fractures are more frequent in adults, and, perhaps, in old men, than in infants; but this is not the case with the smaller animals generally, and particularly with dogs. Five-sixths of the fractures occur between the time of weaning and the animal being six months old; not, perhaps, because of their chemical composition, that the bones are more fragile at this age; but because young dogs are more exposed to fall from the hands of the persons who carry them, and from the places to which they climb; and the extremities of the bones, then being in the state of epiphysis, are easily separated from the body of the bone. When the fracture takes place in the body of the bone, it is transverse or somewhat oblique, but there is scarcely any displacement.

A simple bandage will be sufficient for the reduction of these fractures, which may be removed in ten or twelve days, when the preparatory callus has acquired some consistence. One only out of twenty dogs that were brought to me with fractures of the extremities, in the year 1834, died. Two dogs had their jaws fractured by kicks from horses, and lost several of their teeth. In one of them the anterior part of the jaw was fractured perpendicularly; in the other, both branches were fractured. Plenty of good soup was injected into their mouths. Ten or twelve days afterwards, they were suffered to lap it; and in a little while they were dismissed cured.

It will be desirable, perhaps, to describe our usual method of reducing the greater part of the fractures which come under our notice.

I.—The *humerus* was fractured just above the elbow and close to the joint. The limb was enclosed in adhesive plaster, and supported by a firm bandage. The bones were beginning to unite, when, by some means concerning which I could never satisfy myself, the *tibia* was broken a little above the hock. Nothing could well be done with this second fracture; but great care was taken with regard to the former. The lower head of the humerus remained somewhat enlarged; but the lameness became very slight, and in three weeks had nearly or quite disappeared. Nothing was done to the second fracture; in fact, nothing more than a slight annular enlargement, surrounding the part, remained—a proof of the renovating power of nature.

II.—A spaniel was run over by a light carriage. It was unable to put the left hind leg to the ground, and at the upper tuberosity of the ileum some crepitus could be distinguished. I subtracted six ounces of blood, administered a physic-ball, and ordered the patient to be well fomented with warm water several times during the night. On the following day no wound could be discovered, but there was great tenderness. I continued the fomentation. Two or three days afterwards she was evidently easier. I then had the hair cut close, and covered the loins and back with a pitch-plaster. At the expiration of six days the plaster was getting somewhat loose, and was replaced by another with which a very small quantity of powdered cantharides was mingled. At the expiration of the fifth week she was quite well.

III.—The *thigh-bone* had been broken a fortnight. It was a compound fracture: the divided edges of the bone protruded through the integuments, and there was no disposition to unite. It is not in one case in a hundred that an animal thus situated can be saved. We failed in our efforts, and the dog was ultimately destroyed.

IV.—The *femur* was broken near the hip. I saw it on the third day, when much heat and swelling had taken place. I ordered the parts to be frequently bathed with warm water. The heat and tenderness to a considerable degree subsided, and the pitch-plaster was carefully applied. At the expiration of a week the plaster began to be loosened. A second one was applied, and when a fortnight longer had passed, a slight degree of tenderness alone remained.

V.—The following account is characteristic of the bull terrier. The *radius* had been broken, and was set, and the bones were decidedly united, when the dog, in a moment of frantic rage, seized his own leg and crushed some of the bones. They were once more united, but his wrist bent under him in the form of a concave semicircle, as if some of the ligaments of the joint had been ruptured in the moment of rage. It was evident on the following day that it was impossible to control him, and he was destroyed.

VI.—A spaniel, three months old, became fractured half-way between the wrist and the *elbow*. A surgeon bound it up, and it became swollen to an enormous size, from the adhesive plaster that had been applied and the manner of placing the splints. I removed the splints. On the following morning I had the arm frequently fomented: a very indistinct crepitus could be perceived at the point of the humerus: I applied another plaster higher up, and including the elbow. The hair not having been cut sufficiently close, the plaster was removed, applied much more neatly and closely, and the original fracture was firmly bound together. No crepitus was now to be perceived.

I saw no more of our patient for four days, when I found that he had fallen, and that the elbow on the other side was fractured within the capsular ligament. A very distinct crepitus could be felt, and the dog cried sadly when the joint was moved. I would have destroyed him, but he was a favourite with his master, and we tried what a few days more would produce. I enclosed the whole of the limb in a plaster of pitch, and bound it up without splints. Both the bandages remained on nearly a fortnight, when the fractures were found to be perfectly united, and the lameness in both legs gradually disappeared.

VII.—*July* 22, 1843. A spaniel was frightened with something on the bed, and fell from it, and cried very much. The instep, or wrist, of the *right leg*, before was evidently bowed, and there was considerable heat and tenderness. It was well fomented on the two following days, and then set, and adhesive plaster was tightly applied, and a splint bound over that. *24th.* The foot began to swell, and was evidently painful. The outer bandage was loosened a little, but the inner bandage was not touched. *Aug.* 4. The bandage, that had not been meddled with for eleven days, now appeared to give him some pain. For the last two days he has been gently licking and gnawing it. The splints were removed; but the adhesive plaster appearing even and firm, was suffered to remain. *26th.* Everything appeared to be going on well, when he again leaped from his bed. The wrist was much more bowed, and was tender and hot. Simple lint and a firm calico bandage were had recourse to. *27th.* He is unable to put his foot to the ground, and the joint is certainly enlarging. An adhesive plaster, made by a Frenchman, was applied at the owner's request, over which was placed a splint. The dog soon began to gnaw the plaster, which formed a sticky but not very adhesive mass. Before night the pain appeared to be very great, and the dog cried excessively. I was sent for. We well fomented the leg, and then returned to our former treatment. There was evidently a great deal of pain, but it gradually passed over, and a slight degree of lameness alone remained.

I have great pleasure in adding the following accounts of the successful treatment of fractures in dogs by Mr. Percivall:—

"Hopeless as cases of fracture in horses generally are, from the difficulty experienced in managing the patient, they are by no means to be so regarded in dogs. I have in several instances seen dogs recover, and with very good use of the parts, if not perfect restoration of them, when the accidents have been considered, at the time they took place, of a nature so irremediable as to render it advisable to destroy the animals.

"*May* 4, 1839. A valuable Irish spaniel fell from a high wall, and fractured his *off shoulder*. On examination, I found the os humeri fractured about an inch above its radial extremity, causing the limb to drop pendulously from the side, and depriving the animal of all use of it. The arm, by which I mean the fore arm, was movable in any direction upon the shoulder, and there was distinct crepitus: in a word, the nature of the accident was too plain to admit of doubt; nor was there any splinter or loose piece of bone discoverable. I directed that the animal might be laid flat upon his sound side in a hamper, or covered basket or box, of sufficient dimensions, but not large enough to admit of his moving about; to have his hind legs fettered, his mouth muzzled, and his injured parts covered with a linen cloth wetted with a spirit lotion. *May* 5. The parts are tumefied, but not more, nor even so much as one might have expected. Continue the lotion. 6*th*. At my request, Mr. Youatt was called in to give his opinion as to the probability of effecting a cure. He thought from the inconvenient situation of the fracture, that the chances of success were doubtful; and recommended that a plaster, composed of thick sheep-skin and pitch, cut to the shape of the parts, should be applied, extending from the upper part of the shoulder down upon the arm, and reaching to the knee; and that the whole should be enveloped in well-applied bandages, one of them being carried over the shoulders and brought round between the fore legs, to support the limb, and aid in retaining the fractured ends in apposition. Prior to the application of the pitch plaster the hair was closely shorn off. Thus bound up, the dog was replaced in his hamper, and had some aperient medicine given to him. 8*th*. The medicine has operated; and he appears going on well, his appetite continuing unimpaired. 10*th*. He growls when I open the basket to look at him. On examining him (while his keeper had hold of him), I found the plaster loosening from its adhesion; I took it off altogether, and applied a fresh one, composed of the stopping composition I use for horses' feet. *June* 7. Up to this time everything appears to have been going on properly. The fracture feels as if it were completely united, and, as the plaster continues to adhere firmly, I thought the bandages enveloping it, as they were often getting loose, might now be dispensed with, and that the dog might with benefit be chained to a kennel, instead of being so closely confined as he has been. In moving, he does not attempt to use the fractured limb, but hops along upon the three other legs. *July.* He has acquired pretty good use of the limb. Being now at liberty, he runs about a good deal; halting, from there being some shortness of the limb, but not so much as to prevent him being serviceable, as a 'slow' hunter, in the sporting-field.

"About a twelvemonth ago," continues Mr. Percivall, "I was consulted concerning a blood-hound of great size and beauty, and of the cost of 50*l*., that had been a cripple in one of his hind limbs for some considerable time past, owing, it was said or thought, to having received some injury. After a very careful handling and examination of the parts about the hips, the places where he expressed pain, I came to the conclusion that there had been, and still existed, some fracture of *the ischial portion of the pelvis*, but precisely where, or of what nature, I could not determine; and all the treatment I could recommend was, that the animal should be shut up within a basket or box of some sort, of dimensions only sufficient to enable him to lie at ease, and that he be kept there for at least six months, without being taken out, save for the purpose of having his bed cleansed or renewed. His owner had previously made up his mind to have him destroyed; understanding, however, from me, that there still remained a chance of his recovery, he ordered his groom to procure a proper basket, and see that the dog's confinement was such as I had prescribed. The man asked me to allow him to have his kennel, which, being no larger than was requisite for him, I did not object to; and to this he had an iron lattice-door made, converting it into a sort of wild beast cage. After two months' confinement, I had him let out for a short run, and perceived evident amendment. I believe altogether that he was imprisoned five months, and then was found so much improved that I had him chained to his kennel for the remaining month, and this, I believe, was continued for another month. The issue was the complete recovery of the animal, very much to the gratification and joy of his master, by whom he is regarded as a kind of unique or unobtainable production.

"The fractures of dogs and other animals must, of course, be treated in accordance with all the circumstances of their cases; but I have always considered it a most essential part of their treatment that such portable patients as dogs and cats, &c., should be placed and kept in a state of confinement, where they either could not, or were not likely to, use or move the fractured parts; and, moreover, I have thought that failure, where it has resulted after such treatment, has arisen from its not having been sufficiently long persisted in."

In the opinion of Professor Simonds, when there is fracture of the bones of the extremities, a starch bandage is the best that can be employed. If applied wet, it adapts itself to the irregularities of the limbs; and if allowed to remain on twelve hours undisturbed, it forms a complete case for the part, and affords more equal support than anything else that can possibly be used.

The following case was one of considerable interest. It came under the care of Professor Simonds. Two gentlemen were playing at quoits, and the dog of one of them was struck on the head by a quoit, and supposed to be killed. His owner took him up, and found that he was not dead, although dreadfully injured. It being near the Thames, his owner took him to the edge of the river, and dashed some water over him, and he rallied a little. Professor Simonds detected a fracture of the skull, with pressure on the brain, arising from a portion of depressed bone. The dog was perfectly unconscious, frequently moaning, quite incapable of standing, and continually turning round upon his belly, his straw, or his bed. It was a case of coma; he took no food, and the pulsation at the heart was very indistinct.

"I told the proprietor that there was no chance of recovery except by an operation; and, even then, I thought it exceedingly doubtful. I was desired to operate, and I took him home.

"The head was now almost twice as large as when the accident occurred, proceeding from a quantity of coagulated blood that had been effused under the skin covering the skull. I gave him a dose of aperient medicine, and on the following morning commenced my operation."

"The hair was clipped from the head, and an incision carried immediately from between the eye-brows to the back part of the skull, in the direction of the sagittal suture. Another incision was made from this towards the root of the ear. This triangular flap was then turned back, in order to remove the coagulated blood and make a thorough exposure of the skull. I was provided with a trephine, thinking that only a portion of the bone had been depressed on the brain, and it would be necessary, with that instrument, to separate it from its attachment, and then with an elevator remove it; but I found that the greater part of the parietal bone was depressed, and that the fracture extended along the sagittal suture from the coronal and lamdoidal sutures. At three-fourths of the width of the bone, the fracture ran parallel with the sagittal suture, and this large portion was depressed upon the tunics of the brain, the dura mater being considerably lacerated. The depressed bone was raised with an elevator, and I found, from its lacerated edges and the extent of the mischief done, that it was far wiser to remove it entirely, than to allow it to remain and take the chance of its uniting.

"In a few days, the dog began to experience relief from the operation, and to be somewhat conscious of what was taking place around him. He still requires care and attention, and proper medicinal agents to be administered from time to time; but with the exception of occasionally turning round when on the floor, he takes his food well, and obeys his master's call."[a]

CHAPTER XVII.

MEDICINES USED IN THE TREATMENT OF THE DISEASES OF THE DOG.

These are far more numerous and complicated than would, on the first consideration of them, be imagined. The Veterinary Surgeon has a long list of them, suited to the wants and dangers, imaginary or real, of his patients; and he who is not scientifically acquainted with them, will occasionally blunder in the choice of remedies, or the application of the means of cure which he adopts. Little attention may, perhaps, be paid to the medical treatment of the dog; yet it requires not a little study and experience. I will endeavour to give a short account of the drugs, and mode of using them, generally employed.

The administering of medicines to dogs is, generally speaking, simple and safe, if a little care is taken about the matter, and especially if two persons are employed in the operation. The one should be sitting with the dog between his knees, and the hinder part of the animal resting on the floor. The mouth is forced open by the pressure of the fore-finger and thumb upon the lips of the upper jaw, and the medicine can be conveniently introduced with the other hand, and passed sufficiently far into the throat to insure its not being returned. The mouth should be closed and kept so, until the bolus has been seen to pass down. Mr. Blaine thus describes the difference between the administration of liquid and solid medicines:—"A little attention will prevent all danger. A ball or bolus should be passed completely over the root of the

[a] Trans. Vet. Med. Assoc., i. 51.

tongue, and pushed some way backward and forward. When a liquid is given, if the quantity is more than can be swallowed at one effort, it should be removed from the mouth at each deglutition, or the dog may be strangled. Balls of a soft consistence, and those composed of nauseous ingredients, should be wrapped in thin paper, or they may disgust the dog and produce sickness."

Dogs labouring under disease should be carefully nursed: more depends on this than many persons seem to be aware. A warm and comfortable bed is of a great deal more consequence than many persons who are fond of their dogs imagine. Cleanliness is also an essential point. Harshness of manner and unkind treatment will evidently aggravate many of their complaints. I have sometimes witnessed an angry word spoken to a healthy dog produce instant convulsions in a distempered one that happened to be near; and the fits that come on spontaneously in distemper, almost instantly leave the dog by soothing notice of him.

Acidum Acetum (*Vinegar*).—This is useful for sprains, bruises, and fomentations.

Acidum Nitricum (*Nitric Acid; Aqua Fortis*).—This may be used with advantage to destroy warts or fungous excrescences. A little of the acid should be dropped on the part and bound tightly down. The protuberance will slough off and healthy granulations will spring up. A surer application, however, is the nitrate of silver.

Acidum Hydrocyanicum (*Prussic Acid*).—This is an excellent application for the purpose of allaying irritation of the skin in dogs; but it must be very carefully watched. I have seen a drachm of it diluted with a pint of distilled water, rapidly allay cuticular inflammation. The dreadful degree of itching which had been observed during the last two or three years yielded to this application alone; and to that it has almost invariably yielded, a little patience being used.

Acupuncturation is a practice lately introduced into veterinary surgery. It denotes the insertion of a needle into the skin or flesh of a person or animal suffering severely from some neuralgic affection. The needle is small and sharp: it is introduced by a slight pressure and semi-rotating motion between the thumb and forefinger, and afterwards withdrawn with the same motion. This should always employ a quarter of an hour at least, and in cases of very great pain it should continue two hours; but when the object is to afford an exit to the fluid collected, mere puncture is sufficient. It is attended with very little pain; and therefore it may be employed at least with safety if not with advantage. The operation was known and practised in Japan, many years ago; but it was only in the seventeenth century that its singular value was ascertained. In 1810 some trials of it were made in Paris, and

M. Chenel took the lead. He had a young dog that he had cured of distemper, except that a spasmodic affection of the left hind leg remained. He applied a needle, and with fair success. He failed with another dog; but M. Prevost, of Geneva, relieved two mares from rheumatism, and an entire horse that had been lame sixteen months. In the Veterinary School at Lyons acupuncturation was tried on two dogs. One had chorea, and the other chronic paralysis of the muscles of the neck. The operation had no effect on the first; the other came out of the hospital completely cured. In the following year acupuncturation was tried without success in the same school. Four horses and two dogs were operated upon in vain.

Adeps (*Hog's Lard*) forms the basis of all our ointments. It is tasteless, inodorous, and free from every stimulating quality.

Alcohol (*Rectified Spirit*).—This is principally used in tinctures, and seldom or never administered to the dog in a pure state.

Aloes, Barbadoes.—From these are formed the safest and best aperients for the dog—consisting of powdered aloes, eight parts; antimonial powder, one part; ginger, one part; and palm oil, five parts; beaten well together, and the size of the ball varying from half a drachm to two drachms, and a ball administered every fourth or fifth hour. Mr. Blaine considers it to be the safest general purgative. He says that such is the peculiarity of the bowels of the dog, that while a man can take with impunity as much calomel as would kill two large dogs, a moderate-sized dog will take a quantity of aloes sufficient to destroy two stout men. The smallest dog can take 15 or 20 grains; half a drachm is seldom too much; but the smaller dose had better be tried first, for hundreds of dogs are every year destroyed by temerity in this particular. Medium-sized dogs usually require a drachm; and some large dogs have taken two or even three drachms.

Alteratives are medicines that effect some slow change in the diseased action of certain parts, without interfering with the food or work. The most useful consist of five parts of sublimed sulphur, one of nitre, one of linseed meal, and two of lard or palm oil.

Alum is a powerful astringent, whether employed externally or internally. It is occasionally administered in doses of from 10 to 15 grains in obstinate diarrhœa. In some obstinate cases, alum whey has been employed in the form of a clyster.

Oxide of Antimony, in the form of a compound powder, and under the name of James's powder, is employed as a sudorific, or to cause a determination to the skin.

The *Antimonii Potassio Tartras* (*Tartar Emetic*), besides its effect on the skin, is a useful nauseant, and invaluable in inflammation of the lungs and catarrhal affections of every kind. The *Black Sesquisulphuret of Antimony* is a compound of sulphur and antimony, and an excellent alterative.

Argenti Nitras—Nitrate of Silver (*Lunar Caustic*).—I have already strongly advocated the employment of this caustic for empoisoned wounds and bites of rabid animals. In my opinion it supersedes the use of every other caustic, and generally of the knife. I have also given it internally as a tonic to the dog, in cases of chorea, in doses from an eighth to a quarter of a grain. A dilute solution may be employed as an excitant to wounds, in which the healing process has become sluggish. For this purpose, ten grains or more may be dissolved in a fluid ounce of distilled water. A few fibres of tow dipped in this solution, being drawn through the channel which is left on the removal of a seton, quickly excite the healing action. Occasionally one or two drops of this solution may be introduced into the eye for the purpose of removing opalescence of the cornea. In cases of fungoid matter being thrown out on the cornea, the fungus may be touched with a rod of nitrate of silver, and little pain will follow.

The *Peruvian Bark,* or its active principle the disulphate of quina, is a valuable tonic in distemper, especially when combined with the iodide of iron; the iron increasing with the general tone of the system, and the iodine acting as a stimulant to the absorbents.

Blisters are occasionally useful or indispensable in some of the casualties and diseases to which the dog is liable. They are mostly of the same description, and act upon the same principles as in the horse, whether in the form of plaster, or ointment, or stimulating fluid. Blisters can be kept on the dog with difficulty: nothing short of a wire muzzle will suffice; Mr. Blaine says, that for very large dogs, he used to be compelled to make use of a perforated tin one. The judgment of the practitioner will determine in these cases, as well as with regard to the horse, whether the desired effect should be produced by severe measures or by those of a milder character, by active blisters or by milder stimulants: the difficulty of the measures to be adopted, and the degree of punishment that may be inflicted, being never forgotten by the operator.

We have stated in our work on the Horse, that "the art of blistering consists in cutting or rather shaving the hair perfectly close; then well rubbing in the ointment, and afterwards, and, what is of the greatest consequence of all, plastering a little more of the ointment lightly over the part, and leaving it. As soon as the vesicles have perfectly risen, which will be in twenty or twenty-four hours, the torture of the animal may be somewhat relieved by the application of olive or neat's-foot oil, or any emollient ointment.

"An infusion of two ounces of the cantharides in a pint of oil of turpentine, for several days, is occasionally used as a languid blister; and when sufficiently lowered with common oil, it is called a *sweating* oil, for it maintains a certain degree of irritation and inflammation on the skin, yet not sufficient to blister; and thus gradually abates or removes some old or deep inflammation, or cause of lameness."[a]

Iodine in various cases is now rapidly superseding the cantharides and the turpentine.

Calomel.—Sufficient has been said of this dangerous medicine in the course of the present work. I should rarely think of exhibiting it, except in small doses for the purpose of producing that specific influence on the liver, which we know to be the peculiar property of this drug. In large doses it will to a certain extent produce vomiting; and, if it finds its way into the intestines, it acts as a powerful drastic purgative.

Castor Oil (*Oleum Ricini*).—This is a most valuable medicine. It is usually combined with the syrup of buckthorn and white poppies, in the proportions of three parts of the oil to two of the buckthorn and one of the poppy-syrup; which form a combination of ingredients in which the oleaginous, stimulant, and narcotic ingredients happily blend.

Catechu.—This is an extract from the wood of an acacia-tree (*Acacia catechu*), and possesses a powerful astringent property. It is given in cases of superpurgation, united with opium, chalk, and powdered gum. A tincture of it is very useful for the purpose of hastening the healing principle of wounds. Professor Morton says, that he considers it as the most valuable of the vegetable astringents.

Clysters.—Professor Morton gives an account of the use of clysters. The objects, he says, for which they are administered, are—1. To empty the bowels of fæces: thus they act as an aperient. Also, to induce a cathartic to commence its operations, when, from want of exercise or due preparation, it is tardy in producing the desired effect. Clysters operate in a twofold way: first, by softening the contents of the intestines; and, secondly, by exciting an irritation in one portion of the canal which is communicated throughout the whole; hence they become valuable when the nature and progress of the disease require a quick evacuation of the bowels. The usual enema is warm water, but this may be rendered more stimulating by the addition of salt, oil, or aloes. 2. For the purpose of killing worms that are found in

[a] The Horse, p. 501.

the rectum and large intestines: in this case, it is usually of an oleaginous nature. 3. For restraining diarrhœa: sedatives and astringents being then employed. 4. For nourishing the body when food cannot be received by the mouth. Gruel is generally the aliment thus given. 5. For allaying spasms in the stomach and bowels.

Copper.—Both the verdigris, or subacetate, and the blue vitriol of sulphate of copper, are now comparatively rarely used. They are employed either in the form of a fine powder, or mixed with an equal quantity of the acetate of lead in order to destroy proud flesh or stimulate old ulcers. They also form a part of the ægyptiacum of the farrier. There are many better drugs to accomplish the same purpose.

Creosote is seldom used for the dog. We have applications quite as good and less dangerous. It may be employed as a very gentle excitant and antiseptic.

Creta Preparata (*Chalk*), in combination with ginger, catechu, and opium, is exceedingly useful; indeed, it is our most valuable medicine in all cases of purging, and particularly the purging of distemper.

Digitalis is an exceedingly valuable drug. It is a direct and powerful sedative, a mild diuretic, and useful in every inflammatory and febrile complaint.

Gentian and *Ginger* are both valuable; the first as a stomachic and tonic, and the last as a cordial and tonic. It is occasionally necessary, or at least desirable, to draw this distinction between them.

Chloride of Lime is a useful application for ill-conditioned wounds and for the frequent cleansing of the kennel.

Epsom Salts, or *Sulphate of Magnesia*, are mild yet effective in their action: with regard to cattle and sheep, they supersede every other aperient; for the dog, however, they must yield to the castor-oil mixture.

Mercury.—The common mercurial ointment is now comparatively little used. It has given way to the different preparations of iodine. In direct and virulent mange, it is yet, however, employed under the form of calomel, and combined with aloes, but in very small doses, never exceeding three grains. It is also useful in farcy and jaundice. The corrosive sublimate is occasionally used for mange in the dog, and to destroy vermin; but it is a very uncertain and dangerous medicine.

Palm Oil would be an excellent emollient, if it were not so frequently adulterated with turmeric root in powder. It is far milder than the common lard.

Nitrate of Potash is a valuable cooling and mild diuretic, in doses of eight or ten grains.

Sulphur is the basis of the most effectual applications for mange. It is a good alterative, combined usually with antimonials and nitre, and particularly useful in mange, surfeit, grease, hide-bound, and want of condition.

Turpentine is an excellent diuretic and antispasmodic; it is also a most effectual sweating blister and highly useful in strains.

The Sulphate of Zinc is valuable as an excitant to wounds, and promotes adhesion between divided surfaces and the *radix*.

APPENDIX.

THE NEW LAWS OF COURSING,

As Revised and Enlarged at a Meeting of Noblemen and Gentlemen, held at the Thatched House Tavern, St. James's Street, June 1, 1839.

I. Two stewards shall be appointed by the members at dinner each day, to act in the field the following day, and to preside at dinner. They shall regulate the plan of beating the ground, under the sanction of the owner or occupier of the soil.

II. Three or five members, including the secretary for the time being, shall form a Committee of Management, and shall name a person, for the approbation of the members, to judge all courses—all doubtful cases shall be referred to them.

III. All courses shall be from slips, by a brace of greyhounds only.

IV. The time of putting the first brace of dogs in the slips shall be declared at dinner on the day preceding. If a prize is to be run for, and only one dog is ready, he shall run a by, and his owner shall receive forfeit: should neither be ready, the course shall be run when the Committee shall think fit. In a match, if only one dog be ready, his owner shall receive forfeit; if neither be present, the match shall be placed the last in the list.

V. If any person shall enter a greyhound by a name different from that in which he last appeared in public, without giving notice of such alteration, he shall be disqualified from winning, and shall forfeit his match.

VI. No greyhounds shall be entered as puppies unless born on or after the 1st of January of the year preceding the day of running.

VII. Any member, or other person, running a greyhound at the meeting, having a dog at large which shall join in the course then running, shall forfeit one sovereign; and, if belonging to either of the parties running, the course shall be decided against him.

VIII. The judge ought to be in a position where he can see the dogs leave the slips, and to decide by the colour of the dogs to a person appointed for that purpose: his decision shall be final.

IX. If, in running for prizes, the judge shall be of opinion that the course has not been of sufficient length to enable him to decide as to the merits of the dogs, he shall inquire of the Committee whether he is to decide the course or not; if in the negative, the dogs shall be immediately put again into the slips.

X. The judge shall not answer any questions put to him regarding a course, unless such questions are asked by the Committee.

XI. If any member make any observation in the hearing of the judge respecting a course, during the time of running, or before he shall have delivered his judgment, he shall forfeit one sovereign to the fund; and, if either dog be his own, he shall lose the course. If he impugn the decision of the judge, he shall forfeit two sovereigns.

XII. When a course of an average length is so equally divided that the judge shall be unable to decide it, the owners of the dogs may toss for it; but, if either refuse, the dogs shall be again put in the slips, at such time as the Committee may think fit; but, if either dog be drawn, the winning dog shall not be obliged to run again.

XIII. In running a match the judge may declare the course to be undecided.

XIV. If a member shall enter more than one greyhound, *bonâ fide* his own property, for a prize, his dogs shall not run together, if it be possible to avoid it; and, if two greyhounds, the property of the same member, remain to the last tie, he may run it out or draw either, as he shall think fit.

XV. When dogs engaged are of the same colour, the last drawn shall wear a collar.

XVI. If a greyhound stand still in a course when a hare is in his or her sight, the owner shall lose the course; but, if a greyhound drops from exhaustion, and it shall be the opinion of the judge that the merit up to the time of falling was greatly in his or her favour, then the judge shall have power to award the course to the greyhound so falling, if he think fit.

XVII. Should two hares be on foot, and the dogs separate before reaching the hare slipped at, the course shall be undecided, and shall be run over again at such time as the Committee shall think fit, unless the owners of the dogs agree to toss for it, or to draw one dog; and if the dogs separate after running some time, it shall be at the discretion of the Committee whether the course shall be decided up to the point of separation.

XVIII. A course shall end if either dog be so unsighted as to cause an impediment in the course.

XIX. If any member or his servant ride over his opponent's dog when running, so as to injure him in the course, the dog so ridden over shall be deemed to win the course.

XX. It is recommended to all union meetings to appoint a committee of five, consisting of members of different clubs, to determine all difficulties and cases of doubt.

The following general rules are recommended to judges for their guidance:

The features of merit are—

The race from slips, and the first turn or wrench of the hare (provided it be a fair slip), and a straight run-up.

Where one dog gives the other a go-by when both are in their full speed, and turns or wrenches the hare. (N. B. If one dog be in the stretch, and the other only turning at the time he passes, it is not a fair go-by.)

Where one dog turns the hare when she is leading homewards, and keeps the lead so as to serve himself, and makes a second turn of the hare without losing the lead.

A catch or kill of the hare, when she is running straight and leading homewards, is fully equal to a turn of the hare when running in the same direction, or perhaps more, if he show the speed over the other dog in doing it. If a dog draws the fleck from the hare, and causes her to wrench or rick only, it is equal to a turn of the hare when leading homewards.

When a dog wrenches or ricks a hare twice following, without losing the lead, it is equal to a turn.

N. B. It often happens when a hare has been turned, and she is running from home, that she turns of her own accord to gain ground homeward, when both dogs are on the stretch after her; in such a case the judge should not give the leading dog a turn.

There are often other minor advantages in a course, such as one dog showing occasional superiority of speed, turning on less ground, and running the whole course with more fire than his opponent, which must be left to the discretion of the judge, who is to decide on the merits.

LOCAL RULES.

I. The number of members shall be regulated by the letters in the Alphabet, and the two junior members shall take the letters X and Z, if required.

II. The members shall be elected by ballot, seven to constitute a ballot, and two black balls to exclude.

III. The name of every person proposed to be balloted for as a member, shall be placed over the chimney-piece one day before the ballot can take place.

IV. No proposition shall be balloted for unless put up over the chimney-piece, with the names of the proposer and seconder, at or before dinner preceding the day of the ballot, and read to the members at such dinner.

V. Every member shall, at each meeting, run a greyhound his own property, or forfeit a sovereign to the Club.

VI. No member shall be allowed to match more than two greyhounds in the first class, under a penalty of two sovereigns to the fund, unless such member has been drawn or run out for the prizes, in which case he shall be allowed to run three dogs in the first class.

VII. If any member shall absent himself two seasons without sending his subscription, he shall be deemed out of the Society, and another chosen in his place.

VIII. No greyhound shall be allowed to start if any arrears are due to this Society from the owner.

IX. Any member lending another a greyhound for the purpose of saving his forfeit (excepting by consent of the members present) shall forfeit five sovereigns.

X. Any member running the dog of a stranger in a match shall cause the name of the owner to be inserted after his own name in the list, under a penalty of one sovereign.

XI. No stranger shall be admitted into the Society's room, unless introduced by a member, who shall place the name of his friend over the chimney-piece, with his own attached to it; and no member shall introduce more than one friend.

XII. The members of the Clubs shall be honorary members of this Society, and when present shall be allowed to run their greyhounds on payment of the annual subscription.

XIII. This Society to meet on the in , and course on the following days.

INDEX.

APPENDIX

TO THE EDITOR'S ADDITIONS.

THE END.

www.ingramcontent.com/pod-product-compliance
Lightning Source LLC
LaVergne TN
LVHW052217200926
848481LV00001B/137
* 9 7 8 1 4 2 5 5 5 0 1 2 7 *